# Autistic Company

# Autistic Company

Ruud Hendriks

Translated from the Dutch by Lynne Richards

Amsterdam - New York, NY 2012

The Netherlands Organisation for Scientific Research (NWO) generously
helped to make this publication possible by funding the translation.

Cover illustration: Clock Dial with Moon Phase Disc. Poster Paint on
Paper. © Kees Momma. July 1999.

The paper on which this book is printed meets the requirements of "ISO
9706:1994, Information and documentation - Paper for documents -
Requirements for permanence".

ISBN: 978-90-420-3575-1
E-Book ISBN: 978-94-012-0850-5
©Editions Rodopi B.V., Amsterdam - New York, NY 2012
Printed in the Netherlands

# Table of Contents

# Acknowledgements

I am grateful to Gerard de Vries for his inspiring role during the research that forms the basis of this book. The Faculty of Arts and Social Sciences of Maastricht University, the Department of Philosophy in particular, was and increasingly is the best possible context in which to develop my research interests. The late Lolle Nauta generously shared his philosophical interest in clowns with me, which still keeps me going in both academia and health care practice. In discussing our work, Annemarie Mol showed me how to become an empirical philosopher. The residents and staff members of the residential institution I refer to as W generously offered me the possibility to do my fieldwork. I should like to express my gratitude to Lynne Richards for her translation of my work into English. Sabine Kuipers helped me with the layout. Ruth Benschop shares a life of work and living with me, for which I am very grateful. When I first published my work on autism in Dutch, I was curious what the world would look like from under the butterbur in our garden; now this revised and updated English edition is being published, Mendel, Jelit and Esra remind me on a daily basis to sit down on the ground and watch.

# Introduction
## A Mixture of the Strange and the Familiar

> Autism is a human disorder which offers us
> a glimpse of experience close to,
> and yet perhaps infinitely far from,
> our own perception of ourselves and our social world.[1]

In the nineteen-eighties I was a care worker. I helped to look after autistic teenagers with learning difficulties. I used to set out their breakfasts, tie their shoelaces, wave goodbye to the ones who were off to school, and get the others ready to go to the day centre. After school we sat around the table for a chat. I encouraged the youngsters to state their preferences and say whether they wanted orangeade or lemonade. After supper we watched some television, and then there were bedtime stories before lights out at around 8 p.m. during the week and a bit later at weekends, when some of the kids went home to their parents. We organized some special activities for the ones who stayed with us.

Daily life in the unit - very different though it may have been from what many of us are used to at home - resembled ordinary life. There were, of course, obstacles to be overcome. Just sitting with the others for a while or deciding between two sorts of drink seemed to be too ambitious for some of our youngsters. Any departure from familiar structures required careful planning. Most of the staff had scars around their wrists left by fingernails that had been dug into the flesh - silent witnesses of failed efforts to communicate.

We may have been too busy solving all kinds of practical problems, but at the time neither my colleagues nor I found it particularly surprising that we - pupils and staff - somehow managed to *share* some sort of daily life. It was only afterwards, when I looked at my former position from an academic distance and learned more about autism from various disciplinary points of view, that I started to realize how remarkable this really was. If these were indeed 'children who understand nothing of our world,'[2] how did we manage to get on together?

I was not the only one who developed a fascination for the subject. With public awareness slowly growing since the mid-nineteen-seventies, autism seems to have been barely out of the public eye in many European countries since the late nineteen-eighties, with a peak in attention in the past decade. This public interest was initially sparked off by articles about autistic children in magazines aimed at child rearing and parenting practice. Later there were publications by researchers and therapists which found their way to readers by way of the shelves of bookshops and libraries. Parents of autistic children began to share their personal experiences with the public, following the example of Clara Claiborne Park, who wrote about life with her autistic daughter in *The Siege* - a book first published in 1967. As time went on, the most diverse subjects came in for attention and there was a gradual shift in interest to autistic adults. Having been a regular subject of specialized scholarly research for decades - ever since the pioneering studies of Kanner and Asperger in the nineteen-forties - people with autism started to speak for themselves more often. They made their appearance on TV, in documentary series such as Oliver Sacks's *The Mind Traveller* and in human interest programmes. The new millennium saw huge media coverage, especially in the US and the UK, of a possible 'autism epidemic,' said to be caused by the combined MMR vaccine. Autism became a trope in popular culture, too. Barry Levinson's film *Rain Man* (1988) presented the first opportunity for a mass audience to make the acquaintance of an autistic character. More recently Mark Haddon's prizewinning novel *The Curious Incident of the Dog in the Night-Time*, featuring a hero/narrator with an autistic disorder, became an international bestseller. Nowadays one may come across people with autism anywhere - in the street, in the supermarket, in your local school, in films and novels, and on the internet.

Not that autism is common. Five individuals in 10,000 have an autistic disorder, with reported rates ranging from two to twenty cases per 10,000 and possibly up to three times as many for the broader spectrum of autistic disorders. Autism is therefore a relatively rare condition.[3] So, why is there this recurring interest in autism which, given the rarity of the condition, has to be regarded at the very least as remarkable?

The term 'autism' (from the Greek *autos* - the self) refers to the self-absorbed, inward-looking impression that autistic people make. From an early age, before they turn three, children with this developmental disorder display striking and similar abnormalities in their relations with the outside world. Their social awareness is very limited, they communicate little if at all and they have inexplicable outbursts of rage. The development of an autistic child is not so much retarded as *different*. The qualitative difference is expressed in at least three areas: in social interactions, in communication skills and powers of imagination, and in limited, repetitive, stereotyped patterns of behaviour, interest and activities.[4]

The precise cause of autism is not known, although there are convincing indications that it is a congenital defect. Around three-quarters of these people also have learning disabilities. The condition is three to four times more common in men than in women. So far it has not been possible to identify the physical basis, but given the broad spectrum of symptoms in which the underlying defect is expressed, it seems safe to assume that it is located at a basic (and hence influential) level in the central nervous system.

Autism is a 'pervasive' developmental disorder. The central deficit permeates an individual's whole development, as we read in the revised fourth edition of the *Diagnostic and Statistical Manual of Mental Disorders, DSM-IV-TR.*

These symptoms may explain part of the interest in autism, but the fascination really begins where autistic and non-autistic people *meet*. It is here that we find ourselves in an area of tension. Despite very real obstacles, in all sorts of situations - at home with their families, as pupils in special needs schools, as guests on a TV chat show - autistic people are part of the daily life of the non-autistic people around them. On the other hand, people with autism are so different from others in a number of essential ways that we can legitimately ask ourselves *in which respects* there can be any question of interaction. My aim in writing this book has been to chart something of this 'shared existence' of autistic and non-autistic people, because this teaches us something about ourselves and our social world. As we shall see, when autistic and non-autistic people come into contact with one another the intrinsic character of people's shared existence is constantly under discussion.

What is it, then, that makes an encounter between autistic and non-autistic people special compared with 'ordinary' encounters between strangers? How can one describe the specific nature of such an encounter? It is the popular image of autism that seems to provide the beginnings of an answer.

### The Autist-Savage

The mixture of bewilderment and curiosity with which bystanders react to autistic people is not a modern phenomenon. Although 'early infantile autism,' as it was called, has only been recognized as a separate disease category since Kanner's work, the history of fascination with the 'other' that the autistic person represents, so some people say, goes back much further. From time immemorial, stories have been told about the other-worldly behaviour of people who display anomalies in their social, communicative and imaginative abilities - deficits that sometimes go hand in hand with above average skills in other areas and that from a present-day perspective are typical of what has come to be called 'autistic disorder.'

Uta Frith traces the roots of the attraction that 'autistic' people appear to have exerted on others - in mythology, in fairy tales and in stories about 'changelings.' Rather closer to home she observed the same fascination with 'autistic' behaviour in historical descriptions of wolf boys like Victor, the wild child who was supposedly found roaming in the forest near Aveyron in 1799, and in the legend of Kaspar Hauser. Many of these stories revolve around behaviour traits that, with hindsight, could indicate autistic problems.[5]

Take for instance the myth of the changeling. On clear starlit nights, so this story goes, elves or nature spirits come out to gaze at human children as they sleep. They take the most beautiful away with them. In the child's place these magical creatures leave one of their own children, but the humans are unable to cope with the usurpers. These other-worldly children may look perfectly normal, but they neither speak nor laugh. Instead, as is sometimes seen in young children with autism, they cry incessantly or remain eerily silent. Another parallel is that sometimes, so it was said, these children unexpectedly come out with one or two words, so that they create the impression that they *can* speak but wilfully refuse to do so.[6]

Another example. In the late eighteenth and early nineteenth centuries, the French cultural elite responded with great excitement to the discovery of a boy who, in view of his wild appearance and completely antisocial behaviour, appeared to have grown up outside society. People were unable to agree on the question as to whether Victor, as the boy was called, had been deviant since birth - and for that reason had been abandoned to his fate - or whether his uncivilized state was in fact the consequence of his social isolation. The greatest attention, however, focused on whether Victor could be enticed out of his wild state and be brought up to be a civilized human being. Victor's teacher, the physician Jean-Marc Itard, kept a detailed record of his many years' involvement in Victor's upbringing.[7] After five years of intensive education and guidance, during which Victor learned a number of practical and social skills, Itard abandoned the experiment.

Victor's dexterity, which was noted by Itard, is reminiscent of an 'excellent, purposeful and 'intelligent' relation to objects,'[8] which Kanner observed in the autistic children he described, and which was in stark contrast to their defective ability to relate to people. When he was found, at the age of eleven or twelve, Victor could not talk and he approached people by sniffing them, he became fascinated by certain objects and absolutely had to have things in their proper place - from a modern perspective all typical autistic behaviour traits. Although Victor learned to communicate to some extent and opened up a little to social contact, a development that is by no means ruled out in autistic people, he was nevertheless always an outsider. Unobserved for a moment while his progress was being discussed in Madame Récamier's fashionable salon, so the story has it, Victor escaped into the garden, took off his clothes and climbed, naked, into a tree. Beyond the reach of his benefactors, 'he was finally tempted to descend by the gardener (evidently one of Nature's psychologists), who showed him a basket of peaches,'[9] comments Lorna Wing, who relates this anecdote to the similar experiences of parents who try to teach their autistic child socially acceptable behaviour.

Even if Victor was not raised by wild animals, he certainly grew up in the wild, and the story of his life among people is one of characteristic autistic 'aloneness.' What he may have lacked is *common sense* - a typical deficit in autistic people expressed in their inability to share in the close-knit structure of implicit meanings which are regarded as self-evident but only shared by initiated members of the social community.

Metaphorical comparisons that do the rounds in the context of autism often have something in common, notes W. R. Albury.[10] The people around whom stories like this revolve have usually crossed a border between human society and the realm of nature. A good example is the autistic José, who was described by Oliver Sacks. José is also very close to nature: he lacks the ability to enter into normal human relationships and abstract concepts are beyond him, but he does have an exceptional gift for the concrete, for the particular, which he expresses in drawings in an extraordinary way. 'He grasps the world as forms - directly and intensely felt forms - and reproduces them,'[11] wrote Sacks of José's work. José likes drawing plants, grasses whose species, according to the famous neurologist, he seems 'to recognize, to greet each one as a friend.'[12] Sacks went on to wonder just how lonely and cut off an autistic 'multiverse'[13] - a view of the world that in the absence of the broad context, of meaningful relations, is constructed solely of separate and intensely experienced particularities - actually is.

> For though 'horizontal' connections with others, with society and culture, are lost, yet there may be vital and intensified 'vertical' connections, direct connections with nature, with reality, uninfluenced, unmediated, untouchable, by any others.[14]

Sacks's description dovetails perfectly with the creation of the image of Kaspar Hauser and with the idea that people in the late eighteenth and early nineteenth century had of the 'noble savage.' Kaspar Hauser was a sixteen-year-old boy who appeared in Nuremberg, seemingly out of nowhere, on Whit Monday 1828. To the astonishment of the bystanders, the boy could barely speak, he did not appear to know how to walk and apparently understood nothing of what was said to him. Gradually people started to suspect that he had spent his whole life isolated from the outside world in a cellar, with only a wooden horse for company and a view of four bare walls. In the report he wrote in 1832, the renowned lawyer Anselm von Feuerbach, who saw in the case of Kaspar Hauser 'an example of a crime on the soul of man,'[15] examines the extraordinary power of Kaspar's sensory perception. Tradition has it that Kaspar could distinguish colours in pitch darkness and was drawn to metal like a magnet.[16]

And so there appears the stereotype of the 'autist-savage' who, unlike modern civilized man for whom such an unaffected state is now out of reach, has direct access to nature: to a concrete world and forms of order beyond human concepts and intervention.

There is also a moral side to the notion of the savage child of nature. The effect of Rousseau's ideas about the natural goodness of mankind and the social origin of evil can be seen as an important formative element in the society in which Hauser surfaced. His mentors' interest was not confined to educating the boy, they were also looking for insights that overcivilized society could gain thanks to this 'blank sheet.' With Kaspar as the medium, they hoped to gain access to a lost world of moral purity and innocence. [17]

This same idea of the natural goodness of man and the social origin of evil is projected on the autistic person's characteristic inability to pretend, to lie or to cheat. 'There is something very pure, very touching about them; lying, manipulating, scheming and so forth are simply not part of their make-up,' [18] said the remedial educationalist Van Berckelaer-Onnes in her oration. Around the time of the film *Rain Man*, in which Dustin Hoffman played an autistic man who could not see through his brother Charlie's hidden agenda (in the casino the brother exploited the Hoffman character's extraordinary memory for numbers), the fascination with the moral purity of the autistic person was still surprisingly topical.

A markedly romantic subtext harking back to the noble savage clings to the image of the autistic person. Anyone who ventures to reflect on this nowadays usually hastens to correct this image by pointing out that autism also - and predominantly - has very harrowing aspects. Uta Frith, commenting on the film *Rain Man*, for instance, says that 'we can learn a great deal about ourselves through the phenomenon of autism' as depicted in this story. 'Yet,' she continues, 'the illness should not be romanticized. We must see autism as a devastating handicap without a cure.' [19]

This does not alter the fact that the metaphor of the autistic person as a savage is a telling one. It may not be directly informative about people with autism as such, but it is certainly revealing when it comes to the interactions between autistic and non-autistic persons that I am concerned with here. As in the comparison between autistic people and aliens, a more recent phenomenon, autistic people are repeatedly described as lacking typical human qualities.

> They all identify the autistic person as someone whose defining characteristics are non-human - whether they are those of nature spirits, or wild animals, or extraterrestrials. The effect of this identification is that these metaphors all set the autistic person outside the sphere of the human, not as someone who is different in degree but as someone who is wholly 'Other.' [20]

This tendency to romanticize is less evident in another metaphor used in connection with autistic people, although here again autism is positioned outside people's reach, on the material side of existence. This is the stereotype of the autistic person as a machine-person.

*The Autist-Machine*

Although in most cases autism is coupled with a mental impairment, within the autistic population there are considerable individual differences in intellectual capacity. Some people with autism have a normal or even above-average IQ. It is not a lack of intellect in the general sense of the word that makes autistic people outsiders; it is a specific lack of insight into, of feeling for the underlying context-related meaning that people attach to certain things. Another characteristic of autism is an unbalanced development profile, with weak performance in the social and communicative domain coexisting with above-average skills in areas where there is little call on intersubjective abilities (spatial concepts, for instance). These are described as islets of ability, or peak or splinter skills. They stand out from the rest of the profile, and in exceptional cases are also much higher than the non-autistic norm. These extraordinary abilities are sometimes described as 'savant skills.'[21]

Savant skills may lie in a variety of areas, among them drawing, music, calendar calculation, mechanics, shape recognition and the mechanical memory. A famous case is that of Nadia, who at the age of three drew pictures of horses she had seen in a book with photographic accuracy. But that was not all; she drew the horses from every conceivable viewpoint and in any position she chose. When she was eleven Nadia learned to talk and started to draw less and less; her special talent withered away completely.[22] Another case, described by Sacks, is Stephen Wiltshire, who after seeing a building for a brief period can draw it perfectly, capturing the style and reproducing the right proportions of windows and ornaments. We do not know how the autistic Stephen thinks, the neurologist says.

> But we do know that though he may be lacking in the symbolic, the abstract, he has a sort of genius for concrete or mimetic representation, whether drawing a cathedral, a canyon, a flower, or enacting a scene, a drama, a song - a sort of genius for catching the formal features, the structural logic, the style, the 'thisness' (though not necessarily the 'meaning'), of whatever he portrays.[23]

Autistic savants are also among the subjects of Stuart Murray's *Representing Autism*. One of the contemporary savant celebrities is Daniel Tammet, whose 2006 book *Born on a Blue Day* became an international bestseller. The reception of Tammet's book and his appearance in television shows bear witness to the public fascination with his exceptional mathematical and synaesthetic skills. Drawing on work of Garland-Thomson, Murray argues that autism is 'strangely satisfying' the contemporary conflation of rationality with wonder. 'In a time of rationality and scientific knowledge, it provides the space for wonder and awe, and no kind of autistic figure does this more than the savant.'[24]

Frith was one of the first to point out that the fascination with the combination of fragmentary achievements - intellectual and otherwise - and the lack of social instincts resonates in the popular imagination. It has to be remembered here that this extraordinary combination of characteristics is usually presented as a caricature, but it does nonetheless reflect the unbalanced development typical of autistic people. The archetypal detective Sherlock Holmes, for example, could be the very model of the high-functioning autistic person: an eccentric personality who, unhindered by normal human prejudices and with an above-average capacity for observation and deduction, has a keen eye for things that other people regard as trivial. Holmes's quirky preoccupations, such as that expressed in his 'little monograph on the ashes of 140 different varieties of pipe, cigar and cigarette tobacco,'[25] could be a textbook example of the special and limited pattern of interests that is characteristic of autistic people. The model of the famous detective inspired Mark Haddon in the creation of his character Christopher Boone - hero/narrator with an autistic disorder in *The Curious Incident of the Dog in the Night-Time* - who in his quest for the murderer of the poodle Wellington is following Holmes's example, using a specific forensic (and autistic) style and method.[26]

It is a small step from the logically reasoning detective to the more contemporary myths of the almost-human heroes in science fiction series like *Star Trek*. The android Data, whose human exterior conceals sophisticated electronics, is a positive identification figure for many autistic people. Following his visit to the autistic biologist and engineer Temple Grandin, Sacks raises the question of this identification with the humanoid machine Data.

> 'I can really relate to Data,' she said as we drove away from the farm. She is a 'Star Trek' fan, as I am, and her favorite character is Data, an android who, for all his emotionlessness, has a great curiosity, a wistfulness, about being human. He observes human behavior minutely, and sometimes impersonates it, but longs, above all, to *be* human. A surprising number of people with autism identify with Data, or with his predecessor, Mr. Spock.[27]

As we see, some metaphors for autism are also - or indeed even in the first place - used by autistic people themselves. Jim Sinclair, himself

someone with an autistic disorder, calls himself an 'alien,' although he rejects
the idea that his strange origin makes him inhuman.

> Being autistic does not mean being inhuman. But it does
> mean being alien. It means that what is normal for other
> people is not normal for me, and what is normal for me is
> not normal for other people. In some ways I am terribly ill-
> equipped to survive in this world, like an extraterrestrial
> stranded without an orientation manual.[28]

As a rule people seem to have a sort of sixth sense for the implicit
rules and underlying structure of society. As is evident from their problems
with manners and rules of etiquette and their need for an explicit manual for
social interaction, it is precisely this sense that autistic people lack. They 'live
by the letter,'[29] instead of acting according to the spirit of the unwritten treaty
that binds people. In all its rigidity, autistic behaviour could be reminiscent of
the mechanical regularity of machines. According to Frith, a comparison with
the robot - intelligent, packaged as a human being, but soulless - can at least
make the inflexible and relatively un-socialized behaviour of the autistic
person more understandable.

> Robots carry out jobs that that they are specialized for,
> without concern for wider aspects, with precision and,
> above all, in an unvarying routine. The machine-like
> behavior reminds us of many characteristics of autistic
> behavior: we see repetitiveness, stereotyped movements,
> lack of emotional expression, and lack of spontaneous
> playfulness. . . . The robot metaphor symbolically captures
> the   coexistence   of   the   physical   and   intellectual
> achievements of individuals with autistic disorder and, in
> sharp contrast, their perceived emotional insufficiency in
> personal relationships.[30]

The machine metaphor not only helps to clarify the nature of autistic
behaviour, it also throws light on the difficulty of interactions between
autistic and non-autistic people. Non-autistic people have a tendency to be
wrong about autists in the same way as they often are in their dealings with
computers. In situations that appear to be normal communicational situations
- such as in the exchange with a robot that asks questions and gives answers -
people tend to ascribe to the thing they are talking to all sorts of human ideas
and intentions. In fact there is no question of an empathic reaction; it is
simply a programmed response. Young children who learn to use computers
tend to develop an animistic view of things. They attribute all sorts of mental

capacities to their digital playmate, such as the ability to cheat.[31] This same tendency to search for underlying reasons for behaviour could explain communications problems with people with autism, argues Frith.

> Like autistic people . . . robots have no sense of humor, and are utterly literal in their understanding. But - despite their metal exterior - one tends to forget that they are machines. More often than not people treat robots as if they too are scheming beings. This is understandable if we assume that the attribution of states of minds is pervasive and compulsive.[32]

People with an autistic disorder are not robots, but all the same the stereotype of the autist-machine is revealing. Again, this imagery may not say so much about autistic people as it does about the *interactions* between autistic and non-autistic persons. Anyone who grew up with the idea that disabled people 'are different but still just ordinary people' would be well advised to forget the 'ordinary' when it comes to autism. Much as they may resemble normal people, they still lack what Frith tellingly refers to as 'some elusive but essential humanness.'[33] So what, then, could better express such an essentially alienating experience than a metaphor which refers to the material world? What source offers more fitting analogies to describe this other-ness of autistic people than the mechanistic vocabulary?

Whether these stereotypes are based on natural or artificial models is not really relevant. Obviously there are differences. The autist-savage refers first and foremost to an unmediated contact with a purely material order outside human categories, while the autist-machine denotes a type of thinking untroubled by human emotions. Or, if we focus on the negative side, the metaphor of the savage refers to an inability to be part of human civilization; the image of the machine reflects, among other things, an empathic deficit. The savage metaphor harks back to a distant past, the machine metaphor projects the fascination with autism on to existing and future products of modernity.

But in both cases the autistic person who is being measured against these metaphors is placed outside the world of people-among-themselves, and positioned under the influence of the concrete, mechanically conceived world of non-humans. What predominates is the alienating connotation. And which gulf is deeper, in our view, which opposition more comprehensive than that between people and things? (And yet sometimes there seems to be an echo of a strange sort of yearning in the tales, a sense of kinship with this thing-like other.)

*A Trip to the Park*

When we (average western readers in the early twenty-first century) talk about people, by and large we use terms other than the ones we use when we talk about things. In all sorts of respects we assume an essential difference between people and things. Sartre's famous passage about a man going to the park in *L'être et le néant* [Being and Nothingness] can illustrate this.[34]

A man in the park sees the things that come within his field of vision (the chairs, the grass), but then sees a person. How does this person differ from other objects in the park? Sartre's answer is: if I, the man in the park, were to think that the person who impinged on my field of vision was only a *dummy*, then I could describe this man's appearance entirely with the aid of the time and space coordinates I use when I describe material objects in the park. His appearance would not essentially have changed anything in my universe, the world as it appears from my perspective, except that a thing would have been *added to it* - a thing which at a given moment is located at a certain distance from other objects.

Regarding the other as a *man*, in contrast, means that a simple addition sum is no longer enough to allow for this event. As a result of the appearance of the other as a person, the connection between the objects that I have established is disrupted. Because the other regards the world from his point of view and engages in a relationship with the world that escapes my perception, my world, of which I was the centre as long as I was alone, begins to shift. I realize that the world is not just for me, that it also presents itself to the observation of the other in a way that is inaccessible to me.

Sartre says that this disintegration of my world can be traced back to the fact that a person, unlike a thing, is *free*. You cannot pin a person down. A thing is what it *is*, a person specifically is *not*. 'His existence is the denial of every being, and here nothingness and freedom touch,' is how Nauta puts it.[35] 'Human being is not the same as the rest of being but is distinguished from it by a separating nothingness,'[36] wrote Hazel Barnes. Sartre is saying that a person differentiates himself from the material reality because he does not have to put up with the world as it is. The park where someone goes to look for a friend, for example, becomes, thanks to the 'nothingness' that his consciousness disseminates, the park where this friend is *not*.[37]

> The massivity of being, as one can formulate it with the customary metaphor in EN [*L'être et le néant*], is broken thanks to this 'no.' Cracks and splits that would not be there without the human being appear in it. The destruction that happens in nature is only a shift within the constellation of being. A little less here and a little more there; thanks firstly to the human being the no comes into the world, the nothing makes its entrance.[38]

The park itself does not change because of it. More fundamentally, the nihilating character of the consciousness becomes manifest at the moment when the visitors notice each other. My world, of which I, as a visitor in the park, was the centre as long as I was alone, begins to lose ground under the influence of the presence of the other. When I realize that I myself am also being observed by the other, however, I am forced even closer to the periphery of the observation. Under the influence of the other's gaze I am made a specific part of *his* world. 'Whereas previously I myself was the centre of my world, now I have suddenly lost this centre; my world has been set adrift,'[39] says Nauta. (Until the roles are reversed and the other in his turn becomes aware of my nihilating gaze.)

### *More Like a Doll than a Child*

To emphasize the difference between people and things, Sartre used the concept of 'freedom.' This may sound naively idealistic, but the way the concept is used in Sartre ties in with a distinction that most of us can understand. Sartre's work is only one of the many examples in modern western philosophy where the dichotomy between 'people' and 'things' is interpreted in a specific way and as such constantly recurs, albeit in not always entirely overlapping guises: mind-matter, mind-body, subject-object, representation-world, action-behaviour, and so on. Essential humanness is often conceived of as in the mind, while everything outside it is considered as obeying the laws of nature. *Locus classicus* for the modern definition of such a thinking thing (*res cogitans*) in a universe otherwise subject to geometric laws and knowable in mathematical terms (*res extensa*) is Descartes (1637). As Steven Shapin establishes, this dualism is always a deeply rooted distinction:

> We do not *feel* ourselves to be machines, and Descartes agreed that we are not. We feel ourselves to exercise will, to have purposes, to move our bodies in response to our purposes, to be conscious, to make moral evaluations, to deliberate and to reason (that is, to *think*), and to express the results of our thought in language - none of which Descartes reckoned that machines, or animals, can do.[40]

It could of course be argued that the difference between what I have for the sake of brevity described as 'people' and 'things' is a simplification. Contrary to what is suggested by the conceptual distinction, surely objects in everyday life not infrequently play a perfectly non-problematic role. People can sometimes, or partly, behave like a thing, where the dividing line runs straight through them. In philosophy, although the legacy of this dualism has occupied philosophical minds for three centuries and more, surely there have been numerous attempts to get away from the rigid human-thing scheme.[41] Surely where people did adhere to a human-thing dichotomy, the dividing line was constantly being shifted a little. My depiction of the question as a great dichotomy of people-among-themselves on the one hand and things-in-themselves on the other, tends - hastily added inverted commas around 'people' and 'things' notwithstanding - to miss these nuances. The question arises as to whether my 'naive' division was perhaps set up as a straw man, so that I could overturn it later when it became apparent that the reality is more complex.

It is not, however, my intention to raise such suspicions. The human-thing distinction as I use it is indeed a caricature or an ideal type, but one, all the same, that is actual. When we talk about people, we usually do it in different terms from the ones we use when we speak about things. Wittgenstein formulates this as follows:

> But can't I imagine that the people around me are automata, lack consciousness, even though they behave in the same way as usual? - If I imagine it now - alone in my room - I see people with fixed looks (as in a trance) going about their business - the idea is perhaps a little uncanny. But just try to keep hold of this idea in the midst of your ordinary intercourse with others, in the street, say! Say to yourself, for example: 'The children over there are mere automata; all their liveliness is mere automatism.' And you will either find these words becoming quite meaningless; or you will produce in yourself some kind of uncanny feeling, or something of the sort. Seeing a living human being as an automaton is analogous to seeing one figure as a limiting case or variant of another; the cross-pieces of a window as a swastika, for example.[42]

The human-thing distinction is part of what the philosopher John Searle, using a computer metaphor, calls our 'default position.'[43] Searle says this is not so much about sharing an 'opinion' - surely it does not make sense to ask someone's *opinion* about whether or not the world exists independent of ourselves, our language, thoughts and experiences - but about presuppositions without which all sorts of practical matters would be incomprehensible. These are matters that we usually take as read, things that *precede* common sense.

In the light of the metaphors that do the rounds in the context of autism, however, our normal intuitions are really put to the test. When the child psychiatrist Lorna Wing, referring to the daily personal hygiene routines of autistic children, observes that they lie 'limply like a rag doll' and generally undergo procedures like washing and dressing 'passively, like little dolls rather than children,'[44] this is more than just a manner of speaking. Here she is tinkering with the otherwise self-evident boundary between the realm of the human being and the world of things; with the validity of a framework which, as a rule, one never stops to think about.[45]

### A Stranger in Our Midst

If metaphors have anything to say in the context of autistic people, it is that we may be dealing here with a form of existence that is radically different from what is considered normal for human beings. As an extension of this, these analogies can be conceived as an *expression* of the distance and the powerlessness that can overcome people in their dealings with autists: few seem to be so far away from the familiar, meaningful world of people-among-themselves as people with autism. This gives us the beginnings of an answer to the question of where the fascination with autism we have identified comes from. 'Autism is a disorder which fascinates because it seems to be so essentially a disorder of the human condition,' says psychologist Francesca Happé.[46] It is 'the condition of fascination of the moment,' argues Stuart Murray, with 'the allure of potentially unquantifiable human difference and the nightmare of not somehow being 'fully' human.'[47]

Autism seems to touch on what is considered to be essentially human. Yet, we should not allow this experience to blind us from seeing another side of living with autistic people. People with autism often seem more like ordinary people than the metaphors we have looked at so far might suggest. Albury argues that the context of the human-thing distinction makes an issue of differences between autistic and non-autistic people, whereas possible commonalities are underrated.[48] Surely there are more opportunities for reciprocal contact than thinking in terms of irreconcilable extremes supposes, particularly if we would be willing to accept differences between people, to a certain extent, as a valuable part of existence.

Anyone who has any sort of regular dealings with autistic persons will agree with Albury. For all those who have no choice but to live with an autistic person and for those who choose to spend time with him or her, for those who care for an autistic child or who teach one, for instance, the observation that there really are possibilities of interaction is undoubtedly trivial. They experience the interweaving of their existence with that of the autistic person on a daily basis. Thus, Clara Park, for example, wrote about her daughter: 'Elly only seemed to live in isolation. In fact she lived with us. There were five other human beings in her house. We passed, we spoke, we touched, we provided.'[49] Instead of emphasizing her daughter's isolation, Park lists various ways in which living together every day was structured. In the house where the six of them lived, the space was shared, people talked, contact was made and care was given.

All the same, we must not confuse this *practical* familiarity with autistic people with analytical self-evidence. All things considered, the fact that, one way or another, autistic and non-autistic people do succeed in living together is anything but trivial. Given the manifest lack of common consensual mechanisms on which we normally rely, the shared existence of autistic and non-autistic people - at home, at school, at work - represents a remarkable achievement. Autistic people may well be less strange than the stereotypes suggest, but they are still so different from the rest of us that we can ask ourselves how it is in any way possible for non-autistic and autistic people to get on together. Our familiarity therefore deserves to be approached with the same, if not greater, surprise and curiosity as the strangeness of the autistic existence.

These are the elements that make up the popular fascination with autism. Autistic people differ in important respects from non-autistic people, but at the same time they are part of our everyday lives. They are, admittedly, at a great remove from people, but they are also among them. People with autism, as Sacks puts it, are like 'a strange species in our midst.'[50] It is not the strangeness as such, but rather the combination of distance and closeness, this *mixture* of strange and familiar that makes autism such an intriguing phenomenon. As Freeman Dyson remarked about an autistic girl he has seen growing up:

> It's a marvellous thing to know an autistic child. Her universe is radically different from mine. Concrete social relationships are for her very difficult to comprehend. On the other hand, with anything abstract she has no trouble, so we can talk very easily about mathematics . . . It's a marvellous mixture - strangeness and familiarity.[51]

In a book that deals with the nature of their common existence, the *proximity* of autistic and non-autistic people therefore deserves to be as much a subject of study as the differences between them.

How can bonds be established between people if social relationships remain a mystery to one of the parties? What alternative consensual mechanisms are available if the familiar meaningful world of people-among-themselves has to be largely suspended? What efforts are made in a shared existence and by whom? How is this community formed?

### Choosing Our Words
We have at our disposal a historically developed arsenal of words, manners and rules of behaviour so that we can approach people and things in the appropriate way. Autistic people, however, always seem to confound our expectations about what people are and what things are, or so it would appear

from the image that I have examined here. Our society does not seem to be geared to their participation. At the same time, autistic people, in a non-trivial way, make up a self-evident part of the lives of the non-autistic people around them. Self-evident but not trivial: in the dealings between autistic and non-autistic people the nature of the community of people-among-themselves is constantly being redefined. This shapes the outlines of a shared existence, the first of two themes that are central to this study.

My focus is the nature of the interactions between autistic and non-autistic people. This question will be interpreted conceptually. Although I shall be discussing the ways that autistic and non-autistic people can coordinate their lives, it is not my intention to provide guidelines for good practice. This book should be read as a conceptual study, as a contribution to the repertoire of words and images that can help us to better understand situations in which autistic and non-autistic people come into contact with one another. For, in order to be able to discuss what takes place in the mutual interaction between autistic and non-autistic people, and to assess work being carried out in this area at its true worth, we have to choose our words carefully. That is the second theme in this book.

Not at home in the meaningful world of people-among-themselves, there seems - at least as far as our language is concerned - to be no alternative available to the autistic person other than to be part of a nature that is inhospitable to people, or of a mechanistic order outside the human sphere. For the non-autist, on the other hand, a place among people seems (again - if we can believe the stories) to be guaranteed. The conceptual framework of the human-thing distinction seems to create a gulf which *subsequently* has to be bridged in practice. Of course we could counter that our language confuses us; that the human-thing distinction is a philosophical fiction and that in practice people have always just got on with it and lived together. The question then would be what this practical living together looks like, if we manage one way or another to clear the conceptual barriers out of the way. (To some extent this is already being done by people who write from practical experience themselves, from whom we can take our inspiration for the conceptual detailing).

And still we are not yet there. On the one hand it would be naive to think that, aside from a few conceptual obstacles, there is nothing standing in the way of two-way contact between people with and without autism. On the other, the fact that we have terms at our disposal which we can use to talk about the way autistic and non-autistic people sometimes manage to live together does not automatically disqualify a dualistic vocabulary. The human-thing distinction, I have argued, is not just a philosophical fiction that blocks the view of reality, it is at the same time a certainty that is assumed in the normal course of events.

In practice the dualistic vocabulary plays two roles. On the one hand the human-thing distinction governs what, generally speaking, can be *established*. Mechanistic metaphors, similes and analogies tell us something about 'this uniquely abnormal 'feel' that is a feature of relations with autistic people'[52] and about the effort it takes to live with that difference. In order to express this feeling in words, we resort to or re-invent metaphorical resources that are available to us. Take for instance Rosie Barnes's portrait of her autistic son in her photo series *Understanding Stanley* that features a cactus in a pot, not a child at all. The image of a cactus for Barnes symbolizes the combination of her son's perfectly normal looks and his inflexible mind: 'It looks like nice soft circular shapes, but it's as stiff as a board.'[53]

The thing metaphor thus refers to real experiences of people who have dealings with autists. We talk of wild children, natural talents, robots, artificial intelligence, or picture a cactus, and convey the perceived difference in dualistic terms. With Susan Sontag, however, we can point out that an analogy not only represents, but also has certain *effects*.[54] Narratives have both an epistemological and an ontological dimension: they provide a frame of reference and affect our actions, the decisions we take and the way we perceive the world of autism. They may even affect how people start to see and understand themselves. Images and stories of autism have multiplied, especially since the multimedia revolution. As Ian Hacking points out:

> A 'thick' kind of human being is coming into being, where once there was a 'thin' one. The autistic thin man of yore, or rather the thin child, when not having a tantrum, was a silent self-absorbed creature, alone with bizarre habits.[55]

Contrary to the 'thick, dense or rich' characterizations of personalities with autism that appear in the more interesting, recent (self) descriptions, mechanistic metaphors may be one-dimensional. They may also be harmful. Metaphors that link people with an autistic disorder to non-human things, says Albury, are anything but neutral denominators. They are explicitly exclusive in nature. What is different about autistic people is magnified, and this dilutes the potential emphasis on common features and reduces the chance of integration into a non-autistic society. This defensive attitude can be traced back to what Albury exposes as 'deep cultural fears.'[56] He postulates a social fear of anything that is different, and says that for this reason people try by means of stereotyping to ward off potential danger.

Murray critically argues that popular narratives on autism lead us to believe that there is 'such a space to travel between autistic otherness and full neurobehavioural normality' that there seems almost no alternative to trying to 'overcome' and 'erase' this seemingly 'most enigmatic of conditions.'[57]

> Allowing for autism to be 'incredible' in this way ...
> pushes the condition into the world of fantasy. It makes it
> easier to ignore the social dimensions, the apparently
> mundane questions of schooling or respite care or
> employment options for adults with autism. It keeps things
> at arm's length.[58]

What it is that we are trying to keep at a distance in the case of autistic people is one of the themes I shall return to in this book. For now it is enough to see that the human-thing distinction does more than *represent* the (perceived) difference between autistic and non-autistic people - it also *produces* a gulf.

To sum up: without this human-thing framework that lets us put names to experienced differences and makes them manageable, what happens in practice is just as impossible to understand as it would be if it were squeezed into the dualistic straightjacket. If we want to discuss the interactions of autistic and non-autistic people and want to do justice to both the self-evidence and to the unusual achievement being made here, we will have to try to clear stigmatizing, conceptual barriers out of the way, without detracting from the everyday reality of the human-thing distinction.

### Some Context and Directions

This investigation shares an important starting point with the field of disability studies, where disabilities are not understood primarily as medical impairments but attention focuses on the social world in which disabled people live. The world in which people with a disability live is sometimes even seen as a distinct culture, with its own values, standards and customs.[59] Studies of cultural phenomena like these are based on the methods and insights of the social sciences and humanities. Oliver Sacks's exploration of the world of the deaf in *Seeing Voices* provides a good overview of such contributions to the understanding of the culture of deaf people.[60] Disability studies challenge the predominant medical view on neurobehavioural otherness as a mere *deficit* and imply 'a reconfiguration of what we might think of as a 'working' spectrum of humanity.'[61] Recently, too, there have been calls for a more respectful approach to autism, as a distinct culture with valuable elements within the working spectrum of humanity. Insider voices such as Jim Sinclair's have articulated that call, asking us to 'question . . . our assumptions' by recognizing that autistic and non-autistic people 'are equally alien to each other' and accepting that autistic ways of being 'are not merely damaged versions' of the so-called normal (or 'neurotypical') ones.[62]

I have taken this plea to heart, but nonetheless take a particular position in a number of respects. To start with, *Autistic Company* is not a study of the world in which the autistic person lives, even if it were accessible. What I am concerned with are the forms of living together that autistic and non-autistic people develop in their dealings *with one another*. In the second place, autism is a special case within the studies of other cultures - in autistic people the very ability to take part in what is usually described as the social world or culture seems to be fundamentally impaired. Jim Sinclair writes that 'autism goes deeper than language and culture; autistic people are 'foreigners' in any society. You're going to have to give up your assumptions about shared meanings.'[63] I have therefore looked not so much at the question of how the interactions of autists and non-autists are perceived, experienced, and given meaning by those involved, since that would rule out in advance much of the autistic part of the story. Rather, I have looked at the way this shared existence is actually *lived* in practice.[64]

In the third place, and following on from the first two points - how can a one-sided, non-autistic interpretation of the envisaged interactions be corrected? I pay particular attention to the conceptual snags inherent in the representation of shared existence: how to *conceive* of the special nature of the interactions of autistic and non-autistic people? Our common dualist understanding of the world, it will be argued, seriously delimits our understanding of how autistic and non-autistic people can get on with each other. In this book inspiration for an account that better appreciates what autists and non-autists may actually *share* will be sought in literary fiction.

Although it is one of the most philosophically interesting forms of psychopathology according to Sass, Parnas and Whiting, until recently autism was seldom the subject of discussions in a philosophical context.[65] This has started to change with links coming about between the theory of mind models of autism, advances in the cognitive neurosciences and the philosophy of mind.[66] Although some of these links are addressed here, this study is inspired more by philosophical and anthropological work that tends to move away from mentalist accounts of what constitutes or impedes sharing in human, communal life.

In this study I shall draw on very diverse sources, ranging from literary works and popular imagination to factual writing on autism in scientific literature, from philosophical treatises to everyday empirical details, and from autobiographical accounts to observations on a community for young autistic people with intellectual disabilities. The analysis draws on methods from both the arts and social sciences. Jointly, these constitute a distinct interdisciplinary approach to the subject. As we explore this subject, I shall be commenting above all on the idea that the creation of a communal existence takes place on the level of interpretations and other activities of the human mind.

There is a specific terminological issue concerning the question as to whether it is correct to refer to 'autistic people' or to 'autists.' This question is sometimes answered in the negative because it identifies the person with his deviation from the norm. The preference is therefore for the alternative, deemed to be more humane, of 'people with autism,' which labels the impairment but not the person himself; the two are disconnected so that the person is (partly) protected against being different.[67] This does, however, create the suggestion that autistic difference is something negative and that we already *know* what our non-autistic company has to offer people with autism - the rescue of their personality. Within the autistic community, people even take pride in being different and some have started to call themselves 'autists.' To me, the way we can understand the differences and proximity between autistic and non-autistic people is an open question. For this reason I do not choose to give preference to the term 'people with autism' and will use the terms 'autistic,' 'people with autism' and 'autist' interchangeably.

Finally, some remarks about the structure of this book. I shall look at the need to rethink our concepts in chapter 3. Drawing on the 1989 novella *Vallende ster* [Shooting Star] by the Dutch literary writer and essayist J. Bernlef, this chapter offers a further exploration of the interactions between autistic and non-autistic people. I shall also examine at length the solution that Bernlef formulates for representing a shared existence. Using the same strategy, I will then examine a variety of empirical domains: in chapters 4, 5 and 6 I discuss situations that exemplify the interactions of autistic and non-autistic people on which this study focuses. And I reflect on the question as to *how* these interactions can be described. Each chapter revolves around one of the core problems of the autistic syndrome. They are impairments of, in turn, imagination, socialization and communication. In chapter 7, finally, I shall come back to questions that were formulated in this introduction. But first, in chapter 2, I set out a number of hypotheses and facts about the autistic disorder. I am aiming this chapter particularly at readers who have little background in factual writing on autism. Without this background we can only half understand the fascination with this disorder.

# Given Reality
## Autism - Facts and Figures

The ultimate understanding of autism
may demand both technical advances and conceptual ones
beyond anything we can now even dream of.[1]

When I gave up my job as a care worker to study health sciences and later, when I was able to undertake research into a subject which, up till then, had just been work, social constructivism was very popular. What could have been more obvious than an investigation into *meaning* constructs of autism in our culture? It had a lot in its favour. Existing factual writing on autism at the time occasionally ventured on cultural and historical excursions, but they seemed to be comprehensively influenced by essentialist thinking - a legacy of the struggle for the recognition of autism as a real, existing, congenital impairment. Uta Frith, for instance, dealt with historical case descriptions like the ones found in myths, legends and fairy tales because they seem to suggest that autism has probably always existed independently of socio-cultural influences. From such descriptions we should be able, she wrote, 'to distill those features that are the essence of the disorder beyond our immediate time and cultural context.'[2] Any other history of autism by implication is seen to detract from the reality content of the disorder.

In 2005, in *Constructing Autism*, Majia Nadesan provided an alternative account. She demonstrated in historicizing terms that the way autism could be identified, labelled and approached as a separate, meaningful disorder can be traced back precisely to the time and culture related context of social practices and institutions. She suggests that these views and practices even shape the performance or expression of autistic symptoms. While not rejecting a biological basis for the condition, 'the social factors involved in its identification, representation, interpretation, remediation, and performance are the most important factors in the determination of what it means to be autistic, for individuals, for families and for society.'[3]

Ian Hacking had taken the first, inspiring steps for such a non-essentialist perspective on the dynamics of autism as a psychiatric category. He had argued that, like other psychiatric and psychopathological conditions, childhood autism is subject to certain 'looping effects.' Although autism as pathology works on the 'indifferent' biological (genetic, neurological) level, people with an autism diagnosis are themselves not indifferent to how they are labelled. On the contrary, they may actively find out about the latest scientific insights or may become aware of other changes in the way their condition is culturally perceived. And if they are not themselves aware of and do not care about such changes, specific institutional arrangements that are set up will contribute to the 'making and moulding' of the autistic spectrum. Classification and treatment thus elicit a response from labelled individuals, who may start seeing themselves differently and act accordingly, or they may experience being treated differently and react accordingly. Such adjustments - down to the level of distinct symptoms - force researchers to modify their insights, which may elicit another reaction, and so on. Hacking thus speaks of a 'moving target': the picture is always changing because the classifications interact with those who are being classified.[4]

I take inspiration from Ian Hacking's suggestion as to how to proceed in a constructivist way, without having to detract in any way from the reality of the disorder and the suffering it causes. I do, it is true, want to show that the differences between autists and non-autists within particular practices and manners of speaking are brought home to people. And I want to set out alternative scripts that offer the prospect of more continuity. In that sense my research is constructivist. It shows how debates on autism are simultaneously discussions about essential characteristics of the human condition. But at the same time I in no way want to overlook real perceived, described and measured differences and similarities. I want to do full justice to the experiences of families in which autism is a factor, to the toil of carers at the sharp end and to the fascinating way scientists try to bring structure to the chaotic and obscure reality.

Before I address the question of a shared existence and before I discuss the usability of non-autistic assumptions in our representations, it therefore makes sense to consider a question that precedes this. What does the reality described in the scientific literature look like? What is generally regarded as a given in terms of the autistic disorder, rather than as a product of our imagination, which may say more about 'us' than about the autistic person?

**Classification and Diagnostics**

To the best of my knowledge, the term 'autistic' was first used to describe children with aberrant behaviour in the annual reports of the Institute of Paedology in Nijmegen, Netherlands. Under the heading 'Formalists' in the Behavioural Schematization category, the report for the years 1937-1938 refers to an '(Intelligent) autistic with stereotypical behaviour.'[5] In the following report, 'autistics' appear for the first time as a separate category, characterized by 'excessive self-worth': a 'tendency to *adhere exclusively* to a particular course, as a result of which the individual has too little 'outward' focus and is too much concerned and involved with himself.'[6] The symptoms described correspond closely to later descriptions, of which Kanner's is best known.[7]

*Autistic Disturbances of Affective Contact*

In 1943 the Austrian-born child psychiatrist Leo Kanner (1896-1981), who lived and worked in the United States from 1924 until his death, published what was later to prove a ground-breaking article. In it Kanner described eleven children (eight boys and three girls) who had come to his attention in Johns Hopkins Hospital and whom he classified under a single heading on the basis of painstaking clinical observations. All these children displayed confusing but similar behavioural characteristics, which Kanner grouped under the term 'Autistic disturbances of affective contact' - also the title of his famous article. Taken together, Kanner argued, the common characteristics marked a 'unique' and 'not heretofore reported' syndrome.[8]

From their earliest childhood, these children (all born in the nineteen-thirties) displayed signs of what Kanner called '*extreme autistic aloneness*' - an '*inability to relate themselves* in the ordinary way to people and situations,' which manifested itself in an inclination that 'disregards, ignores, shuts out anything that comes to the child from the outside.' The parents described their children's behaviour in such terms as 'self-sufficient,' 'like in a shell' and 'happiest when left alone.' The affective deficit was not, though, an obstruction to an '*excellent rote memory*,' which meant that the children could retain large amounts of self-contained information (a page from the contents list of an encyclopedia, the twenty-third psalm, etcetera).

Three of the eleven neither spoke nor signed; eight children did achieve speech, but as far as its communicative function was concerned, reported Kanner, there was 'no fundamental difference' between them and the children who could not speak. The talkers had a tendency to store up words they had heard and reproduce them exactly later ('*delayed echolalia*'). They were inclined to repeat personal pronouns literally, so that they referred to themselves as 'you' and another person as 'I.' They had difficulty with the generalization of the symbolic function of language. One boy, for instance, used 'yes' for one thing and one thing only; it was rigidly coupled to the situation in which he had originally learnt it: as a sign that he wanted to ride on his father's shoulders. Aside from an instrumental use to meet their immediate needs, they did not use language 'as a tool for receiving and imparting meaningful messages.'

The children Kanner saw were oversensitive to any 'intrusion . . . from the outside,' including the noise of vacuum cleaners, certain foods and moving objects. They were quick to panic in the event of changes to their environment. They had an '*anxiously obsessive desire for the maintenance of sameness*.' One of the children was beside himself when the family moved house and did not calm down again until all the furniture had been put back in the familiar configuration. Each and every one of the children presented a 'limitation in the variety of spontaneous activity,' expressed in repetitive movements, language and interests.

Whereas the children had an 'excellent, purposeful and 'intelligent' relation to objects,' *people* left them completely cold. It was not so much that they were not aware of the presence of others, wrote Kanner. 'But the people, so long as they left the child alone, figured in about the same manner as did the desk, the bookshelf or the filing cabinet.' The children were 'in ecstasy' when they could exercise control over an object, for example by spinning things round and round, but they never played with other children. 'Profound aloneness dominates all behaviour.' Adults were used as means of getting things done; the hand that had taken something away could be pushed aside 'as a definitely detached object,' but the children's reaction was never a response to the *person* to whom that hand was attached.

It was often extremely difficult to get through to them with a question, and consequently seven of the children had at some time been diagnosed as deaf or hearing impaired. Although they had previously been regarded as feeble-minded, the children seemed to have 'good *cognitive potentialities*' - an observation that was supported by their 'excellent memory' and appeared to be confirmed by their 'strikingly intelligent physiognomics' and physical normality. Lastly, the children came from 'highly intelligent families' and among the parents that Kanner saw there were 'very few really warmhearted fathers and mothers.'

Although he did not rule out a psychogenic factor in the development of the disorder, this last observation (which was later dismissed) did not lead Kanner to conclude that the cause of the children's behaviour should be sought specifically in the environment in which they were brought up. The extraordinary thing about these children was precisely that the affective deficit existed from the start of their lives. Even as babies, these children failed '*to assume at any time an anticipatory posture*' to indicate that they wanted to be picked up, and the parents all recalled how there had never been even the slightest look of recognition. The early occurrence of the disorder was one of the dimensions that led Kanner to make a distinction between this syndrome and all the examples of childhood schizophrenia known at that time.[9]

> The children's aloneness from the beginning of life makes it difficult to attribute the whole picture exclusively to the type of the early parental relations with our patients. We must, then, assume that these children have come into the world with innate inability to form the usual, biologically provided affective contact with people, just as other children come into the world with innate physical or intellectual handicaps. . . . For here we seem to have pure-culture examples of *inborn autistic disturbances of affective contact.*[10]

*Diagnostic Refinement*

Kanner's original definition of what he came to call 'early infantile autism' in subsequent publications was frequently amended over the years. On the basis of clinical material that became available from 1943 onwards, Eisenberg and Kanner concentrated their definition on two essential characteristics: 'extreme self-isolation' (or autistic 'aloneness') and the always present 'obsessive insistence on the preservation of sameness.'[11] This meant that abnormalities in language development were to some extent relegated to the background and regarded as 'derivatives of the basic disturbance in human relatedness.'[12] In their definitions other authors, such as Ornitz and Ritvo in 1968, stressed a hitherto undescribed aspect, a disorder of the sensory stimulation mechanism. Still others drew up criteria which meant that it was conceivable for individuals to be diagnosed as autistic even though they displayed none of Kanner's essential characteristics.[13]

There has also been a good deal of thought about the age when the autistic disorder manifests. According to Kanner, abnormal development from birth was a distinguishing feature of early infantile autism, although he later placed less emphasis on this aspect. Some children appeared to develop relatively normally in the first one or two years of life, after which a loss of capabilities set in. Some definitions omitted the age criterion altogether. An unintended consequence of this was that disorders beginning in infancy were sometimes lumped together with conditions of later childhood or adolescence. Terms like childhood psychosis, childhood schizophrenia and autism were often used as interchangeable diagnoses, and this tendency was sustained by the fact that the term 'autism' was derived from a description of the behaviour of schizophrenic patients.[14]

As a result, the nineteen-fifties and sixties were marked by diagnostic confusion. Looking back, we can see that there were two studies that pointed the way to a broader consensus - the successive work of Michael Rutter and of Lorna Wing, and their colleagues. Both wanted to arrive at a constellation of symptoms specific to autism that would include few if any symptoms that also occur in other disorders, which would at the same time be as general as possible, so that as few children as possible with autistic problems would slip through the net. Although their work is an extension of one another's, Rutter's research pointed in the direction of a relatively narrow definition of the condition; Lorna Wing advocated a comparatively broad approach.

Rutter's investigation in 1966 - with Linda Lockyer in 1967 - was conducted into sixty-three children identified as 'psychotic.' A control group of 'non-psychotic' children was selected alongside the group with childhood psychosis, who had many similarities to children Kanner had studied.[15] Their clinical data were assessed in terms of thirty-four items (speech, ritualistic and compulsive behaviour, motor symptoms, self-harming behaviour, and so forth), twenty-two of which were scored significantly more often in the psychotic children. But two of the items could be scored in *all* the children in the psychotic subgroup: a serious (characterized as 'autistic') dysfunction in relationships with other people, and abnormalities in communication (such as the failure to acquire spoken language, the failure to respond to auditory stimuli, the inversion of personal pronouns and echolalia). Almost all these psychotic children also displayed a fixed craving for repetition.

The study also suggested that the extreme age limit at which the first signs of the disorder should be recognizable had to be set at thirty months: it could be demonstrated that nine of the sixty-three children had developed apparently normally until they were two and a half. Unlike individuals with psychoses that occur later in childhood, these children did not differ from the early onset group in their behaviour or in the prognosis.[16] The subgroup displayed the same unique combination of disorders as the children Kanner had described.

While other diagnostic categories in the realm of childhood psychoses fell into disuse, Kanner's definition proved to be a usable instrument for clinicians, researchers, policy-makers and representatives alike.[17] It had meanwhile become clear, however, that Kanner's original view that autistic people were essentially of normal intelligence and that their abnormal behaviour stemmed solely from their specific disorder had to be discarded. It was found that the IQs of children who were studied varied greatly, autism and mental retardation frequently occurred together and the level of intellectual function coloured autistic behaviour.[18]

According to Rutter, this implied that the child's mental age had to be taken into account in reaching a diagnosis and in scientific research. On the grounds of his mental age alone, communicative language cannot be expected from a four-year-old who functions at a level of six months; to make a diagnosis of autism requires specific, *qualitative* abnormalities that cannot be accounted for by the level of intellectual function. Rutter's influential definition of 1978 encapsulated these views.

> The four criteria are (1) an onset before the age of 30 months, (2) impaired social development that has a number of special characteristics and is out of keeping with the child's intellectual level, (3) delayed and deviant language development that also has certain defined features and is out of keeping with the child's intellectual level, and (4) insistence on sameness, as shown by stereotyped play patterns, abnormal preoccupations or resistance to change.[19]

*Spectrum of Autistic Disorders*

While autistic behaviour proved to be affected by age and developmental level, conversely certain behaviours observed in people with autism can also be found in passing phases in the development of normal and otherwise handicapped, non-autistic children. One example is echolalia. Social impairment, on the other hand, is never seen in other children. Gradually autism ceased to be regarded as a syndrome associated with schizophrenia and started to be viewed as a *developmental disorder* whose course researchers believed they would be better able to understand by finding out about the interaction of forces that impact on normal and deviant development.[20]

Mindful of this interrelation with other characteristics, in 1978 and 1979 Lorna Wing and Judith Gould conducted a major epidemiological study of all the children with communication problems, social impairments or stereotyped behaviours living in what was then the London Borough of Camberwell and born between 1956 and 1970.[21] They included, of course, children with autism or behaviour akin to autism. Children with serious learning difficulties were also selected. Two subgroups were identified within the selection of 914 children in total - a socially able but intellectually impaired group, and a group with social impairments (of whom more than half may also, but not necessarily, have been mentally retarded). The groups were then assessed for their internal coherence.

A significant proportion of the socially impaired children functioned at such a low level that it could not be established whether the impairments they presented were a sign of autism or had to be attributed to the mental handicap. This could be done in the more intelligent but socially impaired children. As well as their social deficit, these children displayed all sorts of problems in verbal and nonverbal communication and imagination. This boiled down to the absence or the mechanical performance of symbolic, imaginative activities, such as 'let's pretend' games. The authors did not find the combination of related problems in social interaction, communication and imagination in any of the socially adjusted children. The presence of this 'triad of impairments' appeared to point to an unconcealed autistic syndrome.

Wing and Gould saw the limitations in socialization, communication and imagination as the core of a whole series of clinical phenomena, which Wing later identified as a continuum of autistic characteristics. Aside from the three central symptoms, Wing described characteristics that were associated with this cluster without being essential. Firstly, children with the triad displayed all sorts of repetitive and stereotyped behaviour. Impairments in other mental functions were also recorded strikingly often, though not necessarily. Wing noted abnormalities in the use of language,[22] in motor coordination, in the reaction to sensory stimuli and in cognitive skills (for instance in the doubly-handicapped, intellectually impaired group).

Wing's continuum of autism spectrum disorders is more broadly-defined than Kanner's syndrome. True, it was possible to identify seventeen children in the Camberwell study with 'classic autism' consistent with the criteria defined by Eisenberg and Kanner in 1956, but according to Wing and Gould these children represented only one of the many forms in which the underlying disorder could manifest itself. Other types could also be identified on the basis of the quality of social interactions - for instance children who were not socially withdrawn and actually tried to approach others, but in bizarre ways. Some children changed type in the course of their development. In the absence of demonstrable biological differences and practical advantages, argued Wing and Gould, demarcation lines in principle between 'classic autism' and milder, related social disorders, were arbitrary. Hence their call for a relatively broad approach that would include all children with the triad, from mildly to seriously impaired.

*Asperger's Syndrome*

Nowadays anyone discussing disorders associated with autism will inevitably refer to the work of the Viennese doctor Hans Asperger (1906-1980). Asperger's *Die 'Autistischen Psychopathen' im Kindesalter*, long overlooked in the Anglo-Saxon world, came out a year after Kanner published his findings.[23] For several years now, there has been a great deal of interest in Asperger's work because he observed behavioural characteristics that were missing from Kanner's work, but are nowadays regarded as autistic. Whereas Kanner's description is now often associated with the 'classic,' low-functioning autistic child, Asperger's report focused attention on the existence of children who were not mentally retarded, had developed good verbal skills and were older, but who were nonetheless autistic.[24]

There are significant similarities between the two observations, which were carried out independently of one another. Both Kanner and Asperger reported problems of social interaction - Asperger described the connection with other people as flat and weak and said that there was an empathic deficit. They both described an impairment in, particularly, nonverbal communication (gestures, body language). Both saw a resistance to change, avoidance of eye contact and unusual, one-sided patterns of interest. The observations diverge where language and motor skills are concerned. Whereas Kanner's children displayed retarded and deviant verbal communication, Asperger noted that his patients had a good command of language, almost like little adults. And while Kanner's children usually had good motor skills and their connection with the world of things seemed to be better than their relationship with people, Asperger's patients were physically clumsy; their relationship with the world seemed disturbed across the board.

Asperger's Disorder has become an official diagnostic category, although the basis of this status is not uncontested. Wing, for instance, does not accept that people who fit Asperger's description differ essentially from the children Kanner saw.[25] She places them, along with cognitively high-functioning classic autistic people, at the milder end of the autistic spectrum. Some children of the Kanner type even develop to such an extent that there is scarcely any discernible difference between them and the Asperger type. Wing holds that a distinction between the two can be useful in alerting us to the range of behaviours through which the underlying disorder can be expressed, but in essence it is the same intrinsic condition that blocks participation in reciprocal social interaction in everyone on the spectrum.

> The central problem, which, by definition, is both necessary and sufficient for the diagnosis of a disorder in this continuum, is an intrinsic impairment in development of the ability to engage in reciprocal social interaction, which is fundamentally different from those described in neurotic or conduct disorders. This can occur on its own, but in most cases it is accompanied by impairments of other psychological functions, some much more commonly than others. The manifestations of the social and other problems vary widely in type and severity, and all kinds of combinations of impairments are seen in clinical practice. Some of these combinations have been named as syndromes, but many have not been assigned a separate identity. Thus the term continuum represents a concept of considerable complexity, rather than simply a straight line from severe to mild.[26]

In sum, the studies by Wing and Rutter and their colleagues are regarded as important contributions to the question as to whether autistic behavioural characteristics display a chance relationship or point to a 'natural entity, a true syndrome'[27] with a shared underlying cause or complex of causes. Someone with autism is likely to have additional behavioural disorders, such as fits of rage or hyperactivity; there may be strange reactions to sensory stimuli (oversensitivity to or a fascination with sounds, smells and touching); the cognitive profile is usually unbalanced (good visual-spatial understanding, low scores on verbal items) - all of this is possible, but not *necessary*. Eating disorders (rejection of certain foods; compulsive eating of inedible things) and sleep disturbances are common; abnormal mood swings (giggling, crying for no apparent reason) and self-harming behaviour (hand-biting, head-banging) are reported; these children may often fail to recognize real hazards but at the same time display excessive fear of innocent objects (for instance, anything green) - each and every one of these symptoms is important in drawing up an individual plan for treatment, but no single one of them is essential.

What was substantiated empirically for the first time in these studies is the claim that the autistic disorder is a genuine, existing syndrome, with at its centre a unique combination of disorders in social, communication and imagination skills, and limited, repetitive and stereotyped patterns of behaviour. That same cluster is still the starting point for diagnosis in current clinical practice. The definition of the autistic disorder in the limited sense, as we shall shortly see, still includes many traces of Rutter's definition; the overarching category of pervasive developmental disorders is almost entirely covered by the spectrum that Wing defined.[28]

### DSM-IV-TR and Diagnostic Practice

Because autism is a developmental disorder, not a fixed condition, the earliest possible diagnosis is extremely important. Early recognition makes it possible to initiate specific assistance, before the child has deviated still further from the normal course of development. The fact is, however, that the diagnosis is seldom made before the second year, often only after a period of distressing uncertainty in the parents. As a result of capacity shortages in institutions and gaps in the available knowledge, there is said to be under-diagnosis, particularly among mentally handicapped children.[29]

No one has yet found a specific biological cause for the constellation of autistic behaviours. There are no biological markers for the diagnosis of autism. We cannot point to chromosomal abnormalities or disturbances in the enzyme system; we have to go by behavioural symptoms and the case history. Autism scales are designed to recognize autism as early as possible and isolate it from disorders that can cause it to be overlooked, such as a mental handicap, and to distinguish it from conditions with a superficial resemblance to autism, such as deafness. Abnormalities in behaviour, which can manifest in many different ways, often only become clear over time, in contrast with normal developmental progress. Parents' unfamiliarity with normal development or doctors' unfamiliarity with autism can also hinder an early diagnosis.

An important step in the diagnostic process is to assign complaints and symptoms to a specific category of disorder. According to the latest edition of the *Diagnostic and Statistic Manual of Mental Disorders*, which is widely used for this purpose, the Autistic Disorder comes into the category of 'Pervasive Developmental Disorders.' This category also includes Asperger's Disorder, Rett's Disorder, Childhood Disintegrative Disorder, and Pervasive Developmental Disorder Not Otherwise Specified (Including Atypical Autism) or PDD NOS.

## Diagnostic Criteria for 299.00 Autistic Disorder

A.  A total of six (or more) items from (1), (2), and (3), with at least two from (1), and one each from (2) and (3):

1.  qualitative impairment in social interaction, as manifested by at least two of the following:
(a)  marked impairment in the use of multiple nonverbal behaviors such as eye-to-eye gaze, facial expression, body postures, and gestures to regulate social interaction
(b)  failure to develop peer relationships appropriate to developmental level
(c)  a lack of spontaneous seeking to share enjoyment, interests, or achievements with other people (e.g., by a lack of showing, bringing, or pointing out objects of interest)
(d)  lack of social or emotional reciprocity

2.  qualitative impairments in communication as manifested by at least one of the following:
(a)  delay in, or total lack of, the development of spoken language (not accompanied by an attempt to compensate through alternative modes of communication such as gesture or mime)
(b)  in individuals with adequate speech, marked impairment in the ability to initiate or sustain a conversation with others
(c)  stereotyped and repetitive use of language or idiosyncratic language
(d)  lack of varied, spontaneous make-believe play or social imitative play appropriate to developmental level

3.  restricted repetitive and stereotyped patterns of behavior, interests and activities, as manifested by at least one of the following:
(a)  encompassing preoccupation with one or more stereotyped and restricted patterns of interest that is abnormal either in intensity or focus
(b)  apparently inflexible adherence to specific, nonfunctional routines or rituals
(c)  stereotyped and repetitive motor mannerisms (e.g., hand or finger flapping or twisting, or complex whole-body movements)
(d)  persistent preoccupation with parts of objects

B.  Delays or abnormal functioning in at least one of the following areas, with onset prior to age 3 years: (1) social interaction, (2) language as used in social communication, or (3) symbolic or imaginative play.

C.  The disturbance is not better accounted for by Rett's Disorder or Childhood Disintegrative Disorder.[30]

The PDD category as a whole (also called Autism Spectrum Disorders, ASD) is characterized by serious and pervasive impairments in social, communication or imaginative capacity, where the level at which the individual functions is not in step with his general level of development or mental age. The simultaneous occurrence of certain impairments in all three areas is required for the specific diagnosis of 'autistic disorder.' The age of onset is also specified. The term 'pervasive' focuses attention on 'the widespread distortion of the developmental process (involving communication, socialization, and thought processes).'[31] It should be noted here that the central disorders are not 'all-pervasive'; there may be islands of skills that remain unimpaired, particularly in visual-spatial abilities. A person may therefore not be identified with his autism: 'A diagnostic label is not able or intended to capture the fullness of an individual.'[32]

*Autism Epidemic?*
*DSM-IV-TR* reckons the prevalence of autistic disorder at a median rate of five cases per 10,000 people, with reported rates ranging from two to twenty cases per 10,000 individuals.[33] When the disorders related to autism are added, the figure, although less reliable, is considerably higher. For a long time, Wing and Gould's 1979 survey was normative for the umbrella category of pervasive developmental disorders; it works out at a prevalence of 21.2 children with the triad per 10,000 inhabitants up to the age of 15, 4.9 of whom have a history of classic autism. Recent epidemiological studies report figures that are around twice as high as earlier estimates. In this context, in 1997 Bryson discusses recent surveys which, working on stringent criteria, report constant numbers of 1 : 1,000.[34] For the broader category of autistic spectrum disorders the most recent studies report a prevalence of 60 per 10,000 individuals, with an estimate of 8-30 per 10,000 individuals with classic autism.[35] The data are taken from studies in Western and non-Western societies and among different social groups.

Reviewing these figures, it is easy to get the impression that we are dealing with a veritable epidemic of autism diagnoses, particularly since the early nineteen-nineties. In his 2007 work *Unstrange Minds*, however, cultural anthropologist Roy Grinker takes the view that while it is true that autism as a series of social and cognitive differences only becomes visible within a particular cultural context, the underlying symptoms must be realistically denoted: 'the same symptoms are found across cultures and, based on what we know about autism in the distant past, across time as well.'[36] The recent rise in diagnoses can therefore be attributed in its entirety to the increasing awareness and visibility of autism in our culture, he argues. Diagnostic refinements and institutional changes, such as the introduction of the label 'autism' as a valid category qualifying an individual for publicly provided special education, play an important role in this. At the same time Grinker strongly contests the tragic and frightening use of the term 'epidemic' that has dominated reports in the media. He turns it on its head by suggesting that the sharp rise in the figures for people with autism is actually good news and a sign of progress:

the newer, higher, more accurate statistics on autism are a sign that we are finally seeing and appreciating a kind of human difference that we once turned away from and that many other cultures still hide away in homes or institutions or denigrate as bizarre. The result of the new rates is that we are fortunately seeing more research, more philanthropy, and more understanding of how families struggle to cope.[37]

Although it is difficult to test the level of cognitive function in communication skills as a consequence of autistic disorder, sophisticated tests (which also measure non-verbal intelligence) are producing stable results. In 'most cases,' according to *DSM-IV-TR*, autism is associated with a more or less severe degree of mental retardation. The retardation is usually within the moderate range (IQs of 35-50), although much depends on the selection criteria.[38] About half of the quarter with an IQ of over 70 achieved normal scores. The higher the IQ, the better the prognosis as far as schools and social functioning are concerned. As we have seen, people with autism often display an unbalanced development profile (notably a good visual-spatial understanding combined with low scores on tests of verbal items). Independent of the IQ score, 6% of autistic people have exceptional talents, even compared with the non-autistic norm. These so-called savant skills are generally visual-spatial or mathematical, although a few autistic people have musical or other talents.[39]

In autism, special skills in a particular area are not a sign of hidden general intelligence. An 'autistic savant,' for example a calendar calculator, may have an IQ of 40-50. Mathematical and visual-spatial skills certainly do not imply social intelligence either. Splinter skills in autistic people are always in contrast to the typical qualitative deficits in social, communication and imagination capabilities. Peak skills seem to be linked to a specific organization of the brain, possibly with a shift in the brain from the left to the right hemisphere, which is associated with visual-spatial skills. Frith consequently does not regard the presence of a special gift as an unaffected remnant of normality, in fact she does not see it as a skill at all, but as a symptom in which the underlying impairment in the cognitive functioning of autistic individuals comes to the surface.

According to *DSM-IV-TR*, the autistic disorder is four to five times more common in males than females. However, this figure varies from 2 : 1 in severely mentally handicapped individuals to 4 : 1 in those with higher mental function. If cases of Asperger's Syndrome are included, the imbalance shifts still further towards male over-representation.[40]

## Behaviour and Development

Qualitative disorders in social skills, communication and imagination, and limited, repetitive and stereotyped behaviours, interests and activities - the very words sound disastrous enough. But how, in concrete terms, ought we to conceive of such impairments? We know that the way the disorder presents may vary according to an individual's age, character and intelligence. As far as age is concerned, the early literature refers predominantly to autistic children, as if there were no adolescents or adults with autism. When autism was first identified, attention was naturally focused on children because impairments were most pronounced in them and this was where the greatest need for answers lay. It was not until the early nineteen-eighties that adolescents and adults with autism were recognized, a development that contributed to our concept of autism as a dynamic disorder that can take various forms.

### Socialization

The social handicap is one of the most obvious and least understood aspects of the autistic syndrome. Eisenberg and Kanner regarded the combination of extreme indifference to the social environment and, in sharp contrast, extreme sensitivity to changes in the physical environment as an essential characteristic of the syndrome.[41] This characteristic imbalance in people with autism can be defined in more detail with the aid of what Wing called 'social recognition.' 'Social recognition,' she wrote, 'refers to the ability to recognize that other human beings are the most interesting and potentially rewarding features of the environment.'[42]

Normally speaking, the first signs of social recognition, such as a preference for the human voice and facial expression above other stimuli, can be observed in the first few weeks of life. Other milestones in normal social development are learning to read meanings and emotions in the faces of parents or carers, the start of reciprocal eye contact and vocal interaction, learning to distinguish between parents and others, bonding from which the world is then explored, achieving intersubjectivity, and the development of a range of social skills appropriate to contact with other children of their own age. This is where things go badly wrong in autistic children.

An impairment in social recognition occurs very early in the development of autistic children. Infants give the impression of disliking being taken out of the cot, and feel like rag dolls when they are picked up. Reciprocal eye contact and contact through facial expression do not start to develop; these babies do not respond to smiles. As a toddler, a child may become more used to people. He may use their presence to get something done, to play or to tickle, and may sometimes become very attached to someone (albeit more out of routine than emotionally). But the child does not really seem involved with the people around him. He does not share his interest in something that has attracted his attention, happiness, surprise or a sense of pride, with anyone else. Baron-Cohen and Bolton refer to an autistic child who never came to his parents to show them where he had hurt himself when he fell over - he was more interested in lining up bricks in a row.[43]

The lack of skills in dealing with others becomes all the more obvious when the child reaches school age. Although some children with higher IQs may have mastered a few social skills, the essential inability to achieve any form of togetherness remains. Despite the fact that the sharper corners of autism do appear to wear down a little with time - children become nicer and more sociable, are less anxious and rigid, and behave better in public - it is unlikely that anyone ever grows out of his autism. The lack of mutual contact remains, as evidenced by an inability to play with others. These children attract fewer contemporaries than normal and appear to be happiest when they are left alone.

Adolescents can sometimes learn social skills geared to safe, recurring situations from which they sometimes even derive pleasure. For instance they may be happy if the whole family is together. Others have a relapse around puberty, with a loss of skills and a return of anxieties that may be even greater than before. Adolescents and adults sometimes long for connection and human warmth, but do not know how to deal with them. Interaction remains relatively poor and asymmetrical as a result of a lack of understanding of the needs of other people and difficulty in interpreting feelings. The social adjustment that some high-functioning autistic individuals achieve comes across as learned rather than intuitive. People with autism lack the 'social fluency' needed to allow gestures, eye contact, body language and facial expressions to play a regulating role in social interaction in the usual subtle manner.

Even aside from the many individual nuances and changes over the years, the social deficit can manifest itself in very different ways. Working on the basis of the quality of social interaction, Wing and Gould suggested a typology that covers the whole spectrum of social impairments.[44] This typology is connected to a certain extent to the level of mental function.

The group Wing and Gould classify as 'aloof' seem to resemble most closely the group Kanner described in 1943. These people display very severe limitations in social interaction; some of them remain indifferent to social approaches under any circumstances, while others only emerge in order to get something done, rapidly retreating to their isolated state. Yet others do like simple physical contact (tickling, romping, cuddling), but are not interested in the social aspects of that contact. Other people seem unable to get through to them in any meaningful way; it is as if they are living inside a bubble. In children of this type their indifference to other children of their own age is particularly striking. Their 'aloneness' is extreme.

Some children of the aloof type later go on to develop a 'passive' style of social interaction. The main characteristic of this group is that they never seek social contact spontaneously. They accept approaches by others impassively and put up no resistance when other people involve them in their activities. They are very compliant and do what other people tell them to. Children of this type will continue to play the part in a game assigned to them by others for as long as the others carry on playing.

A third group does initiate social contact (chiefly with adults), but in an inappropriate way. These people are unable to imagine another person's wants and needs and are mainly concerned with indulging idiosyncratic preoccupations in a stereotypical manner, for example by constantly bringing up prime numbers. They go on and on; nothing and nobody can stop them. Their 'active but odd' behaviour often makes this group less acceptable to other people than the passive group.

### Communication

Abnormalities in language and communication of the kind found in autistic people are probably a consequence of a fundamental deficit in the relationship with people.[45] Autistic people appear to lack the means and motives to acquire a concept of the world that is shared with others. As early as 1943 Kanner observed that even those children who spoke did not use language to communicate meaningfully. Delayed right across the board, the development of communication is particularly seriously impaired in social terms. According to Wing the social aspect of communication involves giving and receiving non-verbal, pre-verbal and verbal social signals, deriving pleasure from conversation, and the ability and desire to talk about feelings and share ideas.[46]

The first communication skills normally develop very early. The baby makes her wants and feelings clear and responds to people and objects with simple, and later more complex, gestures and other non-verbal means of communication (posture, facial expressions). Increasingly this is accompanied by sounds that parents learn to interpret. The child learns to take turns by smiling and laughing back and through mutual eye contact; the first (pre-verbal) indicative use of signals starts when parent and baby look together at something that attracts attention. Round about the end of the first year, babbling and imitating sounds and words make way for one-word sentences, and it is also then that simple instructions are understood. Once a child discovers that she can communicate with other people through language, her vocabulary rapidly expands to around three hundred words by the time she is two. Language develops to produce longer and more complex sentences between the second and fifth years, and by around the age of eight all grammatical constructions are present.

In autistic children the development of communication is impaired from a very early age. As infants, these children appear to be deaf to attempts to approach them by means of sound and speech whereas they react very violently to certain noises. When autistic babies cry, they are often inconsolable. They babble very little, and when they do it is later and less varied. As in the case of crying, expression and intent are lacking. A striking factor is the absence of joint attention, which involves a child's communicating his interest in an object, or his desire to have it, by pointing at it and is an important forerunner of the indicative or symbolic use of language. An individual who has no notion of joint attention will never get much beyond expressing basic needs; anyone who has no interest in shared references will never respond spontaneously when others stimulate him to communicate, even if he does have intact language skills.

If language nonetheless develops, both comprehension and the active generation of language are more severely delayed than might be expected on the grounds of the intellectual level. Even after the age of three, three-quarters of verbal children with autism still exhibit echolalia - the immediate or delayed repetition of sounds and words that have been heard, sometimes completely mechanically, at others used expressively and functionally, but always exactly. Around half of all people with autism go on to develop more or less usable language in the end.[47] The presence of this before the age of five is of immense prognostic value for the level of functioning later.

As a rule, language development is divided into four levels. Sound recognition and formation are delayed in autistic children, but the progress of development is normal. Admittedly, the voice often sounds mechanical and monotonous, but this is part of a wider failure to convey feelings and emotions. The use of the rules of grammar in forming words and sentences is frequently very severely delayed, but in terms of quality develops no differently from the way it progresses in non-autistic children.

One aspect in which people with autism differ quite specifically is the symbolic representation of events and objects in meaningful language (the level of semantics). Although some are able to build up immense vocabularies with which they can describe things in minute detail, autistic people have problems with more abstract or figurative expressions. These children take language very literally; a question like 'have you lost your tongue?' is likely to prompt them to go and look for it. Children with autism have difficulty forming concepts. Instead of taking their observational cue from meaning, as neurotypical children do, even though this sometimes leads to mistakes (such as calling a glass a cup), autistic children make a striking error in the opposite direction: they use the word 'cup' only for the single example that they learned to call by that name. This indicates that they have difficulty understanding separate observations under an overarching category

of meaning that includes 'cups' in all shapes and sizes. This problem seems
to be related to the difficulty with deictic terms - words without a fixed
referent whose meaning varies according to the context (place, time, person).
They typically lead to confusion in concepts like here/there, now/then,
you/me. The transposition of personal pronouns (referring to themselves in
the third person rather than as 'I') is particularly noticeable.[48]

The greatest problems occur on the fourth level, of the social use of
language, where people are expected to follow rules attuned to the person and
the situation. The pragmatic deficit manifests itself in an inability to read the
intent and the expectation concealed behind the literal meaning. Even
verbally gifted autistic individuals have the utmost difficulty mastering the
subtle role play of a conversation and the accompanying agreement between
the speaker and the listener. These are skills like taking account of the other
person's prior knowledge and interests. Autistic people may utterly lose
themselves in details, deliver endless monologues about what preoccupies
them, and only them, and introduce idiosyncratic language. The difficulty lies
not just with content - the form of a conversation also creates often
insurmountable problems. The skills involved here include speaking in turn,
allowing the other person to finish what they are saying, maintaining eye
contact to gauge the other person's reaction, keeping the conversation going
by asking questions and observing the rules of good manners.

The fact that autistic individuals seldom if ever learn to compensate
for their deficit with alternative means of communication, such as sign
language, confirms that in autism the problem is in communication skills and
not essentially a language impairment. They have particular difficulty with
symbolic gestures that seemingly have nothing to do with the meaning. This
contrasts with their ability to grasp concrete or instrumental gestures, such as
pushing someone away, in which there is little interpretative leeway. As with
spoken language, there is a tendency to make gestures as minimal as possible.
Non-verbal interaction (mimicry, outward appearance, body language, eye
contact and the volume, tone and rhythm of the voice) is as severely impaired
as verbal communication. Non-verbal signs can sometimes be learned by
imprinting them as fixed rules. Even then, non-verbal behaviour is likely to
get out of step with the content of the conversation or be inappropriate in the
situation (speaking too loudly in a formal setting, for example, or going to
stand too close to a stranger) and this is impossible to prevent.

*Imagination*
The autistic imagination deficit as expressed in a lack of varied,
spontaneous imaginative play or social imitation play that cannot be related
to the developmental age is closely related to the communication
impairment.[49] Both communication and imagination skills presuppose the
creation of a cognitive space, of an inner language, where words act as

symbols of reality. A conceptual framework is created into which new events, people and things are fitted and on which a person can draw in communicating with the world. Without a system of internal representations and categorizations, observations and perceptions cannot be placed in a broader, meaningful context. This seems to be the case in people with autism, with all that this implies in terms of the way they deal with reality.

Play usually develops in the early months as an infant manipulates things, puts them in her mouth or looks at them; later she will combine objects. Functional play, using a cup to give a doll an imaginary drink, for instance, develops by the end of the first year. In symbolic play (from eighteen months on), which is regarded as an outward sign of inner language, the activity is no longer constrained in any way by the physical properties of the object. Social imitation play starts to appear at the end of the second year, when the child puts herself in the position of another, real or fictitious, person and enters that person's experience by pretending she is the other person. Imitation of parents' facial expressions, a precursor of social imitation, starts in the first few months of life.

In autistic children the development of the imagination takes a radically different course. The autistic interaction with the world is in stark contrast to the rich play of a child developing normally. 'As an observer, one does not smile at the play of young children with autism; one often feels puzzled or confused and experiences the sense that the child is not having fun,' wrote Wulff.[50] Their play is often determined solely by seeking sensory stimuli. A toy car evokes interest because the wheels go round, not because of what it represents. Autistic children are more interested in the taste, smell, colour or tactile properties of things than in their function. Some play in a stereotypical manner, for example with dolls. But imaginative play, in which a stick becomes a gun, is absent. An autistic child, so it seems, would rather put things in a row.[51]

Autistic people can lose themselves wholly in concrete details, without being able to imagine anything by them - something that transcends concrete observation and in some cases negates it: an implicit connection, a made-up plot, a symbolic order, a probable subject, in short *the story around them*. This indicates that the inner language is not developing. There is no shortage of words and actions as such - what people with autism do not have are enough *ideas*.

Autistic children also reveal a lack of imagination in regard to people at a very early age. Here again, one often sees a preference for sensory properties. Imitating facial expression and other non-verbal signals proceeds with difficulty. Parents of autistic children notice that there is no social involvement, for instance in games of peek-a-boo. Imitation does develop in some children, but it remains superficial - an empty copy of human actions with no understanding of the underlying meaning, without the accompanying inner experience. 'There may be repetitive, stereotyped enacting of a role, such as a television character, an animal or an inanimate object such as a train, but without variation or empathy.'[52] In extreme cases it can be described as 'echopraxia' - a hollow and mechanical mirroring of outward actions that appears to resemble echolalia.

If a child fails to develop social imitation, he will also not learn to put himself in the position and mental world of another person. Later in life some autistic individuals do develop an awareness that there is something going on in the inner world of other people, but they do not have the faintest idea of what it might be or how to find out. Sometimes an autistic child will take an adult's face in his hands and stare at it intently 'as if searching for a meaning which eludes him.'[53] Because they cannot make a permanent *representation* of what is going on in the other person, they will not associate outward signs (an ironic look in the eyes, a raised eyebrow) with mental content. This leads to great uncertainty in social interaction. Some autistic people do learn to read the thoughts and feelings of others, albeit in a calculating way rather than in the usual unconscious, empathic manner.

### Limited, Repetitive and Stereotyped Behaviours

Limited, repetitive and stereotyped patterns of behaviour, interests and activities are the last symptom on which *DSM-IV-TR* focuses.[54] Autistic behaviour is characterized by a rigidity that contrasts sharply with the room for manoeuvre that neurotypical children make for themselves. Their need for structure and repetition notwithstanding, they throw themselves wholeheartedly into life as an uncertain adventure. They are curious about new things, want to grow up, want to tackle things they are really not yet ready for. Autistic children do not want any of that. They cling anxiously to familiar habits, rules, routines, sequences and rituals. It is as if their laboriously constructed world crumbles again with each change. As if in the absence of a general overview and symbolic coherence this is the only way they can achieve order and safety. Or simply because this is the way their brains work. Be this as it may, everything has to tally for an autistic child.

Back in 1943, Kanner had already observed a limited repertoire of spontaneous activities in the children he had seen, describing an 'anxiously obsessive desire for the maintenance of sameness.'[55] The resistance to change can be expressed in different ways and crop up anywhere and everywhere: a surprise in food (a new taste, something extra) is not accepted; an irregularity in the floor, a missing puzzle piece, anything down to the tiniest detail that is not the same can upset an autistic child; moving the furniture, a new face in the classroom, buying new clothes and changes in the daily schedule can all meet with fierce resistance. Repetitive behaviour can also manifest itself in many ways, ranging from stereotyped physical movements - fiddling with tassels, spinning everything that is round (wheels, knobs, ashtrays, cups and saucers) - to special preoccupations with switching lights on and off or the arrival and departure times of trains.

In 1979, Wing and Gould also reported unusual patterns of activity in children with the triad. They described these self-selected activities as varied in nature but their range was always more or less restricted and they tended to be repetitive and stereotyped. In 1988, Wing reported that this desire for repetition related to the imagination deficit was also found in non-autistics. The difference lies in the *intensity* of the behaviour; in autistic children, the repetitive compulsion can totally dominate spontaneous activity. An autistic person is so attached to fixed habits that they can completely take over his life. Changes in the environment can cause desperate panic. Breaking rooted patterns can provoke outbursts of rage. The resistance to change is often so extreme that everything and everyone in the vicinity of the autistic person has to adjust to his fixations.

The way the deficit expresses itself in flexible abilities is related to the level of social and cognitive functioning. Some autistic individuals who have serious social and cognitive impairments, wrote Wing in 1988, engage in virtually no spontaneous activities. They are attached to a specific chair or place at the table, always make the same simple movements or adopt the same posture. Others are obsessed with certain sensory stimuli (light, sound, licking everything). They rock back and forth, bang their fists together, wriggle their fingers in front of their eyes or endlessly pace to and fro. A child who functions at this level is 'as it were trapped in his own movements and the sensation they cause. He is so intent on these self-stimulating activities that he can cut himself off from his surroundings.'[56]

In autistic people with less profound impairments one sees more complex movements and preoccupations with more elaborate stimuli, such as a particular tune. The limited repertoire of activities is expressed in collecting or arranging objects. Flapping the arms and hands, jumping up and down, walking on tiptoe and fluttering motions as if the hands are wings are very typical motor phenomena that are mainly seen in a state of excitement.

In higher functioning people with autism repetitive behaviour can take the form of insisting on doing things in a specific way and in a specific order (fixed rituals for going to bed, demanding exactly the same answer to the same question). This is more a matter of compulsion than unconscious behaviour. The initial rigidity does, it is true, diminish as the child gets older and comes into contact with other people and situations that extend his experiences, but the transitions between activities remain particularly difficult moments. At the highest level of development the repetitive behaviour assumes intellectual and verbal forms, such as accumulating facts about physics or taking an exclusive interest in meteorological phenomena. And finally there is also a typically rigid style of problem-solving thinking that fits into this mould.

## Explaining Autism

People with autism develop in a radically different way from other people. The disorder has far-reaching implications for social recognition, communication skills and intellectual freedom of movement. Autism points up what we usually recognize as typical human characteristics. 'We are led to ask: What is so special about persons, how does the normal infant (and child) come to recognize people *as* people, and what has gone so badly awry in autism?'[57] This supposed undermining of the human condition recurs in various explanations for autism that have been put forward over the years. Accepting that autists are not extra-terrestrials, robots or changelings, where does their other-worldly behaviour come from?

### *Environment*

Despite the widespread acceptance of theories that look for the cause of autism in a genetic defect, authors often make room in their summaries for ideas that are now generally rejected. This pre-history often serves as a jumping-off point for modern insights, to emphasize a break with the past. Hypotheses that locate the cause of autism in the child's social and psychological environment rather than in an organic predisposition are discredited. All the same, living on in what is known as the 'refrigerator mother' myth, these ideas are often still a source of confusion even now.

Bruno Bettelheim's 1967 work *The Empty Fortress* is a well-known example. Although Bettelheim did not rule out an organic factor in his explanation, this nuance effectively disappeared in his work, with its strong psychodynamic slant.[58] Bettelheim's work is therefore known as the source of the idea, regarded as disastrous for parents in both emotional and therapeutic terms, that children are *made* autistic. Bettelheim asserted that autistic behaviour was the child's adaptation - a symbolic refusal to become 'I,' made out of sheer necessity - in response to a hostile, loveless environment. The most important factor in this was the mother who, he argued, was weighed down by guilt because she had not really wanted her child. In consequence she sent ambiguous signals. In every case where, according to Bettelheim, this could be established with certainty, 'these conscious or unconscious attitudes were experienced by the child as the wish that he did not exist.'[59] Bettelheim consequently advocated separating the children from their parents as the best treatment strategy - from a modern perspective a wholly erroneous and unforgivable notion.

Contemporary authors have greater difficulty placing Kanner's views. He believed that, alongside a necessary biological predisposition, a psychogenic factor in the occurrence of autism could not be ruled out. Take, for instance, the cool and detached demeanour he noted in parents of the children he studied. These may have been mild autistic traits, which could indicate a genetic component. But Kanner also pointed to the effect such an attitude must have. In a formulation that has been widely challenged, he referred to parents who had themselves been brought up in 'emotional refrigerators' and who now raised their own offspring in 'refrigerators which did not defrost.'[60]

Eisenberg and Kanner described the paradigmatic example of 'the 'emotional refrigeration' that has been the common lot of autistic children.'[61] They wrote of the autismogenic role of the 'mechanization of care,' the 'absence of emotional warmth' and an upbringing along 'scientific' lines, where parents were told to protect children 'from infections' by 'minimizing human contact' and taught that their child was 'not to be picked up for crying, except on schedule.'[62] The case they cited was 'an extreme instance chosen for emphasis'[63] - gross neglect, Eisenberg and Kanner observed, is seldom seen in autistic children.

> But the formal provision of food and shelter and the absence of neglect as defined by statutory law are insufficient criteria for the adequacy of family care. . . . These children were, in general, conceived less out of a positive desire than out of an acceptance of childbearing as part of the marital contract. Physical needs were attended to mechanically and on schedule according to the rigid precepts of naïve behaviorism applied with a vengeance. One can discern relatively few instances of warmth and affection.[64]

These words resonate with the behaviourist context of the thinking about child-rearing in America in the late nineteen-forties. As a child psychiatrist, Kanner was utterly opposed to this school of thought, as his use of the term refrigerator parent in other contexts and his early ideas about the genesis of autism underline.[65] He continued to use the metaphor of the emotional refrigerator until the nineteen-sixties, and in psychoanalytically inspired discussions and in the media his position was initially reduced to this. In fact Kanner advocated an integral study of autism, in its totality of biological, psychological and social dysfunction - an approach he himself described as 'psychobiological.'

> Arguments that counterpose 'hereditary' versus 'environmental' as antithetical terms are fundamentally in error. Operationally defined, they are interpenetrating concepts. . . . Early infantile autism is a total psycho-biological disorder. What is needed is a comprehensive study of the dysfunction at each level of integration: biological, psychological, and social.[66]

Kanner therefore thought it unlikely 'that a single etiologic agent is solely responsible for the pathology in behavior.' Inevitably the 'emotional configuration in the home plays a dynamic role in the genesis of autism' but this is 'is not sufficient in itself' for the occurrence of the disorder. 'There appears to be some way in which the children are different from the beginning of their extra-uterine existence.'[67] This last remark and Kanner's public attack on Bettelheim's work in 1968 was embraced by the American parents' association that had just been set up. According to Albury that made Kanner an acceptable founding father after all.[68]

We find a more recent variant of environmental thinking in the ethological approach of Tinbergen and Tinbergen. They held that autistic children find themselves in a motivational conflict between the vital importance of rapprochement and the establishment of social bonds on the one hand, and avoidance behaviour on the other. Social avoidance behaviour is part of a child's natural survival kit. The authors regarded autism as a form of *learned* behaviour and as an adaptation to an inhospitable environment. As well as pre- and perinatal events, they listed a series of external factors which, they asserted, have an adverse effect on the development of sensitive children shortly after birth - the critical period for establishing an emotional bond between mother and child. Although they did include a biological predisposition in their explanation, these authors stressed what they said was the often forgotten social environment.

> To recapitulate our views on the extent to which 'nature' (genetic predisposition) and 'nurture' (influences from the environment) causes a child to become autistic: while we do not deny that there may well be hereditary components in the causation of the autistic derailment, we assert that these components do no more than determine the degree of vulnerability to pressures exerted by the environment. There is of course no either/or to this; what we claim is that environmental autismogenic factors are at the moment being greatly underrated, indeed hardly given any attention. We further suggest, more specifically, that the responsible environmental factors are largely of a social nature. And since they act primarily through sensory inputs that affect the child's motivational state and through this his behaviour, our interpretation must be classed as being largely 'psychogenic' - 'organic' (structural) defects seem to us to be of minor importance.[69]

The Tinbergens included among potential autismogenic factors the birth of a sibling, an accident, admission to hospital and moving house, as well as such issues as growing up on an estate of high-rise flats or in a similarly bleak environment, increased parental uncertainty in child rearing (because schools were taking more and more out of their hands), career-minded women and the popularity of bottle-feeding. In short, the Tinbergens were concerned with what they perceived as the emotional deficit of modern Western society, with socio-psychological and material changes that ran counter to the human scale of existence. In their view, autism is a disease of civilization.

> Everyone who has lived among hunter-gatherers has seen how much children in such societies learn without being sent to school, and how refreshingly light-hearted and cheerful the atmosphere in such societies is as a rule. *Few members of modern Western societies realize how uncheerful, sour and efficiency-oriented, how much less happy the atmosphere in modern societies is!*[70]

*Predisposition*

In many respects diametrically opposed to the psychogenic school of thought are theories that seek the cause of autism in an organic predisposition. The pioneer in this field was Bernard Rimland. In his 1964 book *Infantile Autism* he compared arguments in favour of a psychosocial aetiology with arguments in support of a biological explanation. One of his main arguments against a psychosocial explanation was that neglected children, even the most seriously neglected of them, did not display the social remoteness that characterized autistic children. In so far as empirical data permitted conclusions to be drawn, an organic defect, possibly in the brain stem, seemed to him to be the most likely cause of autism. In this context, Rimland pointed at, among other things, the preponderance of males in prevalence figures and the fact that children with a physical brain dysfunction (for instance, mentally handicapped children) often showed autistic behaviour or something akin to it.[71] Rimland's biological thesis was to have a significant impact on the future of subsequent research and the treatment of autism.

Not the least of Rimland's concerns was to free the families of autistic children from the stigma with which they had been branded. It was, though, true that some of the 'nurture' thinkers acknowledged that the families themselves were victims too. The presence of an autistic child, they argued, coupled with ignorance on the part of the parents as to how to deal with it, could send the parent-child relationship into a downward spiral. Although their ideas appeared callous when it came to the role of mothers of autistic children, it had to be recognized, according to Tinbergen and Tinbergen, that it was not a question of its being the mothers' *fault*. The craft and skill of parenting, they alleged, was in retreat. Mothers were themselves damaged by the demands made on them by modern Western society.

> Modern society is placing mothers, especially those who have been educated so that they can have intellectually stimulating or demanding work and who yet try to be fully satisfying mothers, in a difficult position. For career women it is hardly ever possible to combine the two tasks successfully.[72]

Although, as we see, some authors explicitly rejected the suggestion, it goes without saying that nurture theories could easily be interpreted as a criticism of the parents, and more particularly of the *mothers* of autistic children.[73] True, even according to Rimland the parents were a unique and homogeneous group in terms of their intelligence and personality (a claim that was later repudiated), but he regarded this not as a sign of psychogenic aetiology but rather as an indication that the formation of personality was dependent - far more than had until then been thought possible - on hereditary biological factors.

The idea that the parents of children with autism must be bad parents is not swept under the carpet in modern overviews. Contemporary authors are very concerned to banish any lingering misconceptions about this and to encourage parents: despite earlier indications that seemed to point in this direction, autism does not occur more often among well-educated parents with good, demanding jobs from better socio-economic backgrounds. Where this connection was observed in the past, it was probably based on selection bias: it was more likely that well-educated parents could find their way to the scarce specialists in this field more easily.[74] The suggestion that the cause of autism had to be sought in an aberrant (distant, intellectual, detached) personality makeup in the parents was also dismissed.[75] The notion that parents feel compelled to adapt to the needs of their child (providing structure, using few words) is a very different matter. In the case of Asperger's Syndrome in particular, there also appears to be a genetic component. The current thinking is that autism affects the whole family - not because there is something lacking in the children's upbringing but as a result of a random, biologically determined fate.

In recent years the biological thesis has been increasingly substantiated on empirical grounds. Although some autistic individuals appear to be physically healthy and of normal intelligence, at population level there appears to be a high degree of correlation with diverse medical conditions. This leads to the conjecture that a biological factor is at work, even if it is not immediately visible or is expressed in other areas. The most important indications pointing to a biological genesis are that autism often goes hand in hand with neurological symptoms (abnormalities in the structure of the brain, EEG anomalies), with mental retardation (three-quarters of the total population) and with a range of other medical conditions (like problems during pregnancy and oxygen deficiency during birth). Twenty-five percent of autistic adolescents develop epilepsy. Autism is also related to genetic abnormalities (fragile X syndrome and tuberous sclerosis), metabolic disorders (phenylketonuria), neurophysiological impairments (raised serotonin), viral infections (congenital rubella) and other congenital disorders. Twin studies point to a genetic component (a high concordance for autism among identical twins, lower among fraternal twins). Blood relatives of children with autism moreover have a significantly increased risk of autism and are also more likely to suffer associated learning disabilities (such as language difficulties).[76]

Diverse as they may be, what the medical conditions seen in autistic people have in common is that they are associated with impairments and defects in the brain. However, the abnormalities are not necessarily coupled to autism; most people with these conditions do not have autism and these impairments are often not found in individuals who are autistic. It is possible that some conditions only cause autism in conjunction with other factors and are only part of the whole explanation. Other complications - during pregnancy and birth, for instance - could be an effect of an underlying defect that also causes autism. This makes it impossible to give a clear-cut answer to the question as to precisely what causes autism.

In sum, it seems that numerous biological factors can contribute to the genesis of autism. The concept of a *final common pathway* has been suggested in order to take this causal complexity into account: autism itself is not a disease entity but a characteristic collection of symptoms that stems from a series of interacting, partly related, partly unknown factors which have in common the fact that they ultimately do damage in areas of the brain that are responsible for the development of communication, social and imagination skills. It is possible that the time at which neurobiological development is affected may be even more crucial than the precise factors involved.

According to this theory, factors that cause autism could do more or less specific damage. In the case of wide-ranging brain damage, as is the case with a mental handicap, there is a good chance that the component which is autism-specific is damaged at the same time (which explains why there is a significant degree of overlap between mental handicap and autism). But in other, rarer cases, there seems to be a specific defect that only damages the capacity for social and emotional bonding. The relative rarity of this form might indicate that the organic cause of autism should be sought in damage to well-hidden, deep-lying brain functions.[77]

*Psychological Theories*

Biological theories assume that one or more defects in the brain are at the root of autism, and that these defects are themselves caused by one or more biological factors. We do not know where in the brain specific damage occurs.[78] Many theories consequently focus on psychological functions that are impaired. Rimland gave this research an important boost. He developed a theory of autism as a defect in the processing of stimuli, stressing the difficulty people with autism have in integrating new experiences with earlier, memorized experiences. Anthony explained autism as an impairment of the input of sensory stimuli and the repercussions this had on the processing of stimuli at a central level. Hutt postulated that in autism there was a chronic state of overstimulation, possibly of the reticular system, and that stereotypes were a defence mechanism against it. According to these cognitivist theories, the affective deficit (which psychogenic theories regarded as primary) and behavioural problems (to which learning theories point) arise out of fear, confusion, and frustration because the child *understands* so little of the world.

The stream of cognitive explanations did not really start to flow until Hermelin and O'Connor's study in 1970. They saw autism as a fundamental disorder at the level of information processing. Experiments showed that individuals with autism were not able to encode stimuli in a meaningful way. Unlike non-autistic subjects, comparative memory tests revealed, the autistic subjects did not derive any support from the *meaning* of material: a random series of words was remembered no worse than a meaningful sentence; disjointed pieces of information were retained just as well as information that was part of a meaningful context. The authors wrote: 'The failure of autistic children in the appreciation of order and of a meaningful structure in the input must be seen as one of our main conclusions.'[79] The research indicated that instead of using meaning in their dealings with reality, the children always relied on the same relatively simple, rigid ordering strategies.

In 1976 Ricks and Wing refined this hypothesis and suggested that these difficulties in processing semantic information sprang from a fundamental problem in *manipulating* symbolic information (as internal language): 'Autistic people do not seem to be able to use their store of concepts in code in order to modify their ideas or to form complicated abstractions.'[80] Children functioning at a very low level sometimes actually seemed to have undergone no conceptual development at all. Others could classify things by size, shape, colour or number. A very few gave signs of being able to make more abstract conceptual distinctions, for example between types of transport, animal species, and even people according to age group. But even in the best cases there were problems - not in the storage of new data, but in the further processing of symbolic data into more abstract ideas (making a reasoned choice, recognizing a hidden meaning and so on).

Although this could not fully explain the abnormal development, the difficulty in forming concepts and making meaningful connections at the level of higher abstraction could explain many of the autistic symptoms. At first, researchers focused chiefly on language-related cognitive impairments, subsequently they thought that many autistic symptoms could be traced back to the general conceptual deficit they described. This theory thus sheds light predominately on the problem of dealing with people and their feelings, where everything comes down to reading subtle, non-verbal signals, and then interpreting them and integrating them into a context of previous social experiences, available as a mental representation. Recent explanations, four of which I shall deal with briefly, either build on or dispute this explanation.

The 'theory of mind' hypothesis put forward by Baron-Cohen, Leslie and Frith in 1985 sharpened the focus of this explanation. According to this influential hypothesis, autistic symptoms derive from a defect in the cognitive mechanism that enables people to represent *mental* events. This ability to form a mental picture of the feelings, wants, ideas, motives, plans and thoughts of others (the 'theory of mind') plays a crucial role in social communication. Anyone who is unable to imagine and to work out what is going on in other people's heads, concealed behind ambiguous outward signs, cannot possibly anticipate other people's actions. In the case of autism, the hypothetical mechanism that gives access to a hidden world of psychological information appears to be damaged. 'The psychological undercurrents of real life as well as of literature - in short, all that gives spice to social relations - for them remain a closed book. 'People talk to each other with their eyes,' said one observant autistic youth. 'What is it that they are saying?'[81] Autistics are the seeing blind: they suffer from *mindblindness*.[82]

An allied explanation for both the deficits and the peak skills that are part of autism was put forward by Uta Frith. Normally, people look for *coherence* in the vast quantity of information that reaches them in order to store the meaning-in-context at a higher level of abstraction. This human preference for 'central coherence' is confirmed, it is suggested, by the fact that the point of a story is easily retained, whereas all sorts of details are forgotten. According to Frith's hypothesis this information processing mechanism is impaired in autistic people.[83] As a result of a weak central coherence mechanism they devote excessive attention to isolated facts; they display a penchant for forms of order that as a rule would escape attention. The price autistics pay for this is that they see the world in fragments and cannot discern any structure in what, to most people, is relevant information because it is meaningful in the light of the broader *context*.

A third approach, proposed by Claire Hughes and James Russell, assumes that the ability to read states of mind is preceded by another skill: a form of capacity for action that enables people to detach themselves mentally from incoming information and decide on their course of action. This is the *executive function*, the entirety of mental abilities that are needed for

> volitional, goal-directed behaviour: inhibition of perceptually triggered or inappropriate responses; planning and embedding of behavioural and cognitive sequences; maintaining an appropriate set and disengaging from an inappropriate one; and monitoring the success and failure of current strategies.[84]

Autism, Hughes and Russell argued, is characterized by an inability to act purposefully or strategically as a result of a disorder of precisely these abilities. This could explain not only deficits in 'theory of mind,' but also the rigid solution strategies and the repetitive behaviour of people with autism.

A final theory put forward by Peter Hobson suggests that people with autism lack the biological predisposition for the perception of the physical expression of human emotions. Autistic children, for instance, sort pictures of human faces chiefly according to the hats the people are wearing; non-autistic children, on the other hand, sort them as a matter of course on the basis of the emotion expressed in the face.[85] These emotional expressions make no impression on autistic children. They do not seem to recognize people as *people*, with whom they can share inner experiences. Because young autistic children get extremely little experience in affective contact with others, they do not develop any sensitivity to other people's feelings. The primary deficit in 'capacities for bodily intercoordination between the autistic child and other people, and more specifically, impairments in the capacities needed to achieve interpersonal affective contact and participation in the emotional lives of others,'[86] argued Hobson, have a far-reaching impact on the cognitive, social, and communication development of children. By regarding autism as an impairment in what can and cannot happen *between* the young autistic child and other people, Hobson offers an alternative to the essentially cognitive approaches described above.[87]

All this, meanwhile, is far from the direction in which the environmental school sought the cause of autism. Nevertheless there is also a degree of continuity: Where the *nurture* approach sees autism as the decline of the essentially flawless subject, because the world of things advances at the expense of the emotional-affective nurturing environment, the *nature* side regards autism as a disorder that frustrates the social-cognitive development of the subject at the outset. But both assume that in autism being human is threatened to its core. In seeking an explanation that fits and a way of dealing with autistic people, we simply cannot get around these questions - what is it that makes people special, how do we recognize one another as such, and what is it that has gone so drastically wrong in people with autism?

## Interventions

A recurring theme in discussions about supporting people with autism is the desire to reconcile the ideal of a meaningful (communicative, social, free) life with the need to provide autistic people with a predictable, structured environment. While the two may seem incompatible in normal life, for autistic children a stimulus-free and controlling environment may well be their only path to developing into a person who can connect with others.

### From Co-Determinant to Co-Therapist

The type of treatment authors recommend is closely related to the explanation they give for autism. Psychogenic theories usually advocated the psychotherapeutic treatment of autism, possibly at the same time as placing the child in care or treating the parents. Along with the causal claims of explanations like this, psychotherapy as a treatment for autism has been shown in a bad light.[88] At the end of the nineteen-sixties, researchers began experimenting with behaviour modification methods based on the principles of the theory of learning. Encouraging results were achieved by means of operant conditioning, which is based on the idea that behaviour can be changed by presenting reinforcement contingent upon the consequences of the behaviour. It was used in the first place to reduce problem behaviour, but also in teaching skills and tackling fundamental autistic deficits. Lastly, in the wake of cognitive explanations, the end of the sixties saw a growing interest in the possibilities of educating autistic children.[89]

In their standard work *Treatment of Autistic Children*, Howlin and Rutter report results that can be achieved with a highly-structured approach to autistic children. They make a distinction between specific autistic and non-specific behavioural problems. The treatment, they say, has to focus on stimulating normal development, reducing typical autistic behaviour and eliminating non-specific behavioural problems. Howlin and Rutter also identify a fourth therapeutic objective - relieving the burden on the family in which the child is growing up, on parents who have to invest a great deal, usually without getting much in return. One of Howlin and Rutter's basic principles is that parents have to be closely involved in their child's education. Parents thus became expert co-therapists.

Howlin and Rutter are well aware that the approach they promote is normatively charged. It means, after all, that we decide it is good for the child to abandon his autistic world. On the other hand, as Clara Park put it, there is not much else one can do in these extreme circumstances. When you are confronted with a child's refusal to embrace life, she wrote about her daughter, any existential hesitation evaporates. 'We had no choice. We would use every stratagem we could invent to assail her fortress, to beguile, entice, seduce her into the human condition.'[90]

*Social Skills*

One of Howlin and Rutter's key therapeutic goals is to promote normal development and reduce typical autistic problem behaviour. As far as the problems of socialization are concerned, this means that parents/carers have to opt for a directive approach at the earliest possible stage. As we have seen, there is nothing else they could do; leaving the child alone simply means that he would become ever more lost. Bringing about social *reciprocity* means taking *one-sided* steps at first (and often later, too). An autistic child has to be put into situations in which he has no possibility of avoiding contact with other people - for instance, a puzzle can only be completed by asking someone for the missing piece. The underlying idea is that 'skilled intervention can result in what is, at first, a mechanical interaction becoming truly social in character.'[91]

Carer and child have a long way to go before that stage is reached. Whereas a neurotypical child naturally learns to apply social rules in everyday life, it is totally different for an autistic child. His education has to focus on teaching him the most elementary skills step by step in order to make him in any way familiar with the social world. This encompasses such seemingly trivial things as dialling a telephone number, saying 'hello' to the person at the other end, and so forth. The emphasis has to be on *using* elements in their social context; they are of little value as isolated behaviours. One way of achieving this is through role play, in which the aim is to simulate social situations.

The problem with this, however, is that real life seldom sticks to the agreement and instead demands the flexible application and interpretation of the rules - needless to say a skill that children with autism lack. Some can get a very long way with the aid of the rule book, but formal rules, no matter how refined they may be, often fall short in practice. It appears that social competence cannot be captured in formulas. Just because someone can dial a number, it does not mean that they know how to begin or end a phone conversation. 'The final product, 'social behaviour,' can also come across to other people as rather odd or stilted, simply because it has been acquired through systematic teaching rather than being learned 'naturally.'"[92]

Rather than making the learning environment more complex and more 'lifelike,' it is possible to take the opposite route by making the world, to a certain extent, *less* complex. For example, setting up the classroom or workplace in such a way that it is immediately obvious what is expected of whom and when, can bring about a significant improvement in social functioning.

Some skills, however, simply cannot be taught. Ina van Berckelaer described how an autistic boy had learnt during social skills training to take turns in doing things. Later he was asked to push a boy with cerebral palsy in a wheelchair. He stopped after a couple of hundred yards, walked around the wheelchair, made eye contact - as he had been taught - and said: get up, it's my turn to ride in the chair now. Here, concluded Van Berckelaer, social skills training had run up against the singularity of the autistic individual.[93]

*Communication Skills*

Howlin and Rutter observe that in the early days of language and communication teaching it was assumed that autistic children could learn every aspect of language if only they practised hard enough. Little attention was paid to individual development or to the qualitative impairment in communication skills. In contrast, the authors regard the communication objective of language as paramount; regardless of the level of language development, the child has to be trained in using it socially. If children with spoken language do not make progress, supporting means of communication have to be mobilized. All that counts is whether something *works*.

Operant techniques, which aim to direct communication behaviour by utilizing the consequences of behaviour, can be used in teaching communication skills. Mechanical and cold as this approach might appear, in the first instance everything possible has to be done to teach the child to respond to language and communication. The child can be led to discover the meaning of simple commands like 'come here' and 'sit down' by *making* him come or sit as soon as the words are spoken. As the training progresses, physical prompts can gradually be eliminated until the child has enough grasp of the words alone. Parents see for the first time that they can influence their child's behaviour; the child himself understands for the first time what is required of him.

Operant techniques can also be used to train the power of expression. This does, of course, assume that there is something to work on. Sometimes the level of functioning is so low that training has to begin by transforming other behaviour into something that has to do with the exchange of sounds. The first building blocks of meaningful language can sometimes be created by physically modelling the shape of the child's mouth, although the individual differences in response are great. Among the highest functioning children, education focuses on teaching conversational skills and training them to introduce a subject, look at the other person, ask a question in response and end a conversation.

Teaching an autistic child communication skills involves connecting with the child's familiar environment so that he is surrounded by the world that has to be named, in other words the world over which the child can potentially wield power, where objects are deliberately placed just out of reach so that he has to make an effort and is induced to communicate. In a totally adapted environment, where carers pick up on the slightest clue and the child is rewarded for the least possible effort, they cease to expect any more communication and eventually, indeed, there is none.[94] Autistic people derive no satisfaction from communication *in itself*, so an external reward is essential to make what has been learned sink in. This reward can often be hard to find because one cannot really praise an autistic child - he is as indifferent to praise as he is to the communication for which it was given.

Howlin and Rutter devote most attention to the role of language in social interaction. At the same time they acknowledge that this is aiming too high for many autistic children. Sign language may perhaps be helpful here, although it is difficult for people with autism to advance beyond concrete, instrumental gestures. For more complex forms of non-verbal communication it is therefore necessary to try to find a link with the visual and spatial predilections of people with autism. Communication systems using prints and photographs resonate with the specific cognitive style of autistic children. At an even more basic level, objects themselves can be used to communicate.

### Ritual and Stereotyped Behaviours

For a long time the rigid, stereotyped behaviours and the lack of creativity seen in autism were taken to be a neurotic, secondary response to more fundamental autistic deficits. On the one hand they can be a way of compensating for the lack of meaning. On the other, the tendency towards rigidity seems to diminish hardly at all when conceptual ability develops. Moreover, the propensity for putting the environment in a (self-created) strait jacket can rarely be eliminated altogether. This indicates a cognitive problem in itself. Be this as it may, Howlin and Rutter assert that stereotyped and ritual behaviours have an adverse effect on the development of the autonomy of the individual and often have a huge impact on the everyday lives of the rest of the family.

Howlin and Rutter suggest some specific methods of avoiding problems of this kind. In people with autism, unlike those suffering from 'ordinary' compulsive and obsessional disorders, preventing the response often leads to greater stress, agitation and sometimes aggression. An alternative approach takes the gradual path, by changing fixed routines little by little and, eventually, to a significant extent. According to this approach, one could alter the fixed route of a walk a yard at a time, although there is then a risk that a new fixation might develop. It is consequently advisable to provide safety and structure in activities from the outset, but at the same time build in small changes and variation so as to make it easier to respond flexibly to changed circumstances.

The more that children lack the skills which enable them to play or occupy themselves with meaningful tasks, the more strongly stereotyped behaviour develops. It can help to deflect routines towards activities that have more to offer in social terms. Medication can sometimes reduce anxiety and stress and go some way towards tempering the ferocity of reactions to changes, and this can make these behaviours more manageable. If one succeeds in altering rituals and obsessions, however, there is a risk that other behaviours will take their place. An interesting theory in this respect is that repetitive behaviour often meets a need, ranging from making the environment controllable to expressing emotions.[95] The implication here is that carers must learn to read the specific function of this behaviour; simply forbidding it is cruel and doomed to failure. It is better to try to alter harmful or disruptive behaviour by offering an alternative form of repetitive behaviour.

### Non-Specific Problem Behaviour
Treatment, argue Howlin and Rutter, does not relate solely to specific autistic symptoms; it can also be directed towards regulating additional, non-specific problem behaviour. This can include self-harming, sleep disorders, eating problems, anxieties, incontinence problems, fits of rage and so on. It is here that intensive support often achieves good results, but at the same time this underlines the relative impotence of bystanders: specific symptoms must largely be accepted as something inextricably linked to the handicap.

In broad outline, the treatment of non-specific problem behaviour corresponds to the approach to similar behaviour in children who are not autistic. Operant conditioning proves particularly useful here, provided it is used in a creative and specific manner geared to the actual individual and situation. Problem behaviour is often linked to getting attention which, without necessarily having caused the behaviour, has become a stimulus for it. If this behaviour is to be stopped, any reward in the form of attention, positive or negative, has to be avoided. In practice ignoring a behaviour is often difficult because at first the behaviour gets even worse, the child can hurt himself or other people, and things can get broken. A parent/carer has to be very strong not to give in under these circumstances, but at the same time unwavering perseverance is crucial to success.

Withholding attention at such times must be coupled with positive attention at other moments, according to Howlin and Rutter. Alternative behaviour can be encouraged by means of positive reinforcement, by praising the child immediately after the desired behaviour or rewarding him by permitting a favourite activity.

Operant techniques are part of a much wider range of means of modifying behaviour. The combination of gradual change and desensitization presents possibilities as a therapy for extreme fears and phobias. The environment can also be adapted in such a way that problems can be avoided and the child can be encouraged to conform to the norm. Protective clothing can prevent self-harming behaviour, a dark bedroom can promote sleeping through, and a lock on the door can bring reassurance.

*Structure*

Children usually develop spontaneously and without effort in interacting with one another and the world. They master social rules, communication and cognitive skills as a matter of course - as soon as they are ready for them, when the circumstances invite them to do so, usually without frantic attempts to teach them any of this formally. Autistic children do not learn spontaneously. They virtually never show any personal initiative, they apparently have no desire to discover the world and they are not curious. They have little if any interest in interacting with other people or in playing. It is therefore not enough to put them in a normal learning or child care environment, however loving and well-meaning it may be. If they do pick anything up there it is mechanical, not because they see the point of it.[96]

'Structure' is the key word in an effective and adapted learning environment for people with autism. In the absence of an inner language - whereby a person learns by fitting new experiences into an existing and constantly renewed framework of ideas - the coherence and organization of the world has to be presented to autistic children from *outside*. The lack of meaningful connections has to be offset by finding regularity elsewhere - not on a symbolic or conceptual level but by making it visible, tangible, explicit. Complex tasks must be broken down into separate, simple steps, with a clear beginning and end. The space in which activities take place must be clearly organized according to its function. A regular, predictable course of activities, a non-verbal approach and a great deal of personal attention are important. A wait-and-see and tolerant attitude, on the other hand, is counter-productive: carers and teachers must approach the child directively and continually initiate active interactions and communication.

Structure can make connections understandable, rules manageable, events predictable. While some would describe this as an admission of weakness, Howlin and Rutter argue that it is precisely this sort of context that gives autistic children a chance to develop. Others held that a child should not be taught what he does not understand, but, wrote Wing, 'the children who make the most progress are the children who are given the opportunity to learn things in an orderly, structured environment.'[97] Providing structure can help autists to live independently and increase their sense of competence and self-worth. However, Guus Beckers, a psychiatrist at Kanner House in the Netherlands, a centre of excellence for autism spectrum disorders, warns against a purely mechanical approach. Every individual has a 'singularity' with all the 'weaknesses that are a part of him' but from which he also derives 'strength.' At the heart of what is being attempted with the residents of a unit known as the Workhome, is 'to discover exactly what motivates him or her.' Treatment is consequently not confined to behavioural therapy techniques - although they still play an essential role - but also tries to find out by 'empathic understanding' what inspires another person.[98]

## Beyond Facts and Figures

Scientific knowledge about autism has increased dramatically since the first researchers in the field published their findings. Competing and complementary theories offer explanations at different levels for the similarities and differences within the autistic condition. Diagnostic potential has been refined over time. We have a better picture of the abnormal development of autistic children and progress has been made in the support provided for people with autism. Nevertheless, preventing or curing autism is not within the realms of possibility. Our insights are still limited.

At the societal level, money and expert help has been made available for the specific care and supervision that people with autism require. The importance of early identification is universally acknowledged and autism is no longer an unknown or mythical phenomenon to the great majority of people. 'Autism is a lifetime disorder, but it's a better time than ever to be autistic,' is how Grinker stressed the achievements of our time. 'A child with a diagnosis of autism has access to more services and educational opportunities than ever before.'[99] This does not alter the fact that often no more than a start has been made on the specific training of carers in the field, and that there are long waiting lists for many essential services while throughput is stagnating. Dilemmas surrounding the permanent integration of people with autism into society require attention.

And so this overview of insights, provisions and achievements has finally brought us to uncertainties, doubts and waiting lists. The lack of scientific certainty about the ultimate cause of autism and other unknowns regarding this 'enigmatic' condition coincide with the tendency to see autism as a metaphor for all kinds of contemporary social and cultural issues. Considering this link we must be aware, says Stuart Murray, of 'very real dangers' that emerge 'if the conception of autism as a metaphor floats completely free from the actuality of the condition itself.'[100]

This means that there is work to do, not just practical but, above all, on the conceptual level, says Oliver Sacks: 'The ultimate understanding of autism may demand both technical advances and conceptual ones beyond anything we can now even dream of.'[101] If we are to respond to this call for conceptual innovation in this book, primarily in order to better understand our shared existence with people with autism, facts and figures are not enough. We must venture into new terrain, which will be introduced in the next chapter by way of the literary imagination.

# On Stage
## The Autist, the Author, his Characters and their Props

> Whoever is lucky or unlucky enough
> to love an autist is condemned
> to a life of wandering and seeking.[1]

After years half-hidden in the shadows of myth and legend, autism has emerged into the spotlight as a regular feature in popular culture - cabaret, commercial film and television dramas and documentaries. Over the years there have also been countless works of literature featuring a character with an autistic disorder. It is thanks to these and other (notably on-line) sources that many people have encountered autism for the first time. Autism clearly appeals to the imagination, but the precise value we can attach to artistic and literary portrayals of autism is less clear.

As a rule, leading academic journals in the field of autism seldom pay much attention to the way autism is treated in cultural terms. The same is true of the literature aimed at and often written by professionals and parents. As Stuart Murray observes in his 2008 book *Representing Autism*, works like these have 'nothing of substance to say about the multiple popular narratives of autism and cognitive difference that surround any parents seeking more information on the condition, despite this being an obvious context in which their search might take place.'[2]

Recently, scholarly work on autism has shown a growing sensitivity to reflections of autism in popular culture and literary fiction. But such sensitivity usually functions merely as a launch pad for research held to be more scientifically sound that should help us in the end to *distinguish* between fact and fiction in a systematic way. Literary fiction and other narratives of autism are often associated with the myths and quasi-scientific false paths from which practitioners of a scientific approach to autistic spectrum disorders have specifically managed to distance themselves in the past. In this book, in contrast, cultural imagination and literary fiction are taken seriously as potent sources of knowledge that provide a crucial way in to a discussion of the shared life of autistic and non-autistic people.

Autism is first and foremost a disorder of the human condition, as various psychological studies have confirmed. But these studies have no answer to my question as to the *terms* in which people think and speak about crucial differences between those with and without the disorder and how to bridge them. Seen from the perspective of the humanities, this is a lack. When we want to talk about the shared existence of autistic and non-autistic people, we must choose our words with care. To do this we have to step back from the preconceptions and ideas that are taken for granted in the thinking about autistic and non-autistic people, without losing sight of the value of familiar terms we use to talk about autism and non-autism.

As far as this last requirement is concerned, my experience in the practice of care for teenagers with autism helped me during the writing of this book to bear everyday reality in mind. Factual writing on autism increasingly brought home to me the reality of living as an autistic person and with autistic people. But the same valuable sources got in my way when it came to letting go of familiar, non-autistic preconceptions and received wisdom. In order to create the conceptual space demanded by research into the shared existence of autistic and non-autistic people, I needed the powers of imagination found in literary fiction - particularly the novella *Vallende ster* [Shooting Star] by the Dutch author and essayist J. Bernlef.

What conceptual potential for discussing the shared existence of autistic and non-autistic people does Bernlef's novella open up? How does he manage to clear away conceptual barriers without losing sight of the reality of the distinction between people and things? In short, how does his book help conceptualize the interaction between autistic and non-autistic people?

### *Vallende ster* - A Reconstruction

Far less known than his famous novel *Out of Mind* (about the inner life of someone with dementia), *Vallende ster* is about an old comedian, Wim Witteman, who had a special bond with his autistic brother, Peter. We meet Witteman at a moment when a serious but unspecified illness has brought his inner world to the brink of collapse and released a flood of memories.

#### *Open House*

As the light fades in his room, an image of the past appears on the terminally ill actor's retina. Witteman remembers how the lights went down at the start of a film he and his brother went to see as children. 'Peter beside me in the dark. Whenever a brightly-lit scene appeared on the screen I could see his face. He was taking everything in - at least that's how it seemed. But what else was going on in there?'[3] At supper that night, Witteman recalls, Peter unerringly copied a scene with Laurel and Hardy that they had watched in the afternoon, by spreading butter on his hand instead of on his bread.

It was the same with language. Peter did not read words, he absorbed them. Literally, it is suggested. Like the times he was allowed to wipe the words off Witteman's slate with a sponge. 'Brows furrowed, he would watch the sponge as it sucked up the letters, look at the sponge into which the letters had vanished, then put it in his mouth. I would try, carefully, to take the sponge out of his mouth.'[4] Like light, the sounds Peter received seemed to be reflected back uncomprehended. He constantly copied what other people said, always with exactly the same intonation but without understanding the meaning. Just like a parrot, someone observed.

Peter mimicked everything he saw. Witteman had a particularly hard time of it: whatever he did, his brother imitated him. Inanimate objects were copied too. Instead of playing with things or using them for a specific purpose, Peter picked up their mechanical properties. 'The sponge falls from his mouth, he can imitate the noise of the spinning-top perfectly and then he starts to spin himself, faster and faster until he falls over with a bang and begins to howl.'[5]

There can be little doubt about Peter's autism. Indications that point this way - Peter's aloneness, his seeming deafness, his visually-driven memory and his echolalia - are confirmed by the official diagnosis that follows his admission to an institution. More important than this, though, is the way Peter's autism is perceived by those around him. To judge by what Witteman remembers, nothing and no one in Peter's world seems to have been concerned about all sorts of boundaries that would normally be regarded as self-evident. All doors were, in a manner of speaking, wide open. And this put at risk the distinction between Peter himself and the world around him.

> He was drawn into either a frenzy of imitations or a stupor
> of circles, of everything that was round and that he could
> use to calm himself down. The world raced through him
> relentlessly and he was unable to record or stop any of it.
> Perhaps he could not keep the world in its place and that
> was why he stayed so motionless, so aloof.[6]

Peter thus represents the precise confusion that Witteman himself is trying to keep at bay now that his world of language and ideas is beginning to disintegrate and his ability to differentiate is under threat.

The condition in which the patient finds himself means that words no longer refer to the world beyond. In a passage suggesting a short-circuit between words and things - 'evidently this is how the connections are at the moment, loose or wired wrong'[7] - Bernlef evokes an impression of life without a protective outer layer that provides context and meaning. The sheep Witteman sees in his mind's eye, the word 'sheep' he says aloud, a sip of water he is given to drink at that instant - they all seem to be in league. In the end it is impossible to tell inside and outside apart, and Witteman experiences (cold, wet) water flowing from (the word) 'sheep.'

Bernlef makes a strong link between the crumbling of meaningful connections and the loss of *language*. Without language which makes it possible to distinguish meaningfully between categories, between the internal and the external world, which makes things nameable and understandable, any grasp on reality disappears. So that he will not fall prey to the chaos he fears governs Peter's life, Witteman clings to the words with which he learned to name the world, to the meaningful order he has known since childhood. He justifies himself to his former colleague, the comedian Henk de Jong, who loathed all the chatter: 'Making sure I don't lose control. Even if no one's saying anything, it's then I must say my lines, lines that are my only salvation now, Henk, a buoy.'[8]

Peter had to do without a script; he just spun in circles. 'And he shouted words. Any words. Without meaning.'[9] After temporary admission to an institution he did not even do that any longer. 'Whatever we tried. He wouldn't say anything. Or perhaps he couldn't anymore.'[10] Without language things lose their meaning, the world blows straight through you. A knot-hole in a plank of wood was enough to trigger a panic attack in Peter. 'He can't talk about anything. The eye in the fence came at him because he didn't know the word knot.'[11]

### A Close Stranger

In Witteman's eyes Peter was balancing on the edge of an abyss - someone who, because he could not talk about anything, had constantly to be protected from the danger of being crushed by the mechanics of the world. This was an ever-present - and literal - threat. Witteman always took Peter outside on a rope to stop him from charging at the wheels of a moving car.

Witteman seemed to be the only person able to get through to his autistic brother - by imitating him or doing something funny. But later they lost the close bond they had as children. The brothers became estranged, the rope stayed in the cupboard and Peter never went out. This was when he no longer spoke at all. After this Peter was compared with an empty room or an unplayed piano and, in his lack of language, with a thing or an animal. 'When he stopped talking we looked past him, like you look past a sideboard or a vase of flowers.'[12] From then on Peter was a stranger in the family, 'as if he was a thing, a doll with a surprised round face, deathly pale and silent. Couldn't say mama any more. Broken.'[13]

Despite his presence, Peter was more not there than there. Family life seemed to slide past him. On the other hand, the silence and emptiness he projected left the people around him anything but unmoved. 'He didn't want to be there. And we couldn't bear to see it.'[14] That Peter was barely there was an almost palpable fact. Witteman remembers how it sometimes got too much for his mother.

'I don't know, maybe if someone's never spoken you get used to it. But if someone has, and then suddenly doesn't any more, then you don't know what he's thinking, then you lose all control. Of yourself, too. I was frightened of him, I became frightened of my own child.'[15]

There were times when Witteman himself could not cope either. Once, when Peter ran away, Wim wished that he would stay away forever. 'He's dead, I think, I wish he was dead, that he'd never come back with his endless imitation.' It gradually emerges as the story unfolds that Peter died young, in a bizarre fashion, by jumping off the roof, and this provokes feelings of guilt in Witteman. 'That look of mother's again, that silent playing on my sense of responsibility.' Because he had stopped bothering with his brother and by taking a chair up on to the flat roof to look at shooting stars may have set him an example that was later to prove fatal, Witteman regards himself as responsible for Peter's fall into the abyss. 'I see myself in the dark glass, small, frightened and guilty.'[16]

On his deathbed he is still plagued by the sense that he could not stop Peter succumbing to the chaos of the world as he saw it. *Vallende ster* can be read as his ceaseless endeavour to repair the broken bond with Peter. But this presents him with a recurring dilemma: Witteman can try to restore the contact and 'enter' Peter's world, but then he would have to embrace his brother's silence. Or he can cling on to his own ability to speak, to the meaningful everyday order, but then be doomed to stay 'outside.' In Witteman's thoughts, in Bernlef's novella, several approaches are considered, each one an attempt to resolve this predicament. Yet, what is the relevance of these attempts to the terms in which we can speak *outside* the novella about the shared existence of autistic and non-autistic people?

*The Artist's Studio*
With an image of a chair that appears on Witteman's retina, the scene shifts from the hospital to Victor's studio. Commissioned by the boys' father, the artist is busy with brushes and paints, making a lifelike portrait, an *image* of Peter. It appears to be an impossible task.

> Funny, said Victor. I've never seen anything like it, eyes that can't be painted. In most eyes there's expression, a sort of melody you can capture with your pencil or brushes if you just look long enough. But with him there's nothing. Water. Or like a cat's eyes, viscous spheres. He's a child who hasn't experienced anything. I would have to paint your brother's face like an empty room. Or like a window looking out on to a cloudless sky. The secret is that there is no secret behind it. That's the mystery of his face.[17]

The problem confronting the artist is that his paints and brushes seem to become useless as soon as he tries to capture Peter's personality. How do you give an impression of an expression that is not actually there? The impossible choice that appears to be facing him is one between two extremes. On the one hand he can decide to keep hold of his tried and tested tools, which means that the radically different character of his model escapes him. The unappealing alternative is to abandon his paints and brushes, his very imagination itself, which may bring him closer to Peter but at the same time takes him ever further away from his commission.

Victor's problem in making an image of Peter is related to the dilemma with which Witteman wrestles on his deathbed. Now that his grip on reality is loosening more and more, it seems that Witteman can experience something of the world in which Peter found himself all his life: lost in a no man's land halfway between linguistic order and everything that lies beyond it. It appears that the broken bond can, at last, be mended. At the same time Witteman is terrified of facing the ultimate implication of this - he will have to give up his anchor in the meaningful world. And so he clings desperately to the words he knows.

The dilemma Peter presents to those around him appears insoluble. And yet Peter's response to Victor's picture of him leads us to suspect that Victor's skill as an artist has brought him very close to Peter for a moment, without his having to abandon his devotion to painting and to his public. 'The odd thing was that he would never look in a mirror, but he did look at this portrait. Sometimes he stroked a white cheek on the canvas. Then his lips moved. But he never said anything.'[18]

In the end the distance that has forced itself between Peter and the people around him is never brought to a head. On the contrary, the detour to the studio is seized upon to bridge the chasm that had opened up. By switching the reader's attention from the terms in which the dilemma is couched - get closer and give up everything that is familiar, or hang on to meaningful coherence and remain at a distance - from these terms to the *practicalities* of the work in the studio - to the handling of materials, of brushes that move across the canvas to a musical melody - the situation on the spot suggests a *way out* of the dilemma that was outlined.

*Treading the Boards*
The longing to restore the bond with Peter resurfaces in Witteman's memories of his career as a comedian. The scene shifts to a stage, where Witteman is struggling with the objects there. Witteman took the inspiration for his act from his autistic brother. Peter's inability to connect things in a meaningful way is Witteman's model for what a comic should be able to do. In Witteman's act, the props around him, like the things that surrounded Peter, so the comparison suggests, can assume any meaning at all.

> I rubbed my finger on tables, chairs, my shoes, and as I did
> it, looking at my finger, I gave them all a new name. The
> table became my girlfriend, the chair was a blanket, my

shoes became eyes with which I winked at the audience, the bowler hat, with feigned astonishment, remained a bowler hat.[19]

Leave nothing obvious - according to Henk de Jong, who was once the other half of a comedy duo with Witteman, this was a skill that the comedian had to perfect. Peter's autistic speechlessness has something almost enviable about it for the comic. 'Nothing behind the words. But in front of them? The distance to them. Henk said that's where we had to get to. Where Peter was all his life.'[20] For, reasoned Henk, in this world without words things lose their familiar meaning, everything is new, everything happens for the first time, and it is guaranteed to go wrong. And that is the way it should be. 'You come on stage and the first thing they have to think is: hope it's all right. And, of course, it goes wrong; it must always go wrong.'[21] Make everything a problem, that is the trick. 'If you know nothing,' that is funny. 'Nothing. Like a newborn baby. Everything new and for the first time.'[22]

But now a dilemma arises for the comedian, too. The longing for the naive state, the blank slate that Peter represents, goes hand in hand with a terrible reluctance. Now that the meaningless world which Henk evidently experienced is coming within reach, Witteman recalls his words.

> A sort of unattainable ideal and at the same time the end of everything, he said, rather mysteriously. He had to have a drink if it happened to him, if he stepped for a moment into that world where nothing had a name or a function yet, where everything stood on shifting sand, every gesture was still without significance.
>
> Like this, this whining in the night that slowly drives you mad. Because that's a certainty, that's how I'll end up, as a madman, as someone who doesn't recognize anything anymore. Don't give up. Talk to yourself, always pull yourself back out of the darkness.[23]

This attempt to restore the bond with Peter also seems to founder within sight of the harbour. And yet the wordless sketches suggest a way out. Witteman's performance as a comedian suggests a means of transport from the familiar context to a world where nothing has a name or function, and back. From the present to the past, too, when the bond with Peter was not entirely lost and Witteman could sometimes get his brother 'out of his circle trance by doing something, something funny; an 'act' you'd call it now.'[24]

*Serious Theatre*

When, later in life and well past his prime as a comic, Witteman is discovered by serious theatre, the search for the bond that bound him to his brother resumes. The role of Pozzo that Witteman plays in *Waiting for Godot*, in which he drags his slave, Lucky, around on the end of a rope, might have been written expressly for him. Then we read how, after the success of *Waiting for Godot*, Witteman is learning by heart a new monologue, also by Samuel Beckett. It is a difficult piece, for now he has to express the tension between silence and text on his own, without the props he had in the past.

> It started when I couldn't get my head round the script. Well, it is difficult, said Jan. Pozzo was a lot easier. You had Lucky, the rope. Now you're on your own. All on your own in the dark. All you've got is the script. You need to break it up. Look on it as a score. The silence is just as important as the words. But that's just it. Where once there were words there is now only noise, far-off, sluggish waves breaking.[25]

Now, just when he has to learn a script in which the silence is as important as the words, Witteman falls ill. On his sickbed he wrestles with shreds of text - frightened, having given up his fellow actors and his props, of losing his script too. Terrified of losing this last straw, Witteman clutches it desperately. And precisely because of this, the thing that it is all about, the silence, threatens to elude him.

But again, the situation on the spot offers a brighter outcome. 'Try it another way,' Witteman recalls the director's instructions as he turns his aching head. Just as it was in the studio and during his performances as a comic, the way out that Witteman's director suggests has to be found in a manner of *doing*, in a movement, rather than in an exact formulation. 'You have to pretend you know nothing,' the director tries again.[26]

> I said, Jan, how can I? I know all sorts of things, apart from everything I've forgotten. You have to concentrate on your not-knowing, said Jan. Until you're just doing. Back to the point of departure, the beginning, the first movements.[27]

Witteman gradually realizes what he has to do if the text and explanation fall short. Almost nothing, a great performance.

> He tries to read the script on the ground in front of him, but it's too dark. He tries to read the stage directions, what he's supposed to do, but it's too dark. Perhaps he hasn't got a

script at all. He just has to be there. To be on the safe side he moves his lips, pretends he's speaking, but inside he is empty.[28]

## To the Bottom

As his grip on the world around him weakens, so Witteman's world increasingly coincides with Peter's. There is nothing for him to hold on to any more. 'The prompter's lips move, faster and faster. It's just like a silent film. I try to read his lips, repeat his words. It's too fast. Can't understand them. How can I slow myself down when everything inside me is running away with me?'[29]

Towards the end the confusion gets worse and worse, everything is accelerated. Before he dies, though, Witteman reconciles himself to the fact that he was unable to rescue Peter from his isolation. Eventually he embarks on an inner dialogue with his mother - a conversation they never actually had - about Peter's tragic death and how no one could have prevented it. Just like anyone else, Peter wanted to be *free*. 'He wanted to float, free of all those objects and words that constantly beleaguered him, amongst which he no longer wanted to drag out his life.'[30]

This idea seems to liberate Witteman, so that he, too, can let go and is at long last able to follow Peter. The clash between words and things, between the desire for contact and the fear of having to give up everything that is familiar in order to get it, comes to an end. All movement is focused inward, the circle is complete.

> Here's the rope. Hold it. Yes, like that. You hold one end, I hold the other. We make a circle. That's the best thing there is. No beginning, no end. Just a vortex, towards walls spiralling inward. Going on for ever. That's how he wanted it. That's how I want it. You hold the other end.[31]

## Philosophical Intent

A broken doll with a surprised expression, a boulder or a blank wall, someone people simply fail to notice, as they would a sideboard or a vase of flowers... For anyone who expected personal memories of a beloved individual, these are shocking images with which Bernlef confronts his readers in *Vallende ster* - images that describe Peter, the autistic boy, in terms of things that people usually never give a second glance. This comparison between a person and a collection of objects is reminiscent of the material metaphors we discussed earlier. The parallel also presents a good starting-point for considering Bernlef's text in a broader context and examining a number of philosophical questions that can arise at the interface between autistic and non-autistic people.

*People and Things (and Animals)*

When we talk about people we generally use different terms from the ones we use when we talk about things. The person/thing distinction is part of what, emulating Searle, I have characterized as our *default position*. In order to deal with people and things in an appropriate manner, we have a historically evolved arsenal of words, conventions and codes of conduct available to us. With borderline cases, however, we are often at something of a loss. Anything that cannot be placed within established dualistic frameworks has to manage without the ready-made examples that regulate the relationships between people and things, and the relations between people (or things) among themselves. Anyone who moves into the no man's land between material and meaningful extremes is in danger of ending up in what we might call an *exemplary vacuum*.

Given the way in which they are spoken of, this also seems to be the fate of autistic people. When it appears that the autistic person is not like us in important respects, so the template that distinguishes between people and things dictates, he will belong to the domain where a scientific vocabulary of time and space coordinates is seen as an appropriate way of speaking. Or conversely, since autists are not things, we have to treat them like ordinary people. Are there no alternatives? 'I'm a sort of animal, you could say, I live more for myself,' I heard an autist say on television.[32] The fact that an autistic boy can identify with an animal is distressing and at the same time instructive: 'a sort of animal' is a telling metaphor for a form of existence that does not seem to fit into the dualistic view of the world. In the light of the way animals themselves are always allocated to categories, however, this metaphor offers little consolation in the end.[33]

Peter, in whom the distinction between self and the outside world seems constantly to hang in the balance, is also in danger of falling victim to this vacuum. Not at home among people, in the family where he was brought up, but equally out of place when he is abandoned to the blind laws of nature, every gesture towards him seems painfully misplaced. 'Perhaps he was an animal,' suggests Witteman, but this just accentuates the futility of his quest for an appropriate comparison.[34] How do you treat someone like Peter in a humane way? How do you establish contact when language does not work? How do you manage to live with an autistic brother and child? How can you love an autistic member of the family?

There is seldom a cut and dried answer to the questions that arise (at least in the novella) in the dealings between people with autism and people without. They fall outside the familiar conceptual parameters. It is therefore not surprising that Witteman should cling on to his *own* organized world: the world of meaningful connections on the one hand and material things on the other, where Peter is still in danger of fetching up on the same side as things. Comparisons that surface as soon as Bernlef's characters try to put into words the difference between themselves and autistic Peter increasingly show that person/thing dualism is more than a philosophical obsession, superseded or otherwise. Every reason, surely, not to sideline dualistic frameworks too quickly even if the picture they present is not as nuanced as it might be.

The *distance* between Witteman and his brother, between the non-autist and the autist, is measured in terms of the person/thing distinction. Few appear, viewed from the familiar perspective, to stand further from the familiar, meaningful world of people-among-themselves than people with autism. But the same figures of speech, as I argued in the introductory chapter, also serve to create distance and point out that the autist is *closer* to our existence than we expected. At locations where these two seemingly so disparate worlds come into contact, there is a possibility that interesting border conflicts may also occur. Which these are can be explained in greater detail against the backdrop of Bernlef's interest in other outposts of the meaningful order.

### Touching a Nerve

Bernlef's oeuvre can be read as a continual exploration of the boundaries of our interpretative order. In his essay 'Two men without a past,' for instance, the author analyses the 'pure spheres' in which the comics Stan Laurel and Oliver Hardy operate.[35] Their helpless clumsiness stems from the fact that they cannot remember anything. The film begins, the men introduce themselves. Stan Laurel's face is a completely blank surface, to him everything is new, is encountered for the very first time. Hardy does remember some things, somehow, but he reproduces the arsenal of rules of behaviour and sentences he has stored mechanically and exaggeratedly, without nuance. The duo find themselves in a sort of hole in memory and are consequently entirely at the mercy of the world's indifference.

Laurel and Hardy point up the relativeness of the meaningful order. The chain reactions they set off wherever they may be remind the audience of how *fine* the dividing line is between human intentions and the contingent mass that surrounds them. It is as though the mechanism has turned inward - and it is something that often makes people laugh immoderately. So long as they do not lose their desire to laugh. 'My uncontrollable laughter is extremely ambiguous,' notes Bernlef in regard to the legendary custard-pie fight in *The Battle of the Century* of 1927.[36] It is laughter with which we desperately try to keep total chaos, the indifference of things at bay. The comic pair touch a nerve: the suspicion, as the Dutch literary critic Anthony Mertens puts it, 'that our powers of imagination are a very fragile prosthesis.'[37]

Nothing that is human is off limits to the comedian. In old age, the process of forgetting, in brain injuries and dementia, recurrent themes in Bernlef's work, language and reality also begin to disconnect. However, someone who has fallen through the thin ice of our interpretations is not written off as a pathological case.[38] Whether it is comics like Laurel and Hardy, whose act - as the Groningen philosopher L.W. Nauta put it - consists in their wilfully rejecting everything that is generally regarded as normal,[39] or people who have to learn to name the world anew because certainties have disappeared into a void, in all these cases Bernlef has presumed a particular familiarity with the twilight zone where a person borders on the world, with the no man's land *between* language and concrete reality.

It is precisely where they depart from the norm that the characters who populate Bernlef's work interface with what are regarded as essential features of human existence. They draw our attention to the fact that while the linguistic spirit, the thin layer of subjectivity, call it what you will, may well meet the demands placed on it in everyday existence, it is anything but the desired foundation on which the essence of people rests. In their vulnerability, Bernlef's characters are closer to us than is often thought.[40] Under normal circumstances we usually do everything we can to suppress our vulnerable side. But face to face with autistic Peter, we find ourselves in rough waters. On the border between people and things, language and matter, strange and familiar, he, too, touches a nerve.

> His eyes wide open. He wanted to copy everything he saw, particularly me. When I was alone with him I sometimes put him in the cupboard in the passage. I couldn't stand it any longer. He always went straight to sleep in the cupboard. I was rid of him for a bit. If someone constantly copies you, you feel you're being made fun of. As if your own movements and words don't come from you yourself any more.[41]

*Film*

The way the 'self' in *Vallende ster* is threatened to its very core can be explored in terms of Samuel Beckett's *Film*.[42] It is no coincidence that the lead in this 1964 film of a scenario by Beckett was played by a vanishingly frail Buster Keaton. (Although Charlie Chaplin seems to have been the first choice. Despite repeated requests - and oh, how aptly - he remained silent.) The year 1922 in which, according to the script, *Film* is set, the emphasis on the empty sound track (the film is silent save for an audible hiss), the black and white images and the direction (particularly of the funny way the protagonist walks) - everything in *Film* refers to the slapstick genre and to silent movies. The viewer knows: important conditions for an expedition to the outposts of the interpretative order have been satisfied.

Dangers that threaten the subject on his journey are presented visually in *Film*. The nervy Keaton - who is 'O' for 'object' according to the directions - proves extremely sensitive to the gaze of other people who menace him in various ways, including through the eye of the camera - 'E' for 'eye' in the directions. O accordingly tries to conceal his face behind his upturned coat collar, but there seems to be no escape. E's gaze continues to pursue him wherever he goes.

The disturbing effect of the gaze once more brings to mind Sartre's story about the visitor in the park. As soon as he realizes he is being observed by someone else, he is forced to the periphery of his perception and feels all the subjective ground sinking under his feet.[43] In *Film*, a similar experience leads O to remove or cover up anything that even remotely reminds him of eyes in the room to which he has fled to escape the unbearable light of day. Unlike Sartre's protagonist, however, O is also terrified by the gaze of *non-humans*. By a cat and a dog, for instance, that keep trotting back in every time he manages to shoo them out, by the goldfish in its bowl and the parrot in its cage, and even by things like the mirror, photographs and the window through which the light enters. Every time that, despite all his precautions, O thinks he is being mocked by a representative of this alien invasion force, he comes face to face with the shaky foundations of his existence. Feeling his pulse, he tries to reassure himself that he has not been swept away, that there is still someone home, someone who is in control.

And now back to *Vallende ster*, where the harassing effect exerted on the individual by the outside world is also conceived in visual terms. Bernlef's characters are stared at by their environment. The look with which Witteman's mother plays on his feeling of responsibility does not leave him unmoved. And Bernlef's comedian shows his audience that people are also stared at by things: two little white punched-out discs scare the life out of the comic in his hole-punch act. Here he exhibits the same sort of sensitivity as Peter, in whom the annexation urge emanating from the world is most fundamentally apparent. The 'fixed glare' of the fence menaces Peter because he does not know the word knot. For their part, characters who do have the words with which they hope to keep the world of inanimate objects at bay avoid Peter's expressionless eyes. They turn their backs on him or put him in the cupboard, frightened of losing control. Witteman's mother admits: 'I avoided his eyes when he sat across the table from me and mechanically consumed his nourishment. Not food, nourishment. . . . When you weren't here I'd sit with my back to him.'[44]

The (non-autistic) linguistic subject narrowly escapes being driven, just like the autist, from the centre of perception to the periphery.

### Mourning for a Stone

Aside from its ontological significance - 'ontological' because the nature of human existence is at issue here - the confusion that can occur when autistic and non-autistic people encounter one another has implications for the relationships between them. 'It must have been terrible to love Peter. Like loving a stone,' Bernlef has Witteman say.[45] Since speaking in terms of affection is usually appropriate where people, and sometimes animals, are concerned, but certainly not stones, Peter is again in danger of ending up in a social and emotional vacuum (and of dragging the people around him in with him). And indeed it did not seem to affect anyone when Peter was no longer there. 'I couldn't cry. Nor could Dad. Mother had taken pills and gone up to bed. How were we supposed to mourn for someone who had left no trace?'[46] Again Peter touches a nerve - for if close family members do not recognize one another as people, as the individuals with whom they can share inner experiences, it eats away at the foundations of communal life - the 'bedrock' of a 'shared form of life' as Wittgenstein calls it.[47]

All the same, Witteman manages to find alternative ways of relating to Peter. Not so much by reclaiming himself or by trying even harder to do his best; his involvement manifests itself more or less behind his back. In spite of his inability to grieve, Witteman saw in the mirror two tracks running down his white-painted face. 'I must have cried without knowing it.'[48] Unnoticed, his body had formulated an answer to the question as to whether he could love someone who was barely there. It makes a crucial difference in a book where parallels are continually being drawn between people and things, a book that seems to be leading to a conclusion in which not just Peter but others, too, are in danger of fetching up on the side of indifferent laws of nature: in the moral sense of the word, too, anyone who finds himself in the no man's land between the centre and the margins of existence is not written off by Bernlef. All these people are indicators of a hidden potential of alternative mutual adjustment mechanisms.

Let me draw up a provisional balance sheet. When people with and without autism have dealings with one another, all sorts of doubts arise. They spring from the distance between the autist and the non-autist in which familiar mutual adjustment mechanisms no longer suffice. Questions and uncertainties also stem, however, from the suspicion that the 'other' which the autist represents is a lot closer to the non-autist than one would think. Peter's proximity impacts directly on the shared fragility of human existence. Witteman may have been rid of him for a while but the question as to what binds him and his autistic brother together is still acutely topical after all these years. For him, for the author and for the reader. Peter raises doubts in *all of them*. And the cupboard in the passage is of no help at all. This is surely a good enough reason to look again at how Bernlef tries to picture the shared existence of Witteman and his brother.

*An Empty Image*

In his thoughts, Witteman leads the reader to places where the artist Victor and the comedian and the actor whom Witteman used to be seek to approach Peter. But on the stage and in the studio they run up against the same emptiness that made the atmosphere in Witteman's home unbearable. The dilemma Bernlef outlines by way of the creative efforts of his characters is that every endeavour to get to know more about autistic reality (and their interface with it) seems to have a drawback. Admittedly, anyone who sticks to the tried and trusted means of representation, to his script or pictorial idiom, does come up with an understandable end product, but he risks losing sight of Peter's individual presence. If he abandons the language of the community, on the other hand, he will find himself on very shaky ground. He runs the risk of having to remain silent, like Peter, or producing a blank canvas instead of a realistic portrait that is understood by his public.

In the context of autism the use of proven means of representation runs up against its limits. Underlying the idea of 'making a picture,' 'gaining insight' and 'giving a description' is a framework akin to the dichotomy between people and the world around them, as we have previously outlined. To explain how people succeed in acquiring knowledge of the world, various epistemological theories identify special properties of the knowing subject that distinguish it from the object. With the epistemological problem of how 'certain knowledge' is possible, the dichotomy of *subject* and *object* is accepted as a self-evident point of departure for analysis.[49]

The overriding importance that characters in *Vallende ster* attach to linguistic ability in monitoring the meaningful order makes them members of the subject family, too.[50] Thanks to his possession of language, the knowing subject on the one hand is considered to be capable of representing in a meaningful way an object outside himself on the other. But, as we have seen, it is the very tenability of this distinction - the distinction between a person and the world around him, between meaningful language and the world of things, which should shore up our cognitive faculties - that is put to the test in dealings with an autistic person.

Here the lack of meaning with which Peter faces his environment and the people around him touches yet another nerve. Suddenly certainties are called into question in an area where one would never have thought such doubts could be possible: the integrity of the representing subject itself is at stake, now that the constitutive distinction between 'self' and a 'reality beyond' is being tampered with. The very people who want to get to *know* the person with autism (or the shared existence of autistic and non-autistic people) better, have brought the wrong tools with them.

The autist reminds the non-autist just how little it takes to be driven from the centre to the periphery of perception by an encroaching world, and how fragile the cognitive faculty regarded as crucial to mankind actually is. It casts the characters that populate *Vallende ster* into immense confusion. If their epistemologically privileged position relative to the world is no longer guaranteed, on what basis can they do their job? Is there still firm ground to stand on? Or will Peter drag them with him into a world 'where nothing has a name or a function yet'?[51] Might they not just as well abandon straight away their longing for (what they share with) the world of the autist, not to mention their desire to report on it in familiar terms?[52]

If we are to be able nonetheless to describe the shared existence of autistic and non-autistic people undaunted by this dilemma (go in or stay out), what we need is a vocabulary that *is founded as little as possible* on epistemological preconceptions. In concrete terms this means that we should avoid as far as possible presenting the efforts of Bernlef's characters in terms of 'observe' and 'depict.' With nomenclature like this, after all, we would fall prey to the temptation to reproduce specific non-autistic assumptions at the level of description. We would be in danger of forgetting altogether about what *connects* non-autistic and autistic people to one another, whereas our whole concern has been to rescue our shared existence from this fate.

In order not to rule out in advance the notion that autists and non-autists *share* more with one another than people without autism usually think, we need a descriptive language that is not too weighted as to what it might be that makes autistic and non-autistic people *different*. If we are to approach the traffic between autists and non-autists in a more symmetrical way, we consequently need a *lean* descriptive language - in other words, a conceptual framework which, without diminishing the everyday reality of the man/thing distinction, has the least possible baggage when it comes to what distinguishes 'us' from 'the world.'

## Representation by Delegation

When it is not possible to acquire an insight and adopt a position on epistemological grounds, an author may be able to create *movement*. The solution that the Dutch philosopher Gerard de Vries formulated for the intellectual who is aware that he has no firm ground to stand on but nevertheless wishes to be heard provides a suitable structure for comparing Bernlef's approach. Similarly, the work of Bruno Latour proves helpful in understanding how Bernlef goes about conducting his explorations without carrying too much epistemological weight.

### Shifting Vocabularies

In De Vries's essay 'Moved Movers,' we meet Claude Lanzmann, director of *Shoah*, a film De Vries cites as an exemplary model.[53] Lanzmann is presented as someone who constantly doubts the lasting validity of his own vocabulary because he has become shackled by other manners of speaking. Since he is convinced that 'what someone notices and experiences is constrained by the vocabulary he has at his disposal,' he wonders what the world would look like if it was described in terms of the other.[54] He is aware that he cannot *begin* a conversation with the other except in the vocabulary that he happens to have at his disposal because he grew up in a particular language community. But he wants to go *further* and will keep his ear to the ground in a different way so as to enrich his own vocabulary and world.

In the interesting cases, the vocabulary the author already has and that of the other who has aroused his interest cannot be measured by a single yardstick. This, at the same time, points up the trickiness of these situations, because it is not possible to simply translate the other's vocabulary into familiar terms. It eludes every recognizable concept. So the author will go in search of new forms to represent the other - not in the epistemological sense of seeking a realistic depiction, but literally: despite his absence in fact, he will want to make 'something' of the other *present again* in the new context. The other vocabulary must not be translated in the linguistic sense; it has to be *shifted* to the context of the author and the readers.

Before anyone who aims to do this can bring about such a transport of vocabularies, he must familiarize himself with self-evident ways of doing things, with the exemplary models by means of which he can learn how to use a new term. As the ultimate bilinguist, the author can then travel back and forth between the different vocabularies and versions of the world so as to report on them in his familiar environment. 'By establishing connections, shifting other vocabularies to his own life form, organizing his texts in such a way such that the differences come to light,' he as it were represents the alien home.[55] He experiments with blends of the strange and the familiar and makes room for the other in his text, and this enables the informed reader to follow in the footsteps of this commuter between two worlds, expand his vocabulary and see another, unexpected version of the world.

Suspecting that in the context of autism he has as little solid ground to stand on as this 'moved mover,' Bernlef, too, chooses this form as his solution. By *organizing* his book in a particular way he puts the narrator, and with him the reader, in a position such that the latter can both be present on the spot (completely absorbed in the story) and maintain an overview.[56] Using a number of situations that serve as *models* for what it is to come into the vicinity of an autistic life form - the comedian's act, Witteman's speechless confusion - Bernlef explores the boundaries of the familiar interpretative order and learns to enrich his initial vocabulary with new, 'autistic' elements. The contrast between the linguistic, meaningful world of people-among-themselves and a concrete world of things beyond it act as a *beacon* for what we can imagine by these autistic and non-autistic extremes. Bernlef deploys the dichotomy of people and things as a point of departure in the search for an unknown 'in between.'

### Sending Delegates

If the conceptual space in which the other exists cannot be known, De Vries argues, it may perhaps be *explored*. Similarly, Bernlef redefines the closing of the epistemological gulf between Witteman and his brother in terms of *transport* between different *places*. If we want to describe the shared history of different places without presuming in advance a hierarchical difference between the two locations, we would be well advised to emulate the philosopher and anthropologist Bruno Latour and concentrate on what goes on *between* positions that can be recognized from a familiar perspective as centre and periphery, or, through epistemologically-tinted spectacles, as subject and object.[57]

Who or what can be found in the no man's land between meaningful and concrete reality? Bernlef does not go exploring himself. Like most of his readers, the author himself is too attached to a linguistic, non-autistic order to let it go without a struggle. At least in part, therefore, Bernlef has *delegated* to others who seem better equipped for it than he is the task of establishing connections between the familiar, non-autistic vocabulary he shares with his readers and the autistic world that Peter inhabits.

In the first place, Bernlef has farmed out this work to his character Witteman. Witteman had a close bond with Peter and plays an important role in bridging the gulf by transporting the reader from the here and now of the hospital to *other places and times*. 'Let's say it was daytime. OK? I get up, dress and leave the hospital.'[58] Although he keeps trying to cling on to the familiar order, Witteman thus paves the way for a motley crew of commuters, who try to chart the interface between an autistic and a non-autistic existence on behalf of Bernlef and the reader - for once we have arrived at a temporary place and time, there is always another character ready to take the baton from Witteman.[59]

Among the messengers whom Witteman, on Bernlef's behalf, sends out to cross the no man's land between language and reality and organize the transport to and fro in his stead is the comedian he once was. We saw how, as a comic, Witteman borrowed all sorts of things from Peter, particularly his inability to make meaningful connections. The autistic boy served the comic as an example when it came to ridding himself of the depth that (wrongly, he discovers) is generally foisted upon people. 'No, I was never that, a person with depth. You find that out here. Doesn't exist at all. It can all be read on my big blank face. Face I copied from Peter. Or borrowed. Temporarily.'[60]

The comedian proves an excellent guide for the reader in the no man's land before the words, where Peter's life is located. From a familiar, non-autistic starting point that enables him to recognize the autist as 'other' - using a vocabulary that the reader knows - Bernlef sends out his delegate, who in turn carries the reader to a brightly-lit stage in a theatre where things lose their familiar meaning and he is submerged for a moment in a strange new world.

Bernlef does not, however, leave the reader on the stage; time and time again he pulls him back. This makes it possible to combine the familiar context and the alienating loss of meaning in a controlled way with a single circumscribing movement. 'Talk to yourself, keep pulling yourself out of the darkness.'[61] From that moment on, the one who has lost control and the one who is reporting on it coincide once more. 'I must stay in charge. We don't work here. I'm my own boss.'[62] The author, Witteman and the comedian he once was again speak with one and the same voice. Following in the wake of Witteman, who was deputed by the author to go beyond his boundaries on behalf of those who stayed at home, the reader is thus constantly returned to the familiar setting of the hospital where the whole expedition began.[63]

The comedian is ideally suited to act as Witteman's (and at a greater remove Bernlef's) proxy. He is a true 'bilinguist,' one might say, were it not that this description is not specific enough and only tells half the truth. 'The bottom fell out of our business when the words came,' is how Witteman's colleague De Jong explained the decline of the profession.[64] The version of the world that the comedian presents in his act as a possible model of an autistic existence is actually characterized by a *disruption* of the linguistic order. Which vocabulary should the comic shift in Peter's case? At the interface with the autistic world which Bernlef wants the reader to share, it remains remarkably quiet. And in so far as Peter does speak, it is doubtful, given the repetitive nature of his language, whether there really is anyone 'at home' who can be addressed as a partner in a conversation.

In order to keep the interface between autists and non-autists as broad as possible, it is necessary to establish a type of connection that is other than a purely *meaningful* one. And it is in precisely this that the strength of the comedian lies; in the wake of this silent witness, the reader who allows himself to be carried along by the unfolding of the story becomes ever more alienated from the meaningful order of normal life.

The gulf between the meaningful order and material reality in which Peter is in danger of being lost proves too wide to bridge in one go. It has to be taken in stages. This means that the comic cannot do the work needed to make contact with Peter all on his own. He, in turn, delegates something. The comedian delegates tasks to *things* on the stage.[65] The props that support him in his act form the last, but no less crucial, link in the heterogeneous series of (linguistic and non-linguistic) elements which always stand in for another in order to take over the task of their predecessor - to change everything and yet hang on to 'something' so as to connect the familiar context of the reader with the world of the other who is autistic.

The more the comic really has to let go of the reins and is forced to surrender (temporarily) his position as the autonomous, representing subject, the more successful this is.

Never thought much about it when I was up on the stage.
You were surrounded by things, you found yourself in a

situation, like everyone else; there was always something. It was as if that chair gave me its arm, not the other way round. The ladder threw itself into my arms like a woman, the vase on the jardinière shouted 'hat,' so I put it on my head. I looked around me. The things came at me of their own accord.[66]

Slowly but surely the reader is led in the wake of the implied author, of the terminally ill Witteman, the comic he once was, to the props on the stage along an ontologically sliding scale - from people to things, from words to matter, from self to other, and back again. It is along this chain of shifts and translations that Bernlef defines an area *between* meaningful and material extremes. The characters he sends out to reconnoitre succeed as they go in reducing the gulf (defined in dualistic terms) to small, manageable and bridgeable proportions. Eventually these are used to create, layer by layer, by means of a series of *translations*, a chain that leads straight through the great distinction between linguistic order and the world.[67]

Bernlef explores a space between meaningful and material extremes which (from a non-autistic perspective) serve as models for non-autistic and autistic worlds. He does it by no longer thinking in terms of either/or, but by filling what is the middle ground for non-autists with new, unexpected *actors* and *activities*. How do we, the readers, learn to enter this space? Little by little. Who or what provides the transport between our familiar world and the alien universe of the autist? The comedian's act. What takes the place of language and represents an autistic world in our midst? A smile drawn on a blank face. What makes a shared existence imaginable? The act performed on the stage. And on that stage Bernlef places Witteman in a new context where, without words, but with objects, movement, gestures and greasepaint, as befits a performer, he *demonstrates* what it is to live 'in the place before the words.'

### Literally Moving

Bernlef makes a form of transport possible by building up in the layered structure of his text a series of different worlds that can be visited in turn. The sickbed where Bernlef has installed Witteman proves to be a good base camp for these expeditions. From his bed Witteman guides the reader along a cord to the past he shared with Peter. 'With my right hand I feel the smooth rope that hangs over the edge of my bed. Rope to which Peter and I were attached, my little brother and I.'[68] What connects past and present, sickbed and outside world, Witteman and his autistic brother is seldom just a verbal or mental affair. An image that appears on the retina, the feel of a cord on the bed - there is always *something* or *someone* through which the transport back and forth is channelled. This is typical of the way the terrain between familiar language and autistic reality is explored in *Vallende ster*. It is also, as we have seen, a happy discovery.

There is no way of making the autistic other present in the context of the reader save for the one that goes via intermediate links, via characters who carry the reader with them to other places and times, and who during this transport inevitably add their own specific overtones to the message. It is the very fact that something is changed every time which makes it possible to bridge the immense gulf between 'people' and 'things.' In order to do justice to the active input of elements, including things, that provide the transport to and fro, I shall follow Latour's lead and, where they intervene in the traffic between autists and non-autists, call this 'mediation.'[69]

The effect of a long series of small transformations like this, in which each mediator as it were stands with one foot still in the meaningful world but the other already in the material reality, does not produce a realistic picture. Bernlef's mediators do not provide pure 'insight' into an untouched phenomenon of 'autism' outside it (I have shown how a description turns out in those terms). In *Vallende ster* Bernlef reveals what is needed to connect words and matter, people and things, familiar and alien elements together in such a way that a form of *transport* becomes possible. It is only thanks to the fact that the lines that have been cast are reeled in again afterwards that the implied author can 'report' on an event that apparently happened somewhere else, beyond observation, his own interpretation and that of the reader.[70]

As we have seen, these are no ordinary travellers that Bernlef sends off. There is more going on between autists and non-autists than sparse and seemingly meaningless language and one-sided interpretation alone. Things form a crucial link in the series of linguistic and non-linguistic mediators that bring Witteman into contact with his brother. It is precisely for this reason that things other than normal users of language have so much more to offer us when it comes to dilemmas concerning the representation of a shared existence than the traditional, knowing subject. In Witteman's wake the reader is therefore repeatedly sent in a direction that offers him more than text alone.

But what if there are only words to explore the bond with Peter? As in Beckett's monologue, when Witteman, having been discovered in later life by the serious theatre, is faced with the task of continuing his quest for the silence between the lines with ever fewer aids. The actor has been deprived here of all the resources (rope, make-up, props), links between himself and his brother, that he had until then been able to use to express the absence of speech on his behalf. 'Nothing to do, nothing to copy. Then I'll just do the trick with the hat again. But there's no hat here. Most things are gone, lost. Must go and look for them.'[71]

The actor stays behind, unmediated - all he has left is his script. Does the monologue bring us back after all to Witteman's powers of interpretation? Again, we need a little trick to avoid this premature return of the linguistic subject. Although there are no longer any props to hand and the other performers have had to leave the stage, even as he studies the extract from the monologue, elements, which in their nature and effect are reminiscent of *things*, act in the place of Witteman. Firstly there is Witteman the actor, who by behaving in a certain way can simulate having no memory of anything, and who in turn switches over to his body, from thinking to doing. Although, paradoxically, this is easier said than done. You mustn't think so much, the director tells him.

> Perhaps you should do it a bit more casually, as if it's all welling up in you spontaneously, as though you've almost forgotten that you're playing a part. Easier said than done. It's easy for a director to talk. Empty yourself, don't think about anything, then the script will come of its own accord, speak itself. That sort of talk.[72]

Then Witteman 'comes up with the idea' of putting his script on boards on the stage. As a material guide, the boards help him to let go of the text to which, compelled by illness, he is increasingly inclined to cling. As when the prompter used to whisper words to the actor that did not come from himself - or as was the case in the comedy act, or when Witteman was doing his military service, to which there are several references - this means an explicit shift in the power to act: from centre to periphery, from subject to object, from internal to external control, from autonomy to heteronomy. With their deathly silent text, the boards *make* the actor *literally move*.

> I suggested putting the script on large boards on the floor in front of me. So Jan Kaltveld came up with the idea (which was actually mine, of course, born of necessity). The whole floor of the stage covered with the text of the play, a sort of jigsaw puzzle. I slowly moved around the stage, from one section of text to another, and shuffling along like this I read the words aloud as if they were names on gravestones.
>
> Text about a man who moves . . . I read about this man. Stooped. What he does. Then I say it. Next I do it. As if I'm reading an instruction manual I can follow to make myself move, steer myself. Text that leads me, shuffling, across the stage.[73]

It is only in the monologue that the potential of the text is exploited to the full. Instead of conjuring up an unmediated insight for the readers,

Witteman, on behalf of the author, reconnoitres the space on the stage, and (out of necessity) exerts himself to the utmost to call upon other resources, so that he can use them to translate the familiar, linguistic order into a change through time and space: in a manual, a puzzle, a script, a direction - these are Bernlef's terms. It is delegation down to the square millimetre. Moving from one section of text to the next, the actor carries his audience with him in his monologue; he carries the reader through a series of linguistic and non-linguistic elements - a *descending* series, one would be inclined to say from a familiar perspective - which are piled up layer upon layer, in order to shift/ translate the message on behalf of their predecessor: from words he cannot remember, by way of things he may not use, past his body that contorts, to the externalizing way the text boards themselves direct him.

### Tracking

All Witteman has left is his text. In this, his fate seems to have a good deal in common with Bernlef's, who himself, in fact, has nothing but language with which to distance himself from the familiar linguistic order. Bernlef, Wim Witteman, the reader: they *all* began their quest for what binds autistic and non-autistic people together with nothing but a text. 'All a man can do is talk. Even when he's silent, it's still a form of talking. It always just carries on. Except not with Peter.'[74] However, because of the way Bernlef *organizes* his novella, because he hands the say from linguistic to non-linguistic actors, he prevents the heterogeneous events at the interface between autists and non-autists from being reduced in the end to interpretations (that belong on the non-autistic side of the equation). Although conceived entirely in words, Bernlef's approach to a shared existence remains *moving* in the extreme.

The author's motives have been sufficiently discussed, but how should we go about reading a text like this? As long as reading *Vallende ster* is seen simply as a question of processing information, as a cognitive matter, it admittedly takes the reader out of his familiar context to inhospitable regions where a disconcerting absence of meaning reigns, but the void is soon filled again with an epistemological vocabulary. By allowing himself to be physically steered by the text, Bernlef's character, Witteman, shows us how it can be done differently. The innovation that allows him, despite everything, to keep following his monologue also provides a guide to *Vallende ster*. The trick he presents to us can prevent a traditional representing subject (this time in the role of implied reader) from sneaking in by the back door - something that we placed in parentheses before so that it would not get in the way when we were writing about a shared existence. In short: following a text involves more than interpretation alone.

What, finally, does this mean in terms of this specific text, the words with which I address myself to the reader? If I want to describe a shared existence I, too, can only do it in the words I have at my disposal. 'Without text he doesn't move any more. He falls silent, as they say in the business.'[75] What applies to the actor (for it is he, speaking to himself here) is equally true of me. By organizing my argument in the same way as Bernlef, I can to some extent circumvent problems that present themselves in epistemological terms as questions of methodology. Like Bernlef, I, too, will not offer an unmediated insight, but in my argument send delegates out and thus let the words do their *work*. But although essential, this is not enough. In order to make the shared existence of autists and non-autists present in a familiar context, the reader himself will also have to get moving.

Anyone who enters a model of an autistic world in Witteman's wake (a model of a world we share with autists), does not do it primarily by *interpreting* the situation on the spot; not even if the situation - as the actor encounters it, for instance - proves to be a text.[76] Tracking the path of someone who leaves virtually no traces is first and foremost a matter of having an eye for tiny indications and material that is easily disregarded.[77] A similar attitude is required to follow the lines that I shall set out. Afterwards, this book (if I get it right) will be an account of (the representation of) a shared existence; the form of reading we have to turn to in the context of this study is in the *first* place a question of collecting traces, following signs, making connections and shifting oneself to another place.[78] 'Meaning' makes its entrance relatively *late* here.

**Following the Trail**

On the basis of Bernlef's *Vallende ster* I have located the shared existence of autistic and non-autistic people between two extremes: between the meaningful world of people-among-themselves and the concrete world of things beyond it. The dualism this suggests is a loaded one. Nevertheless the same contrast between what I have described for convenience as 'people' and 'things' is also a benchmark in places where non-autists and autists have dealings with one another. *Vallende ster* is one such place; for Bernlef's characters, the human/thing duality is a normal part of their everyday reality. In their eyes, autistic Peter, not at home in the world of people they had in mind for themselves and others, is constantly in danger of being sucked into the indifferent maelstrom of things. At the same time, Peter's very proximity also puts the distinction between the 'people' and 'things' to the test. Where autists and non-autists come into contact with one another, the intrinsic character of the community of people-among-themselves is a constant subject of debate.

*Vallende ster* is a product of the literary imagination. The world the author evokes neither aims nor needs to correspond in any way with the reality outside its own.[79] Literature, as the professor of general and Dutch literature Wiel Kusters argues in his article on the autism in *Vallende ster*, can be regarded as a form of 'illusionism' that plucks fruit from 'a wonderful sort of 'desired' naivety in the reader: for as long as he reads, the world evoked by the writer is real and true.'[80] This realistic effect, I should like to add, is not located exclusively in someone's head. Worlds that are constructed one after the other in *Vallende ster* are real in so far as the reader is made to move; in so far as he or she is encouraged by lines that have been set out in words to follow the trail to other characters, places and times.

The literary imagination does not provide a secret performers' entrance to the stage on which autistic and non-autistic people meet, while others have to make do with opera glasses from the gallery. Bernlef does, though, have something else to offer: a literary technique which leaves open those things that are uncertain. This has certain advantages. For in order to speak about what autistic and non-autistic people share, we need a vocabulary that houses as few preconceptions as possible in terms of what we usually think it is that distinguishes them. In order to steer clear of the epistemological rocks, Bernlef places the autist in the context of the reader by means of linguistic manoeuvres. His answer to the question as to how the interactions between Peter and Witteman can be described in a symmetrical way provides clues as to the way a shared existence can also be approached elsewhere.

This approach will take us to places that are exemplary for the border traffic between autistic and non-autistic people. We shall visit various locations where *differences* between non-autistic assumptions and an autistic existence may be expected to lie close to the surface, so that the constraints that stand in the way of a normal way of living together become visible. Then, though, I shall shift the focus, little by little, to places where such differences are less obvious, where the mutual *proximity* of people with and without autism is actually more self-evident; from familiar assumptions to places where an alienating loss of meaning occurs, from dualistic frameworks to a space between the familiar linguistic order on the one hand and concrete reality, the world of things on the other - in search of signs of human habitation.[81]

# Body and Mind Shows
## The Imagination Deficit, Theory of Mind and Atmospheric Turbulence

> It is *difficult* to know something, and to act
> as though you didn't know.[1]

The world of things seems to hold a particularly powerful attraction for people with autism. McDonnell, mother of an autistic child, describes how her young son developed a fascination with light switches, which he turned on and off for hours at a time.[2] Later he was totally consumed by a passion for screwdrivers, then fire extinguishers, electricity cables, grain silos and clock towers. For a long time it was pipes and drains, then weighing scales and thermometers, clocks and his watch, then the weather and meteorology. The collection of things that drew this boy's attention is peculiar enough in itself, but it is his abandonment that really causes concern. Instead of playing, this child seemed to be able to lose himself totally in the mechanical and sensory properties of things. Objects that the parents had always taken to be passive, cold and remote from themselves excited their child and took him to the brink.

McDonnell's experiences as a parent are not unique; the preoccupation with things is a perplexing aspect of the behaviour of children with an autistic spectrum disorder. It is one of the ways in which the deficit in imaginative capacity, or what Wing described as 'an impairment of social imagination and understanding,'[3] is expressed. In autism there is no question of the sort of play we see in normal children: games that involve pretending are not part of an autistic child's play; he uses toys in an unusual, unimaginative way. The child will lick inedible things, constantly sniff everything, become totally absorbed in a rotating object. In her review Sharon Wulff describes the stark contrast with the intricate play of a child that is developing normally:

> A sterile ritualistic quality is seen in autistic play that appears to contribute little, if anything, to the child's pleasure. If left to his or her own devices in a playroom full of toys, the child will more than likely ignore the toys and engage in stereotypic self-stimulatory body movements, such as rocking or hand flapping. If the toys do catch the attention, chances are one will see the child using the toys

in an unusual fashion. . . . It is apparent that autistic play
lacks the pleasurable, rich complexity of normal play.[4]

Perhaps even more disturbing than the autistic fascination with the
material world, however, is the realization that the familiar world of people-
among-themselves appears to leave the autistic person completely cold - a
second way in which the impairment of social imagination and understanding
comes to the fore. 'He literally walks over us, as if we are dead things'[5] is a
frequently heard cry of distress from parents. According to Eisenberg and
Kanner it seems as if an autistic person does not realize that people have
feelings:

> On a crowded beach he would walk straight toward his goal
> irrespective of whether this involved walking over
> newspapers, hands, feet or torsos, much to the discomfiture
> of their owners. The mother was careful to point out that he
> did not intentionally deviate from his course in order to
> walk on others - but neither did he make the slightest
> attempt to avoid them. It was as if he did not distinguish
> people from things or at least did not concern himself about
> the distinction.[6]

An autistic child seems to lump people and things together.
Anticipating what we shall be looking at shortly: the child seems to be blind
to the fact that people - because they conceive of the world (invisibly,
intangibly) *in thought* - occupy a special position relative to the world of
things. In his essay *Mindblindness* Simon Baron-Cohen, with a nod to Nagel,
raises the question of how we should conceive of such a radically different
condition of mind. 'It is probably impossible to imagine what it is like to be
mindblind, in the same way as it is impossible to imagine what it is to be a
bat.'[7]

The autist's imagination deficit in his dealings with people and
things is in stark contrast to the playful manner in which people normally
approach the world. It is hard to escape the impression that chances to
somehow bridge the gulf between the imaginative capacities of autistic and
non-autistic people are remote. And yet that is exactly what the idea of a
shared existence requires one to do. How to close this imagination gap?

**Inside the Mind: Researching Autism as Mind Blindness**
If you watch the play of an autistic child you may well get the
impression that the child is not getting anything out of it. But that is not the
only reason for perplexity. True, the play is characterized by a limited
repertoire of actions and interests, but when one compares this with the

relations with *people* the interaction with the world of things is relatively normal. The occasional individual is really talented, for example in spatial awareness, drawing or calculating; others develop good practical skills like riding a bike or doing a jigsaw puzzle; many have a surprisingly good mechanical memory whereas any insight into meaningful connections always escapes them. This deficit appears to be largely independent of the general level of intelligence. The combination of an intact intelligence with typical deficits in the domain of social imagination and understanding has lead Freeman Dyson to say about Jessy Park: 'I've always felt that this woman, who is now thirty-five years old, whom I've known since she was a little child, is the closest I'll ever come to an alien intelligence.'[8] For a closer look at this 'alien intelligence,' in which not all abilities are impaired, although several crucial ones are, let us pay a visit to the experimental laboratory of the cognitive psychologist.

### Getting to Know the Autistic Mind
Since the studies carried out by Hermelin and O'Connor and in the light of the striking disharmonious development profile, autism has increasingly come to be regarded as an impairment in the processing of meaningful information.[9] Ricks and Wing built on these ideas with the hypothesis that autistic people primarily have difficulty with the mental processing or reprocessing of symbolic information and the formation of a conceptual framework in which data, new or otherwise, can be integrated and assigned or reassigned meaning.[10] This inability to make anything of symbolic data, suggests Wing, could explain the unbalanced development.

> A child who has these problems in pure and mild form would, once he had control of his arms and hands, be able to manipulate objects and in this way experience success in modifying his own environment. He presumably would develop some degree of self-awareness, some limited concepts, and he would have a source of pleasure and interest. However, his experiences would differ markedly from those of a normal child whose early interests centred around human beings rather than objects. The differences might explain the fascination and skill with objects shown by some of the more able children with the triad.[11]

More than twenty five years ago, with their question 'Does the autistic child have a 'theory of mind'?,' the British researchers Baron-Cohen, Leslie and Frith gave a new impetus to psychological research into autism.[12] The authors assume that people with autism suffer from a specific cognitive handicap. People are beings that are capable of thinking about the world; they have an imaginative faculty with which the world can be known. On the evidence of his sometimes phenomenal memory for facts, or his knowledge of, say, the way a light switch works, the autistic person is a normally thinking human being, at least where the symbolic representation of things - of physical objects and events - is concerned. However, the world does not consist exclusively of bodies, light switches and timetables; it is also populated by knowing, representing, signifying beings themselves, by *people* with invisible mental abilities. And it is here, so the hypothesis of the cognitive psychologists has it, that we find the crucial difference between autists and non-autists.

A 'normal' person is capable of seeing himself and other people as beings who, unlike things, have the ability to conceive of the world intellectually. This crucial faculty of the human mind - crucial because it enables us to project ourselves into the thoughts and experiences of someone else - presupposes a capacity for meta-representation. In interactions with other 'mind readers' this results in what Premack and Woodruff in their 1978 study of chimpanzees (from which the term comes) called a 'theory of mind.'

> This model specifies a mechanism which underlies a crucial aspect of social skills, namely being able to conceive of mental states: that is, knowing that other people know, want, feel, or believe things; in short, having . . . a 'theory of mind.' A theory of mind is impossible without the capacity to form 'second-order representations.' . . [13]

The term 'theory' of mind is used because we are talking here about reflecting on invisible (mental) phenomena that we assume underlie people's behaviour, and because on the basis of these 'hypothetical' mental faculties it is possible to explain and predict human behaviour with a fair degree of certainty.[14]

The fact that we are able to form some idea of other people's state of mind makes it possible for us to anticipate their expectations and actions in a flexible way and to develop social skills; the inadequate development of this ability or damage to it would seriously disadvantage someone in social interactions. It would lead to difficulties in identifying other people's feelings and intentions, in recognizing deceit and dishonesty, mutual expectations and so on. The authors assume that it is precisely this capacity for meta-representation that is disrupted in autistic people, resulting in the delayed or incomplete development of the 'theory of mind' and all its attendant consequences for social interaction. Autistic people do indeed seem to be 'blind' to the fact that people occupy a special position in respect of the world of things.

The difficulty of distinguishing that which is specifically human from things is confirmed by the autistic Gunilla Gerland. Gerland describes how as a child she drew houses that looked like people - 'the windows were the house's eyes and the door was the mouth' - because for her 'the difference between people and houses was not obvious.'[15] She had great difficulty in reading people's facial expressions, an early milestone in normal development; faces looked like empty houses rather than expressing something inside. 'Those faces were as lacking in content as furniture, and I thought that, just like furniture, they belonged in the rooms I saw them in,'[16] writes Gerland about people she did not know well. 'The people, the empty faces that I sometimes saw in the gardens outside the houses, I saw as some kind of stage props belonging to the scenery.'[17]

Animals only seem to add to the confusion. The autistic Jerry, for instance, had a particular problem with dogs:

> Animate beings were a particular problem. Dogs were remembered as eerie and terrifying. As a child, he believed they were somehow humanoid (since they moved of their own volition, etc.), yet they were not really human, a puzzle that mystified him. They were especially unpredictable; they could move quickly without provocation.[18]

We can probably hardly grasp just how fundamental it is for autistic people and their families when we 'find that the very things we take for granted as unquestionable in our assumption of humanness or 'objectness' are often not assumed by older autistic children,' says McDonnell. 'With such children, mothers are in the presence (the daily presence) of difference - of a different reality, a reality which is sometimes unnervingly 'other' than our own.'[19]

As well as throwing light on limitations in social contacts, this cognitive impairment could also explain the lack of spontaneous imaginative play. Pretending presupposes the same capacity for meta-representation as socially oriented imagination and understanding. In order to be able to pretend something is so (for example to pretend that a doll is ill), reality and the representation of that reality - or more accurately, what you *know* and a *distortion* of what you know - have to be disconnected. Leslie suggests that underlying such a sophisticated understanding of symbols is the same uncoupling mechanism as the one that supports the realization that people can think - and can think something different from what you yourself think.[20] Pretend play could be an early manifestation of the ability to conceptualize mental states. An impaired capacity for meta-representation could therefore explain the autistic imagination deficit in all its facets.

The problem of impaired social imagination and understanding affects the ability to copy other people's actions with genuine understanding of their meaning and purpose. It interferes with the development of the type of pretend play that involves the imaginative act of putting oneself in the position of another person, real or fictional, and of experiencing their thoughts and feelings, as distinct from empty copying of their actions. It also adversely affects the capacity to estimate what others are likely to know or not to know.[21]

This brings us back to the empathic impairment. The researchers' hypothesis is tested in a simple but effective experiment, the so-called Sally-Anne test. Sally has a marble that she puts in a basket before she leaves the room. While Sally is away, Anne quickly hides the marble somewhere else. When Sally comes back to fetch her marble, the question is where she thinks she will find it. When this plot is shown to normal children aged four and up, acted out with dolls, they have no trouble predicting where Sally will look, even though they know that this is not where the marble actually is. They can call to mind both Sally's (incorrect) *conviction* (a mental state) and the *actual* state of affairs (a physical state) and weigh one against the other. Children with learning disabilities (for instance Down's syndrome) who have a mental age of four and above also have this capacity for meta-representation. People with autism, however, do not. In the experiment conducted by Baron-Cohen and his colleagues, sixteen of the twenty autistic children with a mental age of nine gave the wrong answer by pointing to where the marble really was, although they scored well on numerous questions that tested their knowledge of the actual situation.[22]

We therefore conclude that the autistic children did not appreciate the difference between their own and the doll's knowledge. Our results strongly support the hypothesis that autistic children as a group fail to employ a theory of mind. We wish to explain this failure as an inability to represent mental states. . . . Thus we have demonstrated a cognitive deficit that is largely independent of general intellectual level and has the potential to explain both lack of pretend play and social impairment by virtue of a circumscribed cognitive failure.[23]

On the one hand the 'theory of mind' thesis can explain an autistic person's handicaps and make it possible to understand why our social and emotional life, permeated as it is with mental representations, is apparently completely incomprehensible to someone with autism, without at the same time having to rule out the existence of skills in interactions with and knowledge of physical things and events. In this model, after all, the fact that the autistic person knows how a light switch works or what time the trains run is separate and distinct from his inability to think about mental phenomena.

Aside from insight, an explanation in terms of a deficit of 'theory of mind' provides something to go on in the clinical treatment of people with autism. In the Netherlands, for instance, Steerneman developed a treatment method that responds to this deficit.[24] His social cognition training is made up of different elements of increasing degrees of difficulty that correspond with the building blocks of a 'theory of mind.' It targets things like symbol formation, perception and imitation, and pretending, which are usually present around the second year of life; skills that develop from the ages of three and four (such as learning to distinguish between physical and mental events, thinking in terms of cause and effect, insight into cheating and deception); and metacognition at the standard of a normal six-year-old. The training consists of practical exercises - a session on points of view asks children to draw how the trainer sees an object, in a session on pretending the children play with puppets. But ultimately the training focuses on the 'thinking and knowing' needed to organize and interpret (social) reality; in other words on *cognitive* skills with which the child learns to develop a better conception of what other people are feeling and thinking.

Social imagination, we can say, is an intellectual affair. Within the framework of the cognitive psychologist we get to know the autistic person as someone with a cognitive handicap who does not *know* the difference between the specific properties of people and of things. Training likewise concentrates on the acquisition of cognitive skills. Where the emphasis is placed on 'learning to think about thinking and learning to understand emotions' (as the title of Steerneman's book translates), we always find ourselves in the field of the mind. It is an approach that can be traced back to a language game with specific presuppositions within which the cognitive psychologist's project itself has to be placed. Let us look at precisely what those presuppositions are.

### (Un)Building the Foundations of Psychological Knowledge

When someone reacts to people and things in ways we are unaccustomed to, it is not inconceivable that we will ask him for reasons for his behaviour. If that does not produce the desired response, perhaps because we do not have a common language, we start looking for an explanation. From that moment on, there is a division between the person who represents and the person who is represented - a contrast that increases when it becomes clear that the behaviour that requires explanation itself actually hampers further investigation. 'Traditional assessments rely heavily on verbal responses and a willingness to cooperate; the autistic child is typically suffering from severe communication or language deficits and often has trouble comprehending what is expected of him or her.'[25] As a result, Wulff remarks, autistic children's IQ protocols are often labelled with the red letters CNT (for 'cannot test'). And so a gulf opens up that only further research would appear to be able to bridge. From this point on, methodological questions - What is a reliable instrument to measure differences and similarities? Can play be used as an alternative assessment tool? What counts as clear and convincing evidence? - determine the agenda of the cognitive psychologist to a significant extent.

What makes an autistic person so different from ordinary people? Well, according to the cognitive psychologist's hypothesis, his inability to distinguish people (as intellectual beings) from things (physical phenomena) at the level of representations. The autistic world view is thus, so it is said, radically different from the *dualistic* world view which people as a rule are assumed to hold.

> Normal children of 4-6 years old can make judgments to distinguish physical and mental phenomena. In this sense they can be called ontological dualists. It also shows the same ability is present in mentally handicapped subjects of an equivalent mental age.[26]

In experiments like the Sally-Anne test, which were designed to test the 'theory of mind' hypothesis - particularly the 'false belief' element - this dualistic reality is replicated on a laboratory scale. Simulating a world of purely mental and purely physical entities and events under controlled conditions makes it possible to compare the cognitive abilities of autistic and unimpaired subjects. As a result, the dividing line between people and things - until then not particularly problematic - suddenly becomes very important; something that was taken for granted is made explicit:

> physical entities afford 'behavioral-sensory contact,' that is, they can be acted upon (e.g., eaten, ridden, etc.), seen, and touched, etc. Mental entities, on the other hand, do not afford these qualities.[27]

Follow-up research by Baron-Cohen from which this categorization is taken yet again illustrates the dualistic nature of the work of the cognitive psychologist. One of the fascinating experiments that make up this study tests children's ability to answer questions of the type: which child can eat or touch a biscuit (a physical activity), the child who *dreams* about a biscuit (a mental phenomenon) or the child who (as everyone can see) is actually *given* a biscuit by her mother? - questions that are assumed to allow the researcher to make a distinction between the subject's ability to represent a mental and a physical event.

> We tested the children's understanding of four mental phenomena (thoughts, dreams, pretense, and memories) in comparison to their understanding of four physical phenomena (food, drink, bicycles, and swings). We predicted that if autistic children were unaware of the special nature of mental entities, they would attribute physical properties randomly to either mental or physical phenomena. On the other hand, we predicted that if subjects did understand the distinction between mental and physical phenomena, they would attribute physical properties to physical phenomena alone.[28]

'Are autistic children 'behaviourists'?' wondered Baron-Cohen, when it emerged that only four of the seventeen autistic children tested, as against fifteen of the nineteen normal children, knew the right answers to the questions. The implications of this explanation for our understanding of people with autism and of our (non-autistic) selves are clear: Everyone does psychology, but whereas from the age of three or four children generally share a 'common-sense mentalistic psychology' with other people, people with autism tend to explain human behaviour from a physicalistic or behaviouristic perspective.[29]

The autistic tendency to ontological *monism* sometimes becomes painfully visible in everyday life, too. For instance, in the first volume of her autobiographical work, the autistic life writer Donna Williams wrote that she 'had a doll and wanted very much to cut it open to see if it had any feelings inside.'[30] This suggests that high-functioning individuals with autism may realize that people have something extra, without being able to get a real grasp of what that 'extra' is.

The suspicion that people with autism are 'behaviourists' in the subtleties of social interactions and mental phenomena is confirmed in a second experiment that finds out what ideas the test subjects have about the working of the brain. In the first place normal children between four and six reply that brains are for thinking with, for dreaming and remembering things - in other words mental functions. In the second instance and to a lesser degree they are also able to suggest other functions, such as that brains 'tell you that you have to walk.' Children with autism, however, primarily associate the organ of the mind with *physical* (motor, behavioural) functions rather than (physical and) mental ones.

The results of this study suggest that autistic children treat
mental phenomena as no different than physical ones. It
may be that the physical level of understanding is the only
one available to them, leading them to force all phenomena
into it.[31]

A third experiment tests the ability to make a distinction between
reality and appearance, for example by giving children a piece of fake
chocolate and observing what they do with it. Some autistic test subjects,
long after discovering that the chocolate was made of plastic, stubbornly
persisted in trying to eat it anyway.

The cogency of the cognitive psychologist's claim stands or falls by
the precision with which the experimental setting simulates a dualistic world.
It depends on the accuracy with which the researcher himself distinguishes
between (the representations of) physical and mental phenomena. There is,
for example, a debate about this methodological question between Baron-
Cohen and Lewis and Boucher, in which the validity of the measuring tool
used is being called into question. Lewis and Boucher raised eyebrows with a
publication in which they presented research results that appeared to refute
the 'theory of mind' hypothesis. They claimed that if people with autism are
*encouraged* to do it, they show no less symbolic play (a meta-
representational activity) than functional play. What's more, under these
conditions autistic children are a match in their imaginative play for children
from the control groups. This points to a deficit other than the one Baron-
Cohen suggested on the basis of findings under non-eliciting conditions.[32]

Lewis and Boucher arrived at their findings by placing their test
subjects in an experimental setting and presenting them with a toy car and
something like an old box. The children were then encouraged to do
something with these things; this calls for an ability to pretend that the box
represents something else. When a child in this inviting situation pretends
that the box is a garage (or whatever), this counts as imaginative play. Out of
the twenty-four toy/junk combinations they were offered, the autistic group
had a positive score on thirteen of them, as against a median score of eleven
and fourteen in non-autistic control groups. The functional ability to play was
measured with a toy car and a real toy garage, which did not require pretence.
Here again the autistic group's scores were not significantly different from
those of the control groups. Lastly, it was striking that in the spontaneous
play situation the autistic children underutilized their theoretically unaffected
functional play ability (at most 14% of the total playing time as against at
least 28% to at most 46% in the control groups), something for which the
'theory of mind' thesis has no explanation.

The conclusion that Lewis and Boucher drew - that people with
autism are potentially capable of second order (or meta) representation - was

contested. What Lewis and Boucher elicited is certainly not pure pretence play, wrote Baron-Cohen in a reaction. All they have shown is that autistic children are good at *guessing* what is meant when they are asked to do something with the things.

> For example, in one trial of the elicited condition the experimenter says 'What can these do? Show me what you can do with these?,' handing the child a car and a box. Unsurprisingly, the autistic children of about 12 years old and with a verbal [mental age] of around 5 years old . . . do the only thing they can with the materials: they put the car into the box. (The car being smaller than the box, the box cannot go into the car.) . . . The core of pretence is *creating* imaginary identities or properties for objects. Lewis and Boucher's study has not demonstrated this ability in autism.[33]

Lewis and Boucher simply measured white noise; the error they made, according to Baron-Cohen, was that they confused the representation of physical qualities - the car goes into the box but the box won't go into the car - with meta-representational activities - pretending that the box is a garage. In so doing, he asserted, they had compromised the essential dualistic character of the research design.[34] Because Lewis and Boucher had not distinguished between mental and physical events with sufficient precision when designing their study, not only is the crucial difference between autistic and non-autistic in danger of being snowed under, so too is what separates the researcher from the subject of his research - that is, his ability to envisage the representative *and* meta-representative activities of his test subject and - this time on a level of representation in the *third* order - to weigh them against each other. Like the autistic person, Lewis and Boucher nibble away at the foundations of the researcher's project.

### Humanoid Computing

As time has passed, the 'theory of mind' thesis has also been the subject of discussion in other ways. Despite the force of this explanation, there are known cases where autistic subjects do seem able to imagine what is going on in other people's minds and have successfully completed 'theory of mind' tests. Baron-Cohen, Leslie and Frith themselves noted 'a small subgroup of autistic children who succeeded on the task and who thus may be able to employ a theory of mind.'[35] In a follow-up, Holroyd and Baron-Cohen wondered how far autistic people could get in developing a 'theory of mind.'[36] According to the authors, in the majority of the cases examined (60-70%) virtually no 'theory of mind' can be expected; for a minority (20-30%)

in puberty the development could extend to the 'theory of mind' level that a three- to four-year-old would normally reach. Studies by other researchers indicate that in adulthood a few of these individuals can attain the level of a six- to seven-year-old, who can understand more complex states of mind.

Baron-Cohen presented an explanatory model whereby the development of the normal 'theory of mind' is divided into four hypothetical steps, which makes it possible to discount the variations that were observed.[37] The first component is the *intentionality detector* (ID), which enables children to interpret incoming stimuli in terms of the aims and wishes of an actor. This ability, which makes it possible to understand primitive states of mind in terms of 'will,' develops in the first months of life and appears to be intact in autistic people too. A second mechanism with which, according to this model, the modern human mind is equipped is the *eye direction detector* (EDD), which from babyhood makes children aware of eyes and eye movements in the face of the carer. This ability enables the child to understand primitive states of mind in terms of 'seeing.' This, too, seems to function in essentially the same way in autistic as in normal children.

Atypical function, however, does seem to occur in the next step, the development of the *shared attention mechanism* (SAM), which normally takes place between nine and eighteen months. This cognitive mechanism lets children construct mental triangular relationships, where they learn to imagine that another person and they themselves can both be looking at or thinking about the same object outside them. The shared attention mechanism does not appear to kick in in most children with autism. In consequence the functioning or otherwise of the SAM could be a good predictor of an impairment in the last component, the actual *theory of mind mechanism* (ToMM), which is present around the fourth year and is fed by information from the other components. The ToMM allows normal children to understand not only volitional and perceptional, but also *epistemic* states of mind. In other words, they can represent and integrate into a usable 'theory of mind' not only what another person wants or what he sees, but also what he believes, dreams, knows, pretends, thinks or takes to be true (regardless of whether what the other person mentalizes is actually true). In almost all cases the concept of epistemic states of mind seems to be too difficult for children with autism.

As we have seen, a small subgroup nonetheless seems able to achieve the 'theory of mind' level of a normal four-year-old and possibly even a seven-year-old. Holroyd and Baron-Cohen, however, saw it as an open question 'whether such individuals are showing late development of the *same* processes as are used normally, or are arriving at the same point via an alternative cognitive compensatory route.'[38] Wing also noted that gifted people with autism sometimes seem to be able to recognize the feelings of others, but she suspected that there was an unbridgeable gulf between this and the more natural, empathic way in which non-autistic people share emotions: 'the capacity exists on an intellectual level without empathic sharing of the emotions.'[39] In those cases where autistic people succeed in 'theory of mind' tests and in so far as that success cannot be attributed to a leak in the experimental design, formal rules and logical deduction could explain this phenomenon. This view appears to be supported by what can be gleaned from conversations with such individuals.

For Temple Grandin, for instance, what went on between other children, the swift exchange of meaningful codes and subtle signals which made them seem naturally involved with one another, remained essentially closed to her. 'She can infer . . . [social signals], she says, but she herself cannot perceive them, cannot participate in this magical communication directly, or conceive the many-levelled kaleidoscopic states of mind behind it,'[40] wrote Sacks, who went to see her. This means that without knowledge of the mind she had to work out what most other people have as a matter of course. Sacks put it like this: 'Lacking . . . [this type of implicit knowledge], she has instead to 'compute' others' intentions and states of mind, to try to make algorithmic, explicit, what for the rest of us is second nature.'[41] For Grandin, concretizing connections takes visual forms. 'My mind is completely visual and spatial work such as drawing is easy,' she wrote. 'When I think about abstract concepts such as human relationships I use visual similes.'[42] The imagery of a sliding glass door, for instance, serves as an approximation of social relations and the gentle manners they presuppose. This visual capacity comes in extremely useful in her work as a leading designer of abattoir processes. 'But this sort of simulation or concrete imagery is much less appropriate when she has to do other kinds of thinking - symbolic or conceptual thinking,'[43] wrote Sacks. 'Knowing this intellectually, she does her best to compensate, bringing immense intellectual effort and computational power to bear on matters that others understand with unthinking ease.'[44]

Gunilla Gerland, another example, did, it is true, discover that everything has a content but this did not at the same time give her automatic access to states of mind.

> I am unable to perceive whether people wish me well or ill. Instead, I try to calculate with my intellect, and the result is not always that good. I've realised that people can sense if someone wishes them well or ill. They seem to accumulate some sort of experience of others, which they then use in order to read them. I have no such sense, no special place in which to accumulate those experiences.[45]

However far some autistic people come and however much this has to be regarded as an extraordinary achievement, it still does not make them real mind readers. While mechanical calculation rules and logical reasoning patterns do enable the very occasional individual to simulate a normal life, the result often lacks the natural fluency we find in ordinary encounters. As a human computer, the autistic subject is again in danger of ending up on the object's side, this time *inside* the sphere from which the distinction between people and things normally *originates* and in which it is reproduced - the domain of the mind.[46] While the exact mechanisms with which a few high-functioning people succeed in something approaching a mind reader's life are unknown, it seems that the empathic way that children usually learn to put themselves in someone else's place and the essentially free character of the non-autistic imagination are beyond their reach; longer sums are as far as an autistic person can get. Some do get very close and can almost touch normal existence, but they are still separated from it by an unfathomably deep gulf.

**Exploring Extra-Mental Forms of Imagination**

The cognitive explanation proves to be the laborious result of attempts to simulate a purely dualistic world in the artificial setting of the experiment. Its constructed nature does not detract from the importance and the influence of the 'theory of mind' thesis. The accepted cognitive concept of imagination offers an intriguing explanation for the autistic deficit of social imagination. Parents and others who care will undoubtedly recognize the cognitive psychologist's account. They will admit that autistic people are at a great remove from other people, probably using some of the psychological terms that we have discussed, but they will immediately counter that their loved ones are also *among* us. I have argued before that, given the fact that those consensual means that we normally rely upon are not available, such a shared existence of autistic and non-autistic people must be considered a remarkable achievement by the people around them, but also by people with autism themselves. It is an achievement, I want to argue here, also in terms of imagination. The question arises how we must then understand such an achievement.

*Limitations of Mental Gymnastics*

The dualist language that epitomized the psychologist's and our common non-autistic world view seems to limit our understanding in this respect. First, it invites us to think of human social life, imagination in particular, as an essentially *mental* achievement. Social imagination, the autistic impairment in imagination, and the way out are all located in the sphere of *thinking*. But endeavouring to elicit cognitive feats is ruled out in most cases, because many autistic people lack the intellectual abilities they require. Social cognition training, for example, only achieves results in children with a relatively good starting position (a high IQ and a mild developmental disorder). 'Both verbal and general intelligence is a necessary, but still not sufficient condition for the development of a [theory of mind] T.O.M. Apart from intelligence, the nature and severity of the developmental disorder are factors in the development of a T.O.M,'[47] contends Steerneman.

The cognitive way of circumventing the deficit in social imagination and understanding consequently does not seem helpful as a general strategy. For less gifted and deeply autistic children, in particular, there seem to be few options left when imaginative sources of social life are all located in our mind. But having arrived in the mental realm, there is a curious catch for others as well. For, as soon as we are 'upstairs,' people with autism, intellectually high-functioning individuals included, are denied access to the naturally developing community of mind readers. The cognitive reserves of autistic people, we have seen, are called upon in terms of their *physical* strength; the only conceivable option for them to take part in social imagination is as humanoid computers - a fascination with the idea of autistic savants as human databases or calculators that has dominated the public image of autism since the success of *Rain Man*.[48] Within a dualist framework this sphere of mechanical rules, however, is rendered devoid of meaning and essentially *inhospitable* to people. All the same, people with autism, no matter what their intellectual abilities are, are supposed to also need meaningful human contact. When everything else fails, parents and others who care about autistic children will still try anything to beguile them into living as (imaginative) *human* beings.

How can we avoid these limitations and distance ourselves from an all too familiar dualistic use of language - this time in the guise of a naturally developing community of mind readers on the one hand and autistic computers on the other? For many, finding solutions in their lives with autists is a *practical* affair rather than something about which an 'idea' is formed. For bystanders, the question is usually not how to interpret the other person, but how to deal with the autistic person and his or her lack of imagination in the familiar sense of the word. Although it is true 'that people with autism need carers with a tremendous imagination,'[49] as Theo Peeters, a Flemish expert on autism, put it, precisely because we 'really cannot imagine what a life without this social orientation is like,' we should not in the first place be thinking about a *mental* achievement.

So, what should we be thinking about? How to conceive of human social life, and social imagination in particular, without seeking refuge in cognitive terms? Is it conceivable that imagination has a place in a shared existence of autistic and non-autistic people *without* great feats of cognition or mental gymnastics?[50] Is it conceivable that material objects and physical phenomena play a less restricted, perhaps even humanizing role in it? In order to get away from non-autistic presuppositions in the thinking about the nature of the imagination deficit and how to compensate for it, let us follow Bernlef's example and bring some other actors on stage. More particularly, let us turn the spotlights on some of the practical solutions that have been formulated in the interaction between non-autistic and autistic people.

### Getting to Grips with Things

From the here and now we go back to the early nineteen-seventies. In behavioural studies of the period the relation between people with autism, non-autistic persons and the material environment was the focus of attention. The concern was not so much with explaining the autistic person's behaviour, but rather with determining the influence of people and things on the autistic person's (social) behaviour. This question led on to the examination of how parents and others could make use of the insights that had been acquired to influence the autistic person's one-sided focus (on the world of things).

A widely held view was that things form a barrier between the autistic person and the people around him. When the child is too attached to material properties, this could stand in the way of an inner world of meanings and the formation of relationships with people based on it. Furthermore there are numerous practical reasons for regarding a rigid attachment to objects as detrimental to the development of the child. Sometimes a child drags such inconveniently large things around with him that it limits not just his mental horizon but his physical freedom of movement too. The loss or removal of the cherished object can lead to behavioural problems. And because a child with autism is so often fixated on the sensory qualities of an object, can be wholly absorbed in how it feels, smells, tastes or shines in the light, things can stand in the way of more constructive and educational activities. 'Most of *A*'s day,' for instance,

> was spent wandering round the house (or garden) carrying his attachment object, a cot blanket, and refusing to be involved in any constructive activity beyond basic caretaking. Even during bath time or meals he had to hold on to his blanket and screamed if it was removed from him. Mother had to wait until he was asleep before removing it to wash, returning it before he woke up in the morning to prevent violent tantrums. [51]

Some authors believed that the thing that frustrates the development of the autistic child should be firmly removed from his vicinity. Others warned against such a strategy because of the deterioration it can cause in the child's behaviour. Marchant and her colleagues consequently advocated a very gradual approach.

> The steps would obviously have to be very gradual in order to be unnoticeable to the child and to prevent any catastrophic reactions being induced. . . . Near the beginning of the intervention it was suggested that Mother begin to cut small pieces off the blanket each night when *A* was asleep. This she did for one week and on the next visit the blanket measured only 2 x 8 in. . . . After two months the 'blanket' consisted of 5 threads knotted together.[52]

By gradually reducing the place that things occupied in the life of this little boy, the researchers hoped to avoid a crash and elicit a normal social and instructive relationship between the child and his parents. With the patience of a saint, the mother cut away a few threads every night until there was virtually nothing left of the fabric that separated her from her child.

Things - at least the way they are described in this report - can be cut off and smuggled away to make way for loving people. This clears the field for someone who talks to you and smiles at you, who gives up her time for you, who values you and hugs you - provided that you allow yourself to be lured into a socially meaningful relationship with the world, into an imitation of human gestures and delight in play.

> Our intervention at first was mainly aimed at increasing the amount of interaction between the parents and the child and building up meaningful and pleasurable communication between them. This was established by having a short set time each day when the Mother devoted her time to teaching language comprehension, self-help skills, picture matching and imitation of gestures and use of musical instruments. The child was rewarded for any active involvement by praise, hugs and smiles. After only a few days *A* anticipated these sessions with pleasure, fetching the box of toys and materials and 'asking' for such activities to begin.[53]

These bystanders are not as concerned with what an autistic person knows about people and things as they are with the way he lives. Do things form a barrier between the child and the people around him and should they be replaced little by little? Or is there a role for things in the imaginative interaction between people, just as they occupy a more or less self-evident place in normal social encounters? In the situation discussed here, it would seem that this is not the case. Another example, however, answers this latter question quite differently.

*Pacman, Walkman, Chewing Gum*

In a field experiment by Gaylord-Ross and his colleagues the scene shifts to the school yard of an American high school. Alongside the non-handicapped children in this school there are also a number of autistic boys. It is recess and, as usual, the students are hanging around in groups chatting. The autistic students stand apart; there is virtually no contact between them and the others. During the experiment Mike and Dan, two autistic students, are offered three popular leisure objects - a walkman, a computer game and chewing gum - three objects that it is assumed can promote the social orientation of the autistic subjects towards their contemporaries, without making a great demand on their language skills.

> Because autistic persons characteristically have limited language repertoires, there is an inherent problem in relying on verbal discourse for elaborated encounters. Therefore, we selected nonverbal activities that could be used as a means to promote elaborated social encounters.[54]

The way these therapists approach Mike and Dan is reminiscent of a centuries-old custom that we know from descriptions of the first contacts between explorers and native peoples. Before a word was spoken, and long before the 'savage' became the subject of scientific study, all sorts of small objects like mirrors, beads and native artefacts were exchanged. Not infrequently the manipulation of small things like these was the start of the creation of a new, common language repertoire.

In order to investigate the influence of the simple presence of the things on social interaction, the researchers started by offering the objects without any instructions as to how to use them. The test subjects themselves proved to have very few ideas about what to do with the things and the researchers measured no difference whatsoever. During a separate training session Mike and Dan were then taught how the objects function. They learned, for instance, how to chew gum without swallowing it, but this intervention likewise produced no measurable effect. In the third phase they were taught the social rules involved in the use of the things. Non-handicapped classmates acted as sounding boards for initiatives taken by the autistic youngsters during separate training sessions. Here the researchers were working not only on the communication disorder, but also on a deficit of inner language. To compensate for the absence of a system of internal representations and categorizations, there was a complete, written script that created cohesion between individual elements.

The script lays down for both the autistic participant and his non-handicapped peer how to share chewing gum, gather round a walkman or play a game of Pacman together.

| Autistic student (AS) | Nonhandicapped peer (NP) |
|---|---|
| 1. 'Hi.' | 2. 'Hi,–, how are you doing?' |
| 3. 'Fine.' | |
| 4. 'Want to play Pacman?' | 5a. 'Sure (yeah great)' or |
| | 5b. 'No thanks.' |
| 6. Turns on game. | |
| 7. Hands game to NP. | 8. Plays game until it is over. |
| | 9. Hands game to AS. |
| 10. Reads score. | |
| 11. Turns game off and then on and plays. | 12. Watches while AS plays; encourages him when AS plays |
| 13. Reads his own score at the end of the game. | well. |
| 14. Offers game to NP. | |
| | 15. Plays game or says 'No, thanks, |
| 16. Says 'Bye.'[55] | got to go, bye.' |

Autism would thus seem to be an important test case for the possibilities and limitations of translating words, moral messages and social meanings into material structures, tangible things, visual forms and written rules, and vice versa.[56] According to Peeters, who borrowed the concept from Grandin:

> People with autism have too little inner language or too few inner scripts that allow them to organize their thoughts. And what we do in helping them, I believe, should be seen as offering them external scenarios to compensate for the lack of internal scripts.[57]

During this phase the researchers observed for the first time an increase in the social encounters in the school yard. The learned behaviours were generalized to the morning recess, where the autistic students, armed with a walkman or one of the other objects and trained according to the guidelines in the added script, embarked on social interactions. What's more, the non-handicapped students in the school yard - youngsters who had not been informed or trained - also approached the autistic students more readily.

> It was assumed that the object served as a social 'prosthetic' to facilitate interaction among peers who ordinarily had no common language or cultural base on which to build interactions.[58]

A brief glance at the playground reveals that there is a world of difference between the way autists behave and the way non-handicapped youngsters deal with people and things. In normal social interaction, larded with language and social understanding, leisure objects play a more or less self-evident role. For the person with autism, in contrast, a familiar but limited repertoire of activities and interests is coupled to minimal social interactions and deficits in imagination and communication. In contrast to the experiment of the cognitive psychologist, however, in the given circumstances it is not the 'insight' into the autistic person's impaired cognition that is central, but the fact that bystanders - by doing it - prove that they are able to deal with the way that the autistic students face life.

The approach advocated here is very different from that in the previous example. In this experiment things play a crucial role. Where, through a lack of shared conceptual frameworks, people cannot imagine themselves in the other person's position - with all the attendant implications for social interaction - playthings act as social prosthetics. The accompanying script stands in for the usual (cognitively understood) social imagination and concept forming. Circumventing normal cognitive skills, circumventing ideas, they help to create a concrete image of what it means to play together and take part in meaningful relationships in the school yard. Both autistic and non-autistic children learn to adjust to this construction.

### Getting Off the Ground

The absence of social imitative play is not the only sign of the autistic imagination deficit. It is also expressed in a qualitative deficit of varied, spontaneous imaginative play. Autistic children often seem to be totally engrossed by properties that are concrete, observable, by the shape, colour, taste, smell and texture of the world around them. This relationship with the world - superficial and unvarying from the non-autistic viewpoint - is in stark contrast with the imaginative play of a child who is developing normally. This often makes bystanders long to help this child share in the freedom of normal development.

Peeters describes an example that can illustrate how onlookers tried to break through the dead end of autistic play and enable an autistic child to share in free time and space without saddling him with the constantly changing reference points - cultural codes, implicit assumptions, subtle rules - of a non-autistic existence. The subject was a boy with autistic spectrum disorder who had become totally enchanted by aeroplanes. He was given a toy plane, but did not seem able to do very much with it.

> He got no further than making a 'brrm-brrm' noise and lifting and lowering the plane no more than fifty centimetres. Even in his super-enthralled moments he seemed to be locked into a lack of initiative, purpose and direction.[59]

For bystanders it is often heart-rending to see how an autistic person can be totally lost in limited, repetitive and stereotyped patterns of behaviour, interest and activities. In the case of this boy, whose imagination deficit was expressed in something that really could not be called 'play,' the carers found a way out. Experience had taught them that there was no point in trying to encourage the boy to produce creative ideas of his own. Instead they drew a circuit that he could take his plane around.

> During a practical training session the group of trainees came up with the fantastic idea of visualizing what else he could do with his plane. They drew out and marked with tape a circuit a good forty metres long in the playroom to show that the plane could do more than take off and land in the fifty-centimetre tunnel right in front of his eyes - it could fill the whole play area. This was explicitly shown to him.[60]

This increase in the possible actions that was created by expanding the circuit and visualizing the play space was a hit. The circuit got not just the plane but also an *inner* flow moving; the boy appeared to be really liberated in his play.

> The result was predictable and yet overwhelming. He seemed really liberated, he started to flap his arms, picked up his plane, ran round the whole circuit, started to jump up and down, and then ran round the whole circuit again.[61]

This account suggests that the boy's ability to imagine something in his flight resided not so much in a cognitive processing of reality as in a concrete organization and expansion of the room to play and move. The structuring of the space in which the boy could play with his toy aeroplane did not, moreover, lead to a restriction or conditioning of his existence, but in fact proved to be a crucial step in his personal development. Where it proved

impossible to give his imagination free rein, the material extension of the
number of degrees of freedom provided something to go on.

*Bend It Like Gerland*

In *A Real Person* Gunilla Gerland gives a second example of the
way things can 'get round' the characteristic autistic cognitive style in order
to augment and correct it. In the psychologist's terminology, this specific
style can be described as a rigid and blinkered way of reasoning, as a deficit
of abstraction ability that stands in the way of an imaginative interaction with
reality. As she says herself, Gerland's actions revealed all sorts of fixations,
including a compulsive obsession with curved objects. In order to stop an
unbearable feeling of shivers in her spine, she had to keep touching these
things.

> Curved things were what I wanted to touch. I grasped every
> door-handle I passed. I put the tip of my forefinger just
> where the handle curved. This felt good. I followed the
> banister rail with my hand all the way to the middle where
> it curved, then stopped and rubbed my palm back and forth
> on the curve. I did that every time I went up or down the
> stairs, and always at the same place. I had to do it every
> time to calm my spine. I always finished off my walk down
> the stairs by scraping my nails against the rounded bit at the
> end of the rail. I had great feeling in my nails, just like in
> my teeth, and in some strange way I even had some feeling
> in my hair. [62]

When Gerland's obsession with curved objects is defined in terms of
a fixation, her behaviour appears to be an expression of autistic imagination
deficit. Personal growth or development cannot be expected from this
material quarter, the proper course would seem to be to liberate the autistic
self from the stultifying grip of things. Gerland describes how her father did
indeed see it as his job to stop her. Aside from the pain this caused - these
were after all actions that were essential to Gerland herself - the breaking of
her urge to feel the 'curved hollow base' [63] of bottles and other curved things
simply resulted in new rituals.

From a non-autistic perspective the compulsive obsession with
things is an expression of the autistic person's inability to imagine anything
for themselves. The mechanical side of things is also a symbol of the rigid
autistic relationship with reality. Things depict this constrained aspect
*regardless of their shape*. For Gerland herself, in contrast, shape is of the
utmost importance. Just how much further that importance extends beyond
what must be considered conceivable according to familiar, non-autistic

yardsticks is clear from the following quote. Shape, says Gerland, showed her a way out of her mental prison.

> I still have a bent - I like that word - for curved things, but it's no longer a fixation. It comes out mostly in things like finding I want to make a detour in order to take a road that bends instead of a straight one, or feeling a desire to touch something that is beautifully curved. It is good that I can choose to allow myself a detour, to enjoy that curve, but that I can also choose not to if I think I haven't the time. And I know when it's all right to touch whatever arouses my desire to touch and when not, and I don't find it difficult not to. I think it somehow feels as if my attachment to curves comes from being so 'straight' inside. It's because my nervous system is rectilinear that I need to acquire a curve from outside. As if, when I really need an inner curve so as not to be so rigid, I have to find it somewhere outside myself.[64]

Curved objects let Gerland bend her *idées-fixes* and imagine something herself. Without being dependent on higher cognitive functions on which one would normally rely in this case, things make it possible to conceive in a concrete way - tangible, visible - how inner freedom of movement and personal scope can be achieved in an autistic existence. Things in the shape of curved bottoms of bottles, door handles and bending roads *show* Gerland what it is to imagine something for herself that differs from her linear existence and to deviate from the straight line.

### *Braving the Elements*

A third example of how an autistic lack of inner freedom can be circumvented is taken from the autobiographical *En toen verscheen een regenboog* [And Then There Was a Rainbow] in which the autistic Kees Momma writes about his passion for fine cloudscapes, disturbances of the atmosphere, airstreams and other meteorological phenomena.

> Thunderstorms, cloudy skies and forms of precipitation have always fascinated me. I had a book about the weather, but at first I didn't look at it much. However, one spring, dominated by unsettled weather with great banks of cloud and showers, my interest suddenly grew. Using the book as my guide, I drew lots of types of clouds, observed the different remarkable cloud formations and made a study of them. I thought that colourful phenomena like rainbows

and halos around the sun were beautiful. Over the years I acquired more books about the weather, and once someone brought me pictures of clouds. In time I started to make booklets about meteorology myself, with a lot of drawings of beautiful skies.[65]

As long as we are trapped in a dualistic frame of mind that makes a strict and hierarchical differentiation between mental and physical phenomena, Momma's preoccupation with 'unfavourable weather forecasts'[66] and other meteorological facts seems to be yet another expression of the autistic imagination deficit. Someone who is consumed to such an extent by physical processes has no room left for himself, let alone for others. People like Kees Momma seem need protection from the elements.

But for those willing to see, for autists like Momma themselves, the meteorological detour presents itself as an alternative route - concretely imaginable, tangible, visible - to inner freedom of movement. Where his rigid mind leaves precious little room, Momma takes to the air. At first from a safe distance: observing, reading, drawing. But later on, he seeks out higher ground so as to physically experience the power of the elements. Making use of atmospheric up-currents he explores new places full of imaginative activity. He becomes a glider pilot, a new hobby that he discusses extensively in a later book.

'Wouldn't it be fantastic to glide in total silence high up in the air, on the forces of nature! It would give a feeling of freedom,'[67] writes Momma before his adventure. This may sound like a cliché, but if we look more closely we might also discern a meteorological alternative to psychologically informed ideas about imagination. This alternative route is in line with the aeroplane circuit that was laid out in space and with Gerland's winding roads, but gliding adds an extra dimension. Whereas the situations that were discussed before could be called relatively determined and predictable, the weather adds an element of uncertainty and hence of suspense. The previous cases concerned situations that were mostly man-made or conceived by humans, this time one makes use of 'the untamable forces of nature.'[68]

Gliding can thus be conceived as a metaphor enabling us to escape the dualism of human freedom versus determination by things in our discussion of imagination. On the one hand the person, as in the visualized circuit, is driven by the situation, albeit that in this case a whole range of polymorphic forces - 'silent up-currents'[69], 'weak and frayed up-currents'[70], 'billowing movements in the atmosphere'[71] - impact on the person. On the other hand, considerable piloting skills are required, especially given the possibility of 'severe turbulence.'[72] Whereas the settings described before just started to invite resistance, this trial of force with the elements is a significant challenge for the pilot. Both mentalist and mechanist terms fall short if we want to appreciate the hybrid nature of the inner flow that was propelled by Momma's flight at 7,000 metres over the Alps.

### Experiment with the Self

Without detracting from the desire to come as close as possible to meaningful, non-autistic relationships or denying the specific difficulties autists have in this area, non-autistic bystanders are sometimes faced with the likewise not inconsiderable task of making the move in the opposite direction and putting themselves in the position of an autistic person. Efforts here focus not so much on involving the autist in the world of which non-autistic people dream, but on the question of how to make an autistic world imaginable.

Howard Buten is an American psychiatrist who founded a day centre in a suburb of Paris for autistic youngsters who live at home. Every day the staff of the Adam Shelton Centre take in around twenty autistic children who have been turned away everywhere else because of their behavioural problems. The centre is also unlike other places in the type of activities it undertakes with the youngsters in order to give them a meaningful way to spend the day. Artistic input in the form of music, acrobatics and circus, drama, painting and so forth is an integral part of the centre's approach.

Buten himself is closely involved in the work with the children. His endeavours are aimed at 'understanding' people with autism and becoming 'familiar' with their existence, not so much on an intellectual level but rather through what he calls an 'intuitive' or 'instinctive' way of working. As he put it in an interview with Lebert, 'I want to understand people with autism. On all levels. Emotional, mental, physical, artistic.'[73] In his work Buten tries to build a bridge between the world as it is known by the non-autistic, and the *unknown* way that autistic people see the world.

> I share totally the notion of finding ways (practically and theoretically) to put the two worlds of cognition-sensation-relation - theirs and ours - together, for the mutual enrichment of everyone.[74]

It is difficult to generalize about what this achieves in terms of everyday interaction. There are hundreds of subtle ways in which this familiarity produces something in the reciprocal relationship, says Buten. It is in 'the look in my eyes, to 'know' where to touch them, how far away to stay or how close to come, to know how to make them laugh.'[75] Let me underline that Buten 'does not believe that people with autism can be liberated from their condition, nor does he see this as the purpose of his research.'[76] Autistic people suffer, but not necessarily more than other people. 'They suffer differently,'[77] he says. This suggests that a therapeutic motivation is not the only or, from the moral perspective, the only right motive for associating with people with autism; the *desire* for one another's company is of as great if not greater importance and is certainly no less valid morally.

It is not Buten's intention to cure people of their autism. Likewise, it is not the effectiveness of Buten's endeavour that concerns me here, so much as the specifics of his approach.[78] In an effort to bridge the gulf between them, rather than try to move the autistic person in our direction, Buten tries to put himself into the autistic person's existence.

> He began to study people with autism. And he began to imitate them. . . . 'When they [behavioural therapists in the psychiatric institution where he did his internship] saw how I changed myself into an autistic person so that we could communicate with one another, they forbade me to do it. They said that it would only reinforce the patient's autistic behaviour. Then I said to them: how do you know that?'[79]

The interviewer tells us that Buten began to 'study' the behaviour of people with autism, but this immediately puts us in danger of becoming entangled in the cognitivist vocabulary with which I specifically do not want to discuss what Buten does. When we talk about the work of someone like Buten, terms like 'practice' and 'effort' seem far more appropriate than words like 'knowledge' and 'research': Buten has *trained* himself in an autistic life. He learned to keep silent, tried to forget his status as a reflective, thinking human being, and substituted physical behaviour instead. He took dance lessons and learned to control his muscles such that his whole power of imagination was compressed into movement.

> Despite all the warnings, and completely counter to the prevailing scientific wisdom, he looked at the children's body language, practised it in front of the mirror at home, and took dance lessons in order to develop his muscles into perfect instruments (he still trains at the barre in his small Paris flat every day). Hour after hour he sits beside some child or other, chews on a glove, pushes a felt tip across a piece of paper with an unvarying motion.[80]

The term 'body *language*' is used here to describe the movements that Buten imitates, but even this is perhaps pushing things too far. When he performs his *act*, Buten consists almost exclusively of body and muscles. He seems to be searching within himself for the sense of the autistic existence - 'sense' in the meaning of 'physical experience of space and movement.'[81] A better description, then, is to say that Buten trains his body in order to become familiar with what it is to be autistic at a non-intellectual, intuitive level. Buten says, 'one can imagine how they *feel*, rather than what they think.'[82] It is in his physical performance that his power of imagination resides.

> And so the two of them lie beside each other for a long time, their limbs in almost perfect symmetry, without seeing each other and without making a sound. . . . A play is being performed here. Suddenly there's movement. Buten's hand shoots out, tears a tuft of grass out of the ground, throws it into the air and immediately pulls back. A movement one often sees in people with autism: as if they can only touch things for a moment. Things and people: hot. Only Buten's face remains consistently abstracted, and his body language retains that eruptive awkwardness that characterizes autistic persons.[83]

In time, Buten gradually developed a looser way of mirroring his autistic 'partners.' After a while of doing 'exactly what they did as they did it' he 'instinctively wanted to become like them in general - act just as they acted, assimilate and re-enact their exact repertoire of behaviours, but not necessarily at the same time or in the same order.'[84] To him the effects were clear: 'becoming autistic in the fashion of the person with whom I shared space rendered me more interesting to them' and this, he explains, marked the beginnings of a special relationship between him and his 'extravagant partners in mime' that would spill out into the real world outside of the imitation room. He hypothesizes that if

> the autistic state arises from a complex disharmony in the way the brain treats sensory information, a state which prevents the person from being able to adequately control or make sense of his or her immediate environment, then it would seem possible that by imitating an autistic person thoroughly, in detail and for long periods of time, we could obtain firsthand, *visceral* knowledge of the state in which that autistic person finds himself or herself.[85]

Nowadays, Buten does far less imitating but his empathic skills, he assures us, remained intact. Possibly, his body still 'remembers' or has developed its own forms of 'cross-modal sensory associations' through many years of imitation. Could it be, Buten asks himself, that these 'enable me to 'feel, see, smell and hear' with my eyes what the autistic person I'm looking at feels, sees, smells or hears in his or her body?'[86]

Let me add a philosophical note. Buten exerted himself to the extreme to master the embodied being of the autistic other. He trained hard to make autistic physicality a self-evident component of his own life. Wittgenstein wrote about this self-evidence of the body, which he sees as distinct from the sort of 'reasonable certainty' for which the cognitive psychologist, for instance, is looking, and which is based on *observation* and *research*. The certainty of your body is not based on empirical research but on *action*. You do not answer the question as to whether you are certain you have two hands by looking for sensory evidence, for instance by counting and having a good look at them - something that in normal circumstances would be not just superfluous but absurd, as if you could be in any doubt! - but in practice.[87] The fact that you have two hands is obvious all day and every day in innumerable ways: in the way you run your hands through your hair, grasp the handlebars of your bike, or underline your words with gestures.

It is this sort of self-evidence that Buten has always been seeking. Just as it is obvious from everything a person does that he has two eyes, a nose and a mouth, so Buten expresses in everything *he* does his empathy and his familiarity with people with autism. He shows himself how to be the other person. This physical imagination, writes Buten, should not be confused with a superficial likeness. The pretence resonates, as it were, 'inside.'

> Still, there is a sort of insight that comes naturally and that is essential, as if to imitate them, do what they do, but *inside my head*, whenever I'm with them, each of them individually.[88]

It is what Sacks calls 'an experiment with the self.'[89]

*Clown Act*

Buten's familiarity with the autistic existence is achieved in an unusual approach to people and things. Matter-of-course human behaviours, such as the use of language and the acquisition of knowledge, are minimized in Buten's project; the physical nature of the autistic person is his point of reference. He does not, though, draw his inspiration solely from his association with autists. Buten is also Buffo the theatrical clown-mime, trained at the Ringling Brothers and Barnum and Bailey Clown College, who as a performing artist enjoys a measure of fame in Europe and the United States. Buten occasionally appears as Buffo, although nowadays only in his spare time. While it is true that Buffo sometimes uses a gesture or noise of autistic origins, Buten would never approach the children at the centre as Buffo.[90] All the same, there is a close affinity between Buten's intimate work with people with autism and the public performances of the clown.

According to Bakhtin, the clown in literature has an allegorical function; he is 'not of this world' and, as a commuter between worlds, enjoys certain privileges, such as the right to be 'different,' to stand outside the established order, to transcend categories, to shed light on what is usually concealed behind conventions. He externalizes the difference that is inherent in people. And he does it *in public.*

> Their laughter bears the stamp of the public square where the folk gather. They re-establish the public nature of the human figure: the entire being of characters such as [the clown] is, after all, utterly on the surface; everything is brought out on to the square, so to speak; their entire function consists in externalizing things (true enough, it is not their own being they externalize, but a reflected, alien being - however, that is all they have).[91]

The clown act and the work with autistic people are related in so far as they both require an immense effort to strip everyday life of its self-evident, meaningful content. 'Otherwise [there is] no relationship,'[92] confirms Buten. His work is not, though, about transport to and from a world that people can in general easily form an image of - the gulf is too wide for that. We can at most endeavour to distance ourselves from what is familiar and taken for granted. In this respect things have more to offer us than people, as we have already read in Bernlef, and this includes the realm of the imagination. And it is in precisely these material outposts of existence, as we saw in *Vallende ster*, that Bernlef's comic Witteman knows his way. Not by allowing his imagination free rein, but by *using props in his imaginative act.* Nauta commented on the extraordinary achievements of which a clown in the ring is capable.

> I once saw a clown act where a clown comes into a room and finds a thing that he's never seen before and can't relate to anything he's previously observed. He has no idea what to do with what would normally be called a chair and consequently does not succeed in sitting on it. His achievement lies in the fact that he divests the thing of everything that we take for granted in the way we act. He lifts a corner of the veil concealing the Thing-in-itself.[93]

The clown brings the world of things closer, not only by involving it in actual terms in his act but because he himself reminds us of a thing, that is to say, our own corporality. 'Poses, gestures and movements of the human body are funny in so far as this body reminds us of a pure mechanism,'[94] wrote the philosopher Helmuth Plessner, who based his thesis on Bergson's analysis of laughter: 'Whenever a person appears to us as a thing - as a marionette, doll or clown . . . then the comical situation exists in fact.'

His shoes are too big and his clothes are baggy, his face is made up like a mask or the face of a doll, he is all movement and woodenness: in Buten/Buffo's act we see a person who is doing his utmost to look like a body/thing. For this show to go on, it is best to forget about the psychology. As Bernlef says in an essay about Buster Keaton:

> Keaton's invention was that he operated himself like a machine. Apparently without an inner life - his face gives nothing away, except perhaps melancholy - he approaches machines as a 'clever machine' and ultimately manages to make them do what he wants. . . . With the advent of the spoken word, emotionality, the inner life of characters came into film and psychology was the last thing that a comic [from the silent film tradition] could use.[95]

With the help of bodies and things, Buten learns how to be autistic. Or to put it another way, bodies and things make Buten familiar with the autistic person as someone you can conceive of. Being autistic must be pretty much like this, so Buten's body assures him after years of training. After endless practice, Buten's fingertips, his muscles, the make-up on his face 'know' that this is an autist. It proves to be extraordinarily *hard* to be autistic.

In learning to understand people with autism and put himself in their position, Buten exerts himself to the utmost to distance himself from everything that we take for granted.

> Nothing that we use to cope in our world has significance [in the world of the autistic person] . . . It is this other world that Buten investigates so passionately. Not, though, as someone searching for a suitable lens to look inside. Buten transcends the boundary, he gives up the scientist's detachment. Cuts his anchor in the here and now.[96]

On the other hand, Buten stresses that he does not want to lose himself in their world. Like Bernlef's comic he always returns to our world. In himself: 'I want to maintain the two states of mind - knowing and doing - simultaneously in my work,' he says. 'I 'do' instinctively, then try to 'know' intellectually, using what I've observed in 'doing.''[97] But also externalized in the guise of a clown, for the viewing public. It is precisely this transport between two worlds that enables him to show the stay-at-homes something of what he has encountered over there, in the region 'before words,' and to present an autistic existence in the non-autistic context. To make good the imagination deficit it is consequently not enough when Buten does what he can do like no one else: get under the skin of an autistic person. Because then it is our turn. As Buten explains, 'It is rather up to the audience to 'empathize' with the clown on stage.'[98] It is the whole series of substitute elements that are shown on and around the stage that make the connection possible. Only then is the imaginative act complete.[99]

## Past the Blind Spots

In the cognitive psychologists' project, a debate about what a human being is and what a thing is no longer sounds strange to us. The everyday certainty about what people and things are makes way for a no-holds-barred argument about the precision with which the test simulates the ontological dualism between human and thing.[100] The project of the cognitive psychologist is regulated by a series of closely interrelated dichotomies. According to the rules of the profession, according to cognitive psychological theory, the characteristics of people and things - and, as the extension of that, of representations of mental and physical events, of non-autistic and autistic people, of the researcher and his subject - should be confused with one another as little as possible. To the cognitive psychologist, the behaviour of the autistic person touches on crucial issues: it runs counter to the dualism that enables people to acquire psychological knowledge, in everyday life as much as in laboratory research.

When an event cannot be fitted into our usual way of going about things, this not infrequently leads to doubt. But sometimes there is no time for doubt. Sometimes people, because they are born with autism or because they care for someone with autism, simply try to do something. The shared life that is faltering somehow has to be kick-started again. They show us how to live with the autistic imagination deficit, without having to give up entirely on the desire to share in the freedom of a normal development. They take literally what, paradoxically enough, cognitive psychology already pointed out: in terms of social imagination the world of things has more to offer autists than a 'theory of mind' that strictly distinguishes between people and things. But instead of looking for this added value at an intellectual level, as the researcher is inclined to do, it should in the first instance be sought extramentally, outside of thought - in scripts and circuits, along curved objects and atmospheric waves, a body that contorts itself into all sorts of poses. Rather than calling on cognitive reserves, they show that imagination, and compensation for a deficit in imagination, can also be located in places other than people's minds.

While the researcher knowingly differentiates himself in a world where the distinction between people and things is constantly being reconfirmed, we see in the way that autistic and non-autistic people try to live together in practice an undivided world emerging. Unlike the language game of the researcher, where methodological rules prohibit mingling, the rules of the second, more pragmatic language game allow for a busy two-way interaction between people and things, inside and outside, head and hands, between people with and without autism. Within these contrasting world views we learn to see autism as a cognitive disorder, or as an unimagined way of doing things that can only be achieved with exceptional effort.

On the basis of the accounts related here we could conclude that the researcher and the people who then told us their stories each shed light, in their own terms, on different and complementary aspects of the abnormal autistic imagination: one the cognitive aspect, the other his whole way of being. Going a step further is the suggestion that the familiar, dualistic vocabulary - which puts the mind above the body and, having arrived at this point, the 'theory of mind' above mechanical reasoning - stands in the way of the recognition of the specific, unprecedented forms that the imagination can assume for an autistic person and in the interaction with that person. The language of the psychologist, so the explanation goes, is not too one-sided - it is too *sophisticated*.

Wittgenstein suggested that there is an age difference between the language of knowledge acquisition - for instance cognitive psychological knowledge, which is based on observation and research - and the self-evidence of the body - which plays such an important role in the recorded practice - both in the development of the individual and in the history of the language community. The language that is characterized by the search for reasonable certainty supposedly developed relatively *late*. 'The child, I should like to say, learns to react in such-and-such a way; and in so reacting it doesn't so far know anything,' said Wittgenstein. 'Knowing only begins at a later level.'[101] A parallel with autism can be drawn here. It is not inconceivable that people with a severe pervasive development disorder, specifically autistic children with an additional mental impairment, rarely if ever get as far as *knowing* the world.[102]

'In the beginning was the deed,'[103] thus Wittgenstein quotes Faust, who seems to have found an energetic pupil in the clown. This opens up the intriguing possibility that an *early* language game, as dictated by curved objects or by what happens in the school playground, draws closer to what goes on in an autistic existence than the cognitive psychologist's conceptual arsenal. The mistake that the latter makes is that he reduces a way of living that is alien to him and to most of the rest of us to a purely cognitive deficit: according to his theory, autism can be wholly explained by defective meta-representation. But what *precedes* this (defective) cognitive faculty (in the development process), everything that self-evidently belongs to the life of and with an autistic person instead of presenting itself as a case of doubt, cannot stand any more detailed explanation or foundation. The possibility that there is a specifically *autistic* form of imagination - an imaginative capacity which precedes the modern, mentalistic variant of it and which could play a role in a shared form of life - is simply inconceivable in the dualistic agenda. It is precisely because of our non-autistic mind's propensity that the existence of such an autistic gift for imagination all too easily escapes us.

Autistic people and those acquainted with them manage to find those nooks in the imaginative realm, the relevance of which easily eludes ordinary people. When it comes to our ideas about imagination, people with autism show *us* around. Or, to mirror the visual metaphor of Baron-Cohen: autistic people point at a non-autistic blind spot. Instead of always directing our gaze inward and, content with our own interior, pointing to the autistic mind blindness, it seems wise to join the autistic person in looking out: to the variety, the potential, the richness of the world outside the mind. Look up, for instance, at the sky.

# On Words and Clocks
## The Socialization Deficit and Temporal Ordering in a Community for Young Autists

> 'Socialization technology': technology primarily
> aimed not at efficiency and time-saving,
> but at prolonging time: sitting at the table,
> enjoying the companionship. [1]

*Monday 20 June, late shift*
Sitting at the table at five o'clock in the evening. It is quiet,
with just the occasional brief remark. A kitchen timer rings.
David, a big lad, seventeen, sprinkles chocolate flakes on a
piece of bread and butter and starts to eat. As soon as he
finishes his bread, he picks up the timer standing in front of
him on the table and hands it to the care worker. She sets it
to ten minutes. David waits. He waits, in absolute patience,
for it to ring. As soon as it does, David continues his meal.
When the last bite has been swallowed, he gives the timer
to her again and the whole ritual is repeated. Mealtime goes
on this way until four slices of bread have been eaten,
three-quarters of an hour has passed, and it is time to clear
the table. While the others are leaving the table, David
moves his chair over the floor compulsively. Then he
leaves, too. [2]

My ethnographic fieldwork in a facility for mentally handicapped
youngsters with autism, whose ages ranged from eleven to twenty, seemed to
go very well. I had worked with young autists for years as a *groepsleider* - or
care worker[3] - so it did not take me long to get to know the day-to-day life of
the unit. This had certain advantages, but there was also a drawback - I was in
danger of falling short as an ethnographer. The anthropologist learns to
recognize the minutiae of what is regarded as normal and a matter of course
in a community precisely by allowing himself to be initiated into the local
customs as a relative outsider. I was not enough of a stranger. For the four
months I was a guest there several days a week to carry out participant
observations, I was continually inclined to anticipate ways of doing things
that I accepted as self-evident. It was consequently a long time before I
realized the extent to which the way people normally adjust their behaviour
and expectations to those of others seemed to have been blocked during this
meal.

The absence of social rapport I recorded during this meal is bound up with an autistic lack of insight into the rules underlying social intercourse. People with autism can often make no sense of meaningful human behaviour, which in its ins and outs can only be properly understood by someone who grew up and was socialized in the language community. For it is here that the conventions of reciprocal social interaction have their roots.[4] Depending on the severity and manifestation of the social disorder, autistic children grow up, when one compares them with normal children, in a more or less all-encompassing social vacuum. The social disorder is usually more serious if it is accompanied by a mental handicap, as was the case in the unit where I carried out my research, but even in mentally gifted individuals, where there is often a remarkable improvement after the age of five, these problems persist. Lorna Wing identified among this group 'an overwhelming difficulty in acquiring and understanding the multitudinous rules of social life and developing empathy with others.'[5]

One can expect that the socialization deficit would lead to major problems of adjustment in situations where people with and without autism cross one another's paths. Social integration problems can crop up anywhere and everywhere; we will concern ourselves here primarily with problems relating to mutual agreement on *time*. Contrary to what we expect of people, none of the residents in this community could tell us, for instance, what time it is. More importantly, symbolic concepts of time seem to be almost entirely incomprehensible to them. They have no sense of what 'wait,' what 'in a moment' or what 'tomorrow' mean.

> The problems with time are not related to telling time by the clock, which some people with autistic disorders are able to do well. The difficulties lie in comprehending the passage of time and linking it with ongoing activities. This often shows itself as an inability to wait. . . . Some begin to scream if made to wait more than a second for their food, for a walk, for a ride in the car or for anything else they want. . . . One of the most obvious examples of confusion with time is the way in which those with enough speech continuously ask for reassurance about future events and when they will happen. . . . Another aspect of this problem is the lack of awareness that an event, once started, will come to an end. . . . The fear generated by being lost in time also explains why there is often such a strong adverse reaction to any unpredicted change in the expected timetable.[6]

In dealings with autistic people one cannot take it for granted that the progress and succession of events and phenomena will be understood in a common language. All the same, as I only gradually began to realize, time does not pass unnoticed in the life of the group. In practice you cannot escape from the fact that events last for a given length of time, that meals have to be eaten at a certain time, that you have to go to school in a little while, and that now and again you have to wait. This means there is a constant, implicit requirement for residents to keep track of the time in spite of their handicap. The question is how such a temporal order is to be achieved. How can one bridge the gap between socialized and relatively under-socialized people? What work has to be done on the front line and who has to do it? And how are we to describe this work?

**The Art of Waiting**
      A tried and tested ethnographic method is one in which the researcher, by taking part in the world in which his research subjects live, endeavours to become familiar with the way people interpret their world.[7] The right approach to the way people give meaning to their world is to listen to what *they* have to *say*. However, a characteristic feature of autism is an inability to share in the interpretative world and give meanings to things; particularly in mentally handicapped people with autism there can be an accumulation of communication difficulties. Consequently, entering into a conversation with an autistic person has to be seen as highly problematic. It makes sense, therefore, to look through the eyes of those who are closest to these silent kids, the care workers, and to describe dealing with questions of time on the basis of *their* accounts and interpretations. At least, to start with.

*Confusion of Sounds*
      As I learned from the care workers, things that are self-evident to non-autistic members of this small community are anything but obvious to the autistic youngsters who live there. David, for instance, seemed unable to grasp the meaning of a seemingly simple instruction like 'wait a moment.' Because, I was told, 'David's a true autist.' And autistic people are known, among other things, for their inability to deal with questions of time.

> David doesn't know what waiting is. Because what's waiting? How long does it take? You can try to explain it to him a hundred times... When we wait for a train, we know it will come. But I think that in autism there's a completely different concept of waiting, that they do know something about waiting, but...[8]

Imprecise concepts like 'tomorrow' and 'soon' are very difficult for this group to comprehend. This emerged one evening, for instance, when David was allowed to help with the packing for the group's holiday later that week. When it came to bedtime, instead of going upstairs to bed he started getting ready to leave for the holiday. Now. Right away.

David's incompetence in time-related situations can be regarded as typical of the autistic inability to discern order and coherence in matters that go beyond the level of literal, concrete connections. The unit's introductory folder explains how this comes about.

> Autistic people do not seem to understand the world. They are incapable of ordering affairs spontaneously, of putting them in a certain order, particularly if things are at all abstract. They do not appear to catch on to the meaning of things and events.[9]

The characterization of the autistic syndrome as an inability to *give things meaning* explains why it is so difficult to teach someone like David appropriate table manners. It explains why you cannot talk to him about something as obvious, at first sight, as the length of a meal - something that, on further consideration, presupposes considerable skill in sharing symbolic messages. In practice this leads to adjustment problems. Every day the care workers discovered again that there was no point in giving David meaningful looks as he sat at the table or bombarding him with complex messages such as 'David, please wait a moment. It's not very sociable if you gobble all your pieces of bread down one after the other like that.' The term the care workers used here - *gezellig* - is a peculiarly Dutch concept with a huge emotional charge. It evokes a cosy, convivial atmosphere, with associations as broad as snugly-drawn curtains, flowers on the table, the whole family drinking coffee together, talking about the weather, and avoiding delicate subjects like the infamous black sheep of the family.[10] This assumes social recognition skills, consideration for the people around you, familiarity with the unwritten rules of the local community - the very things that people with autism lack.

One was unlikely to hear the staff suggest psychologically-informed explanations for autistic behaviour, however. When and if they did look for explanations it was at the level of the individual: David doesn't know what waiting is. Conversely, the lack of a common framework made it hard for the care workers to imagine themselves in the residents' position and see how they perceive life. When it came to interpreting the behaviour of someone like David, care workers were consequently left groping in the dark.

> The hardest thing is that [these boys are] so difficult to understand. Why does [someone] suddenly backslide?

Then you really want to talk to them but you can't get through to them. Everybody feels the same; you want to talk, to say, 'Please, just tell me what the matter is.' I think that's the most difficult thing. Their world is so different from ours that I can't empathize with it at all.

This, in broad terms, defines the gulf between the residents and the care workers. People with autism do not know what waiting is - they cannot really talk about the past, nor can they look forward to things that are going to happen.[11] People who are not autistic, on the other hand, see that the concept of time that they had regarded as obvious is in fact anything but self-evident. However, they are too attached to their own view of the world to be able to put themselves into this timeless state. One would be tempted to think that the atmosphere in that unit must have been really unsociable.

And yet, as I have said, time did not pass unnoticed in the everyday life of the group. If the daily routine is to proceed with any degree of order, expectations and behaviours have to be geared to those of other people *no matter what*. When care workers talk about the problems they encounter in practice, they are therefore much more concerned about the question of how *to solve* them. The difficulty here is not just the lack of social recognition; this problem is compounded by the fact that the usual methods of bringing up children, which are based very largely on a shared concept of language, do not work with autistic children. The trouble with speech is somewhat similar to the trouble with time: 'It cannot be seen or felt . . . it has no visible, tangible form and has gone as soon as the words have been uttered.'[12]

Anyone faced with the task of bringing the meal to a satisfactory conclusion, let alone anyone who tries to make the time that the group spends together companionably last for a little longer, cannot possibly get around this. As one of the care workers explained:

I found that the hardest thing at first - getting your message across clearly to the residents. Because you tend to make your sentences much too long. To them language is just a confusion of sounds; they understand little if any of a good deal of it. . . . So then you have to readjust.

*Concrete Connections*
David does not really understand ordinary language, so the care workers have to readjust. This is an important principle in looking after the autistic youngsters in the unit. But sometimes any word is one too many, and so other ways have to be found. Difficult as it is to put oneself in the position of someone like David, experience - sometimes years of it - teaches carers that there are means other than speech of making clear to him what 'waiting'

is. Something known as 'socialization technology' has a part to play here as a way of extending the time that residents spend together.[13] The kitchen timer is a good example of this sort of technique. It shows how the staff tried in a down-to-earth, non-linguistic manner to cope with the autistic deficit in questions of time. Specifically, David would have bolted all his slices of bread down much too fast, and agitated mealtimes would have been inevitable, had the timer not provided him with an anchor.

> I don't know exactly how this works, but you can solve [problems to do with waiting] by saying, 'when the timer rings, the time's up,' or 'when all the sand has run through the hourglass, the time's up.' So that you make the passage of time very concrete.

Linguistic concepts like 'wait a moment' were of no use when it came to organizing the progress and succession of activities at the unit. 'You might as well talk to the wall,' observed one of the care workers. So words were replaced with less ambiguous physical signals. Rather than overwhelm David with abstract information that presupposes reasonable skill in sharing symbolic meanings, the care worker set ten minutes on a timer.

> Well, the trick is that you have to... externalize might be too facile a way of expressing it, but it's almost a matter of taking the kind of connections that we make so easily in our brains and making them tangible or material.

The residents in this unit needed a lot of 'clarity,' according to the staff. If implicit connections are cast in concrete (visible, tangible) forms and hidden meanings are made as explicit as possible - by using charts and calendars, for instance - autistic people may, perhaps for the first time in their lives, perceive that things are not governed by chance. As we read in the introductory folder:

> The concept of structure is related to what we would like to call the essence of autism: not seeing the relations, the meaning, the sense of things. Structuring then refers to all activities that are meant to clarify those connections, for instance by making them simple and explicit, by making them visible using means which sometimes look ridiculously naive to us.[14]

The key to the successful translation of things that are obvious to most people - 'ordinary human life with everything that belongs to it' - into autistic terms appears to lie in generating explicit rules of behaviour that people with autism can learn by heart. The unit's approach was inspired by the TEACCH programme, about which its creator Gary Mesibov says:

> Our intervention techniques are designed to make social situations and expectations as clear as possible for our group members. We often generate social rules where they are not ordinarily specified, even if they are less than perfect. Autistic people need rules in situations where actions are guided by judgment and subtle cues from other people. Although concrete rules often do not work as well as good judgment, they are better and more adaptable for autistic people than having no rules at all.[15]

Sometimes, though, rules like these are still not enough, and other ways of providing something to hold on to have to be found. This is certainly essential in dealing with mentally-handicapped autists; the hidden structure has to be made even more obvious. In these cases staff often use pictures or objects to make things clearer. For instance, Rick, one of the residents, did not seem to have the smallest notion of what he was supposed to do with his day. From the moment he got up, he started to ask, in his own particular way, 'Still not bed time?' In his case a regular routine did not provide a sufficient anchor, so the care workers decided to empty a cupboard and put in it a wash cloth, a breakfast bowl and other things that would indicate in a more direct way than language what was coming next.

Often, however, the only way to teach a child social skills is to get him to *feel* or experience how something should be done. Youngsters with autism often lack facial animation; they seem to be wearing a totally expressionless mask. This leads other people to think that autists do not *have* any feelings and to turn away from them, which in turn means that these children do not get the social and emotional experiences they need to develop into fellow human beings. To break this vicious circle, carers can try to physically produce expression in the child's face. It may seem rather peculiar, wrote Wing, but 'a session in which the child's face is moulded into expressions while he watches a mirror can be helpful.'[16] He can be made to smile, for example, by pushing up the corners of his mouth as if they were made of clay. In this case the aim is to impress social recognition directly *on the body*.

> Some aspects of appropriate social behaviour can be taught, even though they are used in a mechanical way. Eye contact does tend to improve with increasing age but it can be encouraged. Provided this does not cause distress, the

child's head can be gently held to attract their visual
attention when talking to them. . . . Positive signs of
affection within the family can also be taught. Instead of
allowing the child to accept a hug and a kiss passively, their
own arms can be guided to return the hug.[17]

I saw this physical guidance in action when a new resident - a boy
who seemed barely aware of the strange faces surrounding him - came into
the unit. Whereas the others were 'at least a bit engaged with the people
around them,' in Martin's case this was 'very vague.'

Before I could get an idea of whether he would really start
to recognize people. . . . When you see the way he looks, I
thought that's really going to be tricky. Where do you start?
Go right up to him and say hello, hold his face and get him
to look at you for a moment, give him a little stroke, and
keep doing it all the time, when he's having his bath or
you're getting him ready for bed.

In David's case, direct intervention like this was not necessary and a
structured approach appeared to work well. Thanks in part to the fact that
there was a timer on the table and the staff confined themselves to providing
specific, timer-like structures, everyone knew what they had to do at any
given moment. As unachievable as it initially seemed to be, meals were eaten
in what the care workers called a 'congenial' atmosphere. For that, in the
final analysis, is what sharing a meal is all about. 'It is here that the exclusive
selfishness of eating is linked to a routine of coming together, with a habit of
encounter, that is only seldom achieved through higher, intellectual causes,'
wrote Simmel as early as 1910 in his classic work on the sociology of the
meal. 'People who do not have a single special interest in common can meet
one another at the shared meal.'[18]
    As a rule, mealtimes provide an opportunity to get together, but in
families with an autistic child this is often a touchy issue. 'Some of the
children will not eat with others but may eat if given meals on their own.
Some will take food left for them if they are allowed to eat while moving
around,' wrote Wing. She reflects on the dilemmas facing parents and carers
without losing sight of the benefits of 'encouraging more conventional eating
patterns' - such as waiting until everyone else has finished - so that a child
can also derive some pleasure from a meal involving the whole family.[19]
    But what if these youngsters do not see the *point* of sitting down
together to drink lemonade, to mention one of the simple social activities of
everyday life in the unit? These are activities which have their point in an
invisible social nature that will not instantly mobilize autistic people. How

can one make the reason clear, if the 'why' is so difficult to understand? Again, the answer seems to lie in a translation of intrinsic ends into a visible, more tangible goal to aim for. 'A conceptual, social why is replaced here by its observational equivalent: to see the final goal is sometimes enough.'[20]

Replacing a reason 'why' with a specific, visible goal appears, however, to be easier said than done, although it may very well be the other way round: our linguistic habits, our tendency to search for hidden meanings, may be precisely what often prevent us from *seeing how* to adjust. Perhaps we can get a glimpse of the difficulty ordinary language-users experience in doing this mirrored in Wittgenstein's observation that 'people who are constantly asking 'why' are like tourists who stand in front of a building reading Baedeker and are so busy reading the history of its construction, etc., that they are prevented from seeing the building.'[21]

Care workers, unlike tourists, are not transitory passers-by who try to compensate for a lack of meaningful experience by going into something in depth. Their experience - sometimes over many years - has taught them to consciously forget about the 'why' and recover or reinvent the evident form. It is precisely this that makes the kitchen timer such a discovery. The timer acted as a social prosthesis at the table, as a form of socialization technology that provided the residents with an anchor when they took part in the social life of the unit. The care workers were aware, however, of the local and temporary nature of the form of sociability that can be achieved at the table. 'The boys are very bound up in themselves,' one of them observed.

> In a mealtime situation they know that they're all together now. But then again, what's together? I actually do think they've realized 'I'm not alone now, it's not just me.' But when they leave the table each one goes to look for his own things again. They have to learn that the things here belong to everyone, not just them; learn to share things, I suppose.

This observation seems to confirm Hirschman's hypothesis that an apparently selfish activity like eating and drinking brings people together in a particularly enjoyable way - much more than the consumption of consumer goods.[22] This, says Hirschman, is because real consumables like food and drink make it possible to satisfy your appetite time and time again, without its becoming boring. A surfeit of consumer goods, in contrast, leads people to try to get more of what they already have (comfort), and hence to boredom and a 'joyless economy.' Hirschman also derives from Simmel the insight that the consumption of food does not simply satisfy private needs, it also has a *public* dimension: 'commensality' or in other words the extension of the community at table. In this way, perhaps, it may become sociable after all.

*Between Clocks and Jokes*

When we analyse the care workers' interpretations, we can infer that the boys they were looking after really needed structure. This does not mean, though, that life in the unit had to be pre-programmed from beginning to end - far from it, there was a great deal more than that to working with this group. Sometimes the staff made a point of *departing* from the customary patterns. There was, for example, the time when David liked his dinner so much that, by way of an exception, he was allowed a second helping. It is a good idea to compromise the structure a bit now and again, the care worker told me when I asked for an explanation. Structure is not an end in itself, I was assured, but an essential adjustment that can serve as a springboard for teaching social behaviour. 'I'm not trying to make them like us,' remarked one of the others. It was about teaching them skills 'so that life becomes easier for them, more fun, better.' As Lorna Wing wrote, 'when a child appreciates and is helped by a timetable, it can become a repetitive routine that must not be changed under any circumstances.'[23] By introducing controlled and planned changes into the regular daily programme, care workers can try to ensure that routines do not become set in stone.

But, as experience shows, the degrees of freedom staff can permit themselves in their dealings with these boys are still limited. 'This may well end in tears,' said Irene, the care worker, as she calculated the risk of her unexpected gesture in giving David a second helping for once. Care workers always have to distance themselves from the self-evident, accepted things of everyday life and, instead, confine themselves to simple, unambiguous actions. As one of them said about her bond with one of the residents: 'He knows where he is with me, as I do with him, and that makes for a degree of calm and the opportunity for more pleasant contact. I feel that acting consistently benefits the bond between us.'

Staff, in other words, see as it as their job to develop a reductionist attitude, a stable background the boys they look after can always fall back on. However, the perceived needs of the residents and the care workers do not always coincide. Abandoning familiar conventions proves very difficult to do. On the one hand, it is all too easy to think that 'just being strict' is the same as providing a formal structure. Take the situation when Rick was made to leave the table.

*Thursday 16 June, early shift*
Mark, one of the care workers, has cooked a hot meal. I think he has done a good job. And so, it seems, do most of the residents, but one of them, Rick, refuses to eat. It is not the first time this has happened. Rick has been so locked up in his compulsions of late that he cannot seem to find a way out of them. I watch as he kneels on the floor, licks the

ground incessantly, taps his neighbour on the shoulders and asks Mark if he may leave the table. Another member of staff, who is keeping an eye on the meal from the back of the room, calls out, 'Oh Rick! Mark went to a lot of trouble to cook a nice meal and now you don't want it! That's not very nice for Mark, is it?!' The remark does not seem to have any positive effect. Instead Rick's behaviour becomes ever more compulsive. In the end the staff see no option but to send Rick into the other room, if only so as not to spoil the meal for the others.

The fact that Rick was made to leave the table seems to point to a structured approach by the book. But the firm words used here, for example that it is 'not nice' to refuse a meal that someone has taken the trouble to cook, were no doubt as impenetrable to Rick as remarks about sociability were to David. The care worker seems to have relapsed into an old-fashioned strict or authoritarian approach, which - because he was calling upon a shared meaningful reality - was radically different from the kitchen timer approach.

On the other hand, there was an insidious temptation to interpret the residents' behaviour as if these were intentional acts, as if they were 'doing it on purpose.' It is remarkable how often the care workers were in danger of forgetting the difference between the residents and themselves and tended to treat their charges as competent members of the language community.

Even in people who work with autists you often come across ideas like 'He doesn't want this' or 'He's putting pressure on us.' Those are all assumptions I think we might very well make, and perhaps autistic people could have something of this kind too, but theirs will be radically different. We constantly attribute *our* concepts to people with autism; thinking that it will be the way *we* think it is.

Given the specific needs of the residents, patterns and routines in the unit were in some ways more conventional than one might expect. This is not really surprising - it is very hard for care workers to distance themselves from everything that they have always taken for granted because of their socialization as non-autists. It can be described as a real *achievement* when staff succeed in bridging the gulf that separates them from the residents, when they manage to reconcile the two forms of governing mutual relations that are at stake here - the regularity of the clock and the conventional order of the language community. This is an achievement by socialized people who, by constraining their actions in a timer-controlled straitjacket, have learned to deal with the relatively undersocialized in their midst.

We should not underestimate the effort that this demands of those concerned. As we can infer from the work of the sociologist of science and technology H.M. Collins, it takes blood, sweat and tears to learn to behave with mechanical regularity. It takes *creativity* to suppress meaningful human actions and put machine-like behaviour in their place, says Collins, and this very constraint could explain how it is possible for man and machine not to be totally alien to one another in their interactions[24] - a counter-intuitive conclusion that can shed new light on care workers' achievement in dealing with autistic residents (without wishing to brush aside the efforts that autistic people make in their dealings with non-autists).

> The staff who work in the unit are not 'rigid,' they are 'flexible' care workers adapting themselves to the rigidity, the 'other cognitive style' of people with autism. Helping people who suffer from a lack of imagination requires an awful lot of imagination.[25]

In other words it is evidently very difficult for people *not* to work on the assumption of shared meanings. One the care workers explained:

> You can't help dealing with them from your own background and the life of normal children. You try to see whether they like the things we like. Take Saint Nicholas' Eve [a Dutch family tradition], they have no idea what that's about. All the same, we have a party for them. And you should have seen David, his face lit up when he saw *Sinterklaas*! If you never try anything, it's such a dismal business.

Being as regular as a kitchen timer, applying rules, is not enough to do a good job in residential care for autistic people. There also has to be some scope for fun and warmth, as one care worker put it.[26]

> At first, I was horrified by the whole programme. So much structure, so many rules - it isn't workable. Everything had to be structured: fixed mealtimes, a separation between the dining room and the living area, and so on. It went so far that a resident would actually go in the shower exactly a quarter of an hour before her parents came, so that she would be finished and dressed at the precise moment they rang the doorbell. So empty and cold, it was too much for me. I thought, 'I won't be working here for long.' In the

end, it wasn't half as bad as I'd feared and there was some room for *gezelligheid.*

The effort care workers say it takes to rein themselves in also has an important moral dimension. Someone who adapts to the autistic need for fixed points to hang on to - by speaking only in very short sentences, for instance, or by not speaking at all but actually guiding the child physically - is quite often viewed with suspicion by outsiders.

> To outsiders who do not know about the real difficulties of autistic children, physical manipulations of this kind can look like robotic control, a mechanistic approach, a kind of animal training. Whereas it is in fact a direct adjustment to the difficulties of the child himself.[27]

The moral indignation is not confined to outsiders, however. If the residents' lives are made up solely of monotonous, repetitive routines, the staff themselves see this as lacking in human dignity.

> To my mind, that would be like something out of a science fiction comic: a robot in the kitchen who programs life on the other side. But I think, no, you're dealing with *people* here. I think that autistic people have feelings too, although it's different, I believe. But you do it for yourself, too, I think: you have to enjoy working here.

As 'humans,' in any event, the care workers found it difficult to cope with the restrictive demands that working with autists imposes. They built in scope for play as a matter of course. I saw the way they enjoyed chatting to the residents, larking around and laughing with them; teasing and jokes were also a normal part of everyday life in the unit. One day, for instance, Ellen, an experienced care worker, saw David sitting in school. She waved some packets of soup she had just bought and called out, 'Look, David, soup!' Ellen knew as well as David, who was highly fixated on soup, that he could not leave the classroom. Powerless, he responded by pointing and shouting 'ooh, ooh!' I asked Ellen why she did such a thing. She tried to explain her motives for teasing him like that. 'I don't know why I did it - because I wouldn't have got a reaction otherwise?' Sometimes the interactions between staff and residents do not actually differ that much from life outside the unit.

Theo Peeters believes we should not generalize when it comes to scope for play in autistic children. 'There are people with autism who can learn to appreciate certain forms of teasing,' he argues. And if it can be done, then why not? But, he adds, 'It is also for the carers, to keep themselves going, they really do need it.'[28] Teasing is something that binds people together, even when caring for people with autism. At least when carers get round to it. The Dutch publicist Lydia Rood, writing about her autistic brother in *The Book of Job*, says that teasing one another tends to be typically something that brothers and sisters do. 'Carers are simply too busy; getting an autist to behave in a socially acceptable manner is a full-time job. Carers provide emotional calm. Brothers and sisters tease.'[29] She tried, for example, to kid her brother Job that an outing had been called off. 'The greatest triumph was not if he believed us. The victory came if he started to laugh. Then Job was one of us. Making jokes means letting go of order.'[30]

Teasing and making jokes in interacting with autistic people runs counter to the dominant image of autism in the public media, in which the tragic nature of the condition, the vulnerability of the sufferers and the desperation of carers dominate. Stuart Murray remarks on this in relation to Haddon's *The Curious Incident*, which is very funny indeed. This is because of Christopher's 'oblique take on the world,' which is immediately evident from his warning that it will not be a funny book because he does not understand jokes. It is this counter-intuitive scope for humour that makes Christopher's story so human.

> For many, there is nothing funny about autism, but anyone
> who has an association with the condition knows this is not
> true, and to deny a relationship between autism and humour
> is to deny it a basic humanity.[31]

Nevertheless, as the staff made clear to me, there are risks involved in this sort of cosy approach towards people with autism. There is a very real danger in ignoring the differences between autistic and non-autistic people - one risks being uncaring, even hurting autistic people, precisely by treating them as fellow human beings. Such unintended indifference to the otherness of autistic people proceeds from its own unquestioned assumptions about universal human needs. These presuppositions about what humans really need are projected on to the other in his or her best interests. In the case of autism, however, naive humanism may end up being cruel.

A dilemma therefore resounds through all these real-life stories. As far as questions of time are concerned, someone like David would seem to be more at home in the silent, mechanical world of things than in the meaningful world of people-among-themselves. This places a heavy demand on the adaptability of the people around him, for while doubts may crop up in the everyday life of the community, the question as to whether these youngsters might be no more than automata simply does not arise. Care workers consequently have to navigate between fixed structures and an ideal conversational situation, between alarm clocks and jokes, between the assumed needs of the other and their own interpretation of what good care and a meaningful life are.[32] Faced with a choice between providing no anchor points at all and the alternative - a very paltry one from a non-autistic viewpoint - of a precise, clock-governed routine, the latter option is infinitely preferable. This is why, despite the limitations inherent in it, there was a timer on the table.

## Objects as Temporal Nodes

What makes social life tick in a unit for young autists? In answering this question, I have so far relied solely on the care workers' accounts. In some ways, we may infer from these stories, people with autism derive more from material objects than they do from people. In contrast to the care worker's life - where linguistic ordering comes first and the timer is no more than a useful aid in communicating temporal messages - objective structures often provide the only anchor points in the lives of autistic residents. My approach reveals, in short, that to really be involved with autistic young people one has to distance oneself from familiar presuppositions about what it means to be 'close to' another person. But how much distance is enough? Does the vocabulary I have used thus far allow us to detach ourselves sufficiently from the self-evident perspective of a non-autistic existence?

### Creating Distance

It seems inevitable that things which are taken for granted in non-autistic life will colour our understanding of the communal life of the unit, but to prevent these assumptions from being accepted as the only possible yardstick, it is crucial to distance oneself from familiar, non-autistic contexts - not just in practice but at the conceptual level, too. Of course it is precisely by depending on a familiar, interpretative background that deviations from the norm are made visible in the first place. But the same perspective also takes sides in what it is supposed to study: the interpretative vocabulary is biased in favour of the linguistic and the meaningful, and thus remains close to the terms in which only *some* of those involved in the social life of the unit - the care workers - understand the unfolding of events in the group.[33] We must create more distance between ourselves and their interpretations. We can nonetheless best address this by going back to their *practice* once more.

We have seen how the care workers used their own interpretations as the starting point but ran into difficulties with residents, for example during meals. In practice, therefore, concessions were made, for instance by putting a kitchen timer on the table. But as soon as the care workers started to *reflect* on their work, they put things into linguistic contexts - for instance, by pointing out that they found it difficult to structure the life of the unit in line with the model of material objects, or justifying their approach by saying that the timer was just a means to a higher ideal. What I want to do now is pick up the thread at the point where the care workers ran up against their conceptual boundaries. At the point where they put the timer on the table but couched their action in familiar terms, it becomes interesting for me to go *further*. In doing this I shall enlarge and exaggerate the practical situation in which things play a central role, at the same time as abandoning the linguistic frameworks with which things are usually surrounded.[34]

In concrete terms this amounts to a description of processes of temporal ordering in the unit in a way that does not focus on the stories or the intentions of the care workers, but puts material objects at the beginning of analyses, rather than as a coda. I conceive of things not as passive means in the care workers' hands, but as narrative nodes around which other elements - care workers, residents, words, gestures, organizations, objects, bodies - are temporally centred. Temporal order, then, is no longer seen as an elusive concept grounded in the linguistic community, but as a result of a (partly) material practice of ordering.[35]

This approach is not validated by asking if members of the community being studied recognize themselves in this analysis, although this is not excluded either. I shall ignore the epistemological status of the claims of the care workers and others who speak on behalf of the residents (as a more or less faithful representation of the autistic other) and take their claims literally instead. I shall magnify the material dimension of what they say and use that as an analytical framework in which to describe social interactions in the unit again.[36] This may allow us to learn something about how temporal matters are handled in this unit for autistic youngsters, and the role played in this by people and things, without automatically taking a non-autistic perspective. Readers may be surprised by what could be seen as an *exaggeration* of their 'own' (non-autistic) interpretations of an 'autistic perspective.'

Just as Bernlef carried his readers, in the comedian's wake, to the stage where the props were in charge, so I want to transport my readers to other characters, places and times. For there are so many places in the world besides the head of a care worker.[37] As far as the facility for young autists is concerned, we shall start on the ground floor.

### Downstairs, Midday

Spatial characteristics provide a constant, stable background for temporal order in the everyday life of the unit. For instance, during the day all activities (mealtimes, recreation, drinking lemonade) are centred on the ground floor. The youngsters only ever go upstairs to shower or go to bed - in other words they are only there first thing in the morning and at night. A gate has been installed at the foot of the stairs, so that they can be closed off to stop residents who do not comply with the spatial separation of day and night from going up. When we enter the unit for our first brief reconnoitre, we ignore the closed gate to the stairs on our left and walk straight ahead into the living room: it is getting on for noon.

Downstairs in the sitting room we find some apparently insignificant objects that have a considerable impact on everyday life in the facility. The sofa, for instance, plays a crucial role in the way David's day is organized. It looks like a comfortable place to lie. Better than the table, for instance, because of its shape and upholstery. What's more, the care workers are happy for the sofa to be used for this purpose. David can often be found lying on the sofa. When he gets home from school, for instance, before the residents have their drinks, and during the summer holidays, when there is no school. The staff describe him as 'a specialist in lying down.'

> *Wednesday 20th July, early shift*
> 'I bet they're starting to get bored,' says one of the staff members after glancing around the unit during a short visit. It is a sweltering day. Outside in the garden Robert is on the swing. David has installed himself on the sofa. He lies half on his side, with his head resting on one elbow and his left leg pulled up along the back of the sofa while the right sticks out under the arm rest. He is still wearing his shoes. From this position he looks around now and then, watching what is happening in the garden and elsewhere within his field of vision. But most of the time he just looks straight ahead and lies there. 'Well, as long as David can lie down, he's happy enough,' responds Irene, the care worker, through the half-open door of the kitchen, where she is preparing a meal.

Here time takes shape. Not an abstract concept of time concealed in the visitor's head and projected on to David's behaviour, nor an intrinsic quality of events as they unfold themselves on the sofa, but a temporal effect of interactions that develop around the sofa and involve a wide range of elements - among them David lying there, the summer holidays, the warm weather, Robert swinging in the garden, the care worker in the kitchen and the visitor's look and comment. For a moment these few elements constitute the loosely-knit fabric in which a specific plot can be read[38] - a brief history which describes the phenomenon of boredom as an empirically observable practice.

Some of the information reaches us through the visitor's words, but these same words threaten to obscure other, non-linguistic parts of the phenomenon we are studying: actors that do not reside in the care worker's head or the linguistic community, and are in danger of being underestimated because of their silent, non-symbolic nature. However, it is precisely these 'minor' details and the unobtrusive part they play that are of interest to us in exploring the micro-physics of temporal actions. Together these elements form a small, mundane and local network, in which, loosely at first, a coherent order of time is bred; a network from which the product only *seems* to be able to detach itself easily once it has been given a name. 'Boredom' is the linguistic outcome of the specific way temporal order is constructed here.

It is probably no coincidence that it is a relative outsider who finds himself translating the shared performance of David and the sofa in terms of its possible meaning - 'boredom.' The visitor, after all, is not as informed about the physical structure of the facility and its characteristic, tangible logic. The joint venture of David-and-the-sofa has a completely different effect on those who are more familiar with everyday life in the unit. The sofa - conceived as a node in the organization of the shared form of life in the facility - having first cast David in his role of a specialist in lying, now allows care workers to spend their time elsewhere in the unit - in the kitchen, for instance - without having to worry about David, because he is lying on the sofa. And so we see how a slightly different configuration may result in a radically different form of time; an effect that translates into a certain praxis rather than interpretations or words.

How, finally, does the sofa impact on the life of David himself? For although it was never put there to play this part, David and the sofa take total possession of one another. The result, unarguably, is that David lies down. But perhaps it also means that he is left in peace. The sofa that previously stage-managed the care workers' consent by providing them with an opportunity to use their (precious) time for other things forges a link that is stable enough to affect life in other places as well. The whole constellation allows David to be on his own for a while. But that, too, is just imposing a familiar meaning on the act of lying on a sofa. In practice one just has to learn to live with the fact that David spends all his time lying down.

> There are some things you can get... like David. The lad lies there all the time, and you take that into account - that's just how David is. But there are some things you simply cannot understand - why do they do these things? That's what makes them autistic.

Lying down is David's specialty; it is also a specific example of what Murray calls 'autistic presence' - a form of autistic subjectivity that cannot be defined further and resists any attempt to reduce it to familiar categories of meaning. Lying down belongs to David. And maybe there is not much more to be said.

*Upstairs, Evening*

Although autistic residents have difficulty understanding symbolic concepts of time, and care workers are often groping in the dark when it comes to understanding what drives the residents, time does not pass by unnoticed in the everyday life of the unit. Temporal regularities can develop around seemingly insignificant objects like a sofa. If such a material node succeeds in creating sufficiently strong links between enough other elements circulating in the facility, fragile temporal structures that enable residents and care workers to share daily life may hold for a while. This is how time is realized in concrete terms in the unit - which sounds more tranquil than it is. Let us go upstairs to highlight another phenomenon which may be observed in everyday life in the unit: the occurrence of clashes in time.

*Friday 19th August, late shift*
On his way to the bathroom Robert comes to a sudden halt right in front of the bathroom door. He places his feet with great precision along an imaginary line on the floor. With one foot he lifts a corner of the bathmat lying there. He almost goes into the bathroom, but comes straight out again. This is repeated several times. Meanwhile he looks over his shoulder with a strange tension in his body. Arms tightly folded across his chest, he swings his upper body from time to time, as if he is hugging himself in glee. Then he pushes the open door of the bathroom firmly against the doorpost around the corner. Seeing how it fits? Again. His feet again, the bathmat again. At long last he enters the bathroom.

A small bathmat and the particular geometric characteristics of the doorposts in the corner between the bathroom and one of the bedrooms rejoice in Robert's attention. Conversely, we might say that the bathroom setting prepossesses Robert in its favour by inviting him to develop a special fascination with its localized material logic. Robert 'has a weakness' for angles, straight lines, the resistance of materials and tense physical movements. This thraldom should not be seen as a quality intrinsic to Robert, nor to autistic people in general, but rather as a propensity that is generated in part by the local circumstances in which he finds himself. An unusual proclivity perhaps, but not as long as it is confined to the limited situation I have just outlined.

The rituals performed in the privacy of the bathroom figure in a very different plot when care workers arrive on the scene. Given the institutional context in which they are anchored - a context in which school hours, the end of the shift and the need for everyone to have breakfast at the same time play an important role - the fascination with the possibilities of the bathroom that they develop is very different from Robert's. In the temporal logic of institutionalized life, a visit to the bathroom had better not take hours. And so these opaque acts taking place in the bathroom doorway translate into what care workers call 'Robert's constant dawdling.'

A situation like this, in which different fascinations are linked with diverging temporal orders, often occurs in practice - sometimes as a form of peaceful coexistence. In other circumstances, however, a case of this kind can easily lead to conflicts. This is particularly true of situations in which care workers and residents move around in a space where shared temporal coordinates (carried by objects, words, sounds, gestures, etc.) are missing, but they still have to manage things together. Institutional frameworks often settle the matter in the event of conflicts, but this is not always the case.[39] For instance, care workers might also have felt compelled to go along with the state of affairs created by the combined forces of the doorpost, the bathmat and Robert. After the former (bathmat and doorpost) had succeeded in engaging the latter in their specific material logic, it proved very difficult to escape the course of time organized by these often underrated, non-linguistic constituents of the social life of the unit.

The specific form that temporal order assumes when care workers are enmeshed in this network is called - in their own vocabulary - 'waiting.' Waiting patiently until Robert's temporal routine is - temporarily - broken when he finally enters the bathroom. A forced exercise in 'patience' which may eventually make care workers 'hurry' - whether they want to or not.

*Downstairs, Afternoon*
Like Robert in the bathroom, David was completely enthralled by the material logic of the furniture in the dining room.

*Friday 8th July, late shift*
David comes in while I am clearing the table. He picks up a chair and places it diagonally so that he can get to the legs easily. He wipes the bottom of one leg with his hand. He examines his hand and removes the dirt he has wiped off. He then wipes the dust off the other legs. He puts the chair down with a bang, repeats this several times, and pushes the chair to within about six inches of the edge of the table. He seems to want to position the chair as accurately as possible. He shifts it to and fro by a few millimetres until it is, as far as he is concerned, in exactly the right place. Then he holds his hand close to it for a moment, as if he is measuring the chair or maintaining its balance. I can tell from his body language that he is getting ready to leave.

But before he does, he comes back to the chair, picks it up
again, slides it back and forth and holds it in its place again.
Then he runs out.

David's behaviour testified to a fascination with flat surfaces, an
absence of crumbs and dust, and precise positioning. An unusual fascination,
perhaps, but not so strange that the care workers did not recognize it as
something they might share.

Sometimes we make a joke of it - if you work with autistic
people long enough you start to get like them. But I think
that there's something like it in everyone. For instance, I
have to have everything in the cupboard - mugs and so on -
in line. And Robert's plate has to be on top because it's
smaller than the others. It's just compulsive.

One of the care workers remembered how at first he 'was very
happy they had a structure like this, so that you knew what you had to do,
could do, and was allowed to do.' Even so, the care workers sometimes tried
to keep David from performing his ritual around the chair at the table. In the
specific context of institutionalized care for autistic people - a network in
which the organizational activities centre on specialist expertise on autism
rather than the furniture, the residents or the care workers who have learned
to live with these 'tics' - it seemed only reasonable to break the pattern of
David's 'rigid behaviour' from time to time.[40]

Because if you don't, you get autists who have serious
difficulty with the very structures they've invented, or with
the care workers whom they compel to go along with them
in a structure from which there's no way out. This is why
we think it's important to teach them that things may
happen differently every now and then.

There is not much scope for having fun in the configuration we now
see emerging. In this set-up David is cast as the 'classic' autist. In his role as
a patient he appears as someone with no sense of time, which explains why
he escapes into what can then be defined as 'compulsive' and 'stereotypical'
behaviour. From now on, David's fascination is presented as marginal or
pathological. Care workers, on the other hand, are cast in the opposite role in
this scenario, as competent members of the interpretative community. For
them, the heterogeneous performance of the chair, David and the dining table
translates into what only *they* are deemed to recognize as a (meaningful) *sign*
of David's actual condition: his lack of temporal understanding. It is this

condition that may have led him to seek refuge in a reiterative form of time, in 'endless repetition' - a pattern in which he seems to be completely locked up, as only the care workers can see.

> Yes, they do the same things almost every day. Roughly the same movements, and so on. You don't often come across this in other units. I think that if you were to observe them for a week and write down exactly where a resident goes, what he does - while the things he uses may very well differ, I think you'd find that he would do the same basic things every day in exactly the same way.

The care workers themselves were thus saying that they had good reasons that justified their therapeutic interventions in David's routine. In practice, however, they were often just as *gripped* by their urge to break the patterns of repetitive behaviour that developed around various material nodes as residents like David or Robert were fascinated by doing them.

> Like Robert with that footprint there - a bare patch in the lawn - he always has to step on that spot when he passes it. Only if you say, 'keep going, and don't stand on it!' he won't. But I think that if you gave him half a chance he'd go back and do it anyway.

*Downstairs, Morning*
To achieve unity in the social passage of time it may be necessary to translate diverging, clashing fascinations into a single coordinated action - something that is not always easy in daily life in a residential unit for young people with autistic spectrum disorder. Sometimes, however, it may be possible to cast an actor in the role of *mediator* between care workers and young autists and thus reconcile their apparently incompatible interests. This responsible task may be delegated to a person, but it can also be assigned to a non-human actor. Sometimes it may actually be better to involve an object, especially when words are not up to the job. For instance, a small device, the kitchen timer, succeeded in aligning all the clashing elements at the breakfast table and in joining their unruly forces for a moment of shared existence. The timer regulated the pace at which David ate, thus providing a satisfactory response to the care worker's fascination with orchestrating participation in the meal by all the residents. At the same time it established boundaries to what 'waiting' is and what is 'enough,' so that David could also be cast in his compliant role.

The timer had become a central actor in the organization of meals - a piece of socialization technology around which other actors, care workers and residents, could be temporally gathered. The translation that delivered this outcome involved transforming the colliding interests and diverging roles into the harmonious participation in the meal by everyone. This change, however, could only be achieved by making the newly-cast actors believe or experience the notion that, although they were *all* playing new roles (thus feeding one other's fascinations), they would still be able to indulge their own compulsion as they had before - if not even better. The successful translation made it seem as if nothing had changed at all apart from the resident's compliance with the new rule. The inconspicuous object that successfully mediated between different and competing positions was retrospectively transformed into an *intermediary* and regarded as a passive *means* in the hands of the successful care worker.[41]

Responsibility for success or failure, however, is not as easily attributed to the constituent elements of the network as an account like this, with hindsight, would have us believe. What this account overlooks is the fact that for temporal structures to be achieved all the entities that go to make up the timer routine have to have cooperated, in one way or another, in conducting mealtimes in a new way. Without seamless cooperation between the care worker who had to set the timer, the device itself and the resident who reacted to it, the whole mealtime would have come to grief. The strength of the links between all the constituent parts was continuously tested, for instance when care workers deliberately 'forgot' to set the timer. As a rule David would protest and urge the care worker to use the clock. Sociality is a locally produced effect; shared temporal routines will not last a minute longer than the fragile networks from which they are built. But the link between David and the timer routine usually proved strong enough to get the care worker back in line.

The care workers were important drivers of social integration at the table, but certainly not the only ones. Irene liked the educational aspect of working with this group. When a new resident arrived, she soon saw the results of the staff's efforts to teach him to eat with a fork. 'When you see that Martin is using a fork himself after just three weeks, I think that merits a little round of applause for us.' But didn't the fork itself deserve a round of applause too? The cutlery played a mediating role, to some extent unconnected with the care workers' intentions. The regulation of eating behaviour by cutlery casts the selfish act of eating into a social form, says Simmel.

> Eating with the fingers . . . creates a direct link between the individual and the food, and is accordingly an expression of unbridled desire. In so far as cutlery enforces some distance between the individual and this desire, eating is cast in a communal form, promoting the coming together of several

people, which does not exist when people eat with their fingers.[42]

Control during the meal appeared to be distributed around the table and could not easily be attributed to a single responsible actor. This was reinforced because the new configuration of temporal order in the unit left none of its constituent elements untouched. As soon as the kitchen timer was introduced into this new, unusual context, it interacted with its setting and started to reconfigure it. Almost nothing remained *unaffected* as the care workers and residents began to gear their mealtimes to the clock, to learn to pass it over, reach out for it, sometimes ignore it, and react to its signal. The temporal order that unfolded in this interaction between staff, residents and object had its own irreducible logic. And so it came about that one morning, Mark, one of the care workers, found that he missed the timer. He had become so used to its physical presence that, like it or not, he was really quite put out after David moved to another unit and the timer went with him.

> I missed the wretched thing! I really missed that timer! I sat there the first morning, and what I always used to do was butter the bread for Jason as soon as the timer went off for David. And my first thought was: when do I have to butter Jason's bread? This was at breakfast. It was so weird. I thought, that damn timer!

**More than Convention**

Efforts have to be made on both sides in dealings between people with autism and those without. Instead of just asking autistic people to adjust, society must also provide scope for an autistic way of life. The unit for mentally handicapped young autists is wholly geared to the residents' needs. One cannot, however, expect people who have been raised in the ordinary social world to relinquish their certainties at a stroke. It is therefore not surprising that an assessment of the question as to how to provide temporal anchor points moves between two familiar poles: while a strictly clock-based organization of life may not be ideal, because as a rule it is downright limiting, it is always preferable to the only conceivable alternative, which is to force autistic people to live without any structure, thus ruling out any possibility of their participating in the world of people-among-themselves.

It may be that an approach to autistic people based on things, as a poor alternative to socialization among other people, really is the best that can be done. When care workers share their experiences with us, we have to acknowledge that in some respects non-human actors such as kitchen timers have more to offer people with autism than (other) people do - predictable behaviour and absolute regularity. These are traits associated with material objects that care workers can attempt to simulate - counter-intuitively and only with great difficulty - in order to involve the residents in social life. The framework that is constructed in the care workers' accounts thus provides both a benchmark for action and an argument with which to refute outsiders' criticisms and allay their own qualms about the moral propriety of the methods used in the unit. There is a clear moral dimension behind a socialization model that is grafted on to physical manipulation, routines and material structures.

Nevertheless, the care workers' frame of reference also proved to have shortcomings. Within this framework, for instance, it was difficult to escape a tendency to conceive of the specific way that care workers, kitchen timers and residents related to one another in general and familiar terms - for example by ascribing events as they developed in the unit entirely to the care worker's intentions, efforts or mistakes. Conversely, the residents' active part in the process of temporal ordering and the transformative power of other non-linguistic elements of life in the unit were underestimated. These latter, as we have seen, were regarded solely as a means of overcoming the indeterminate nature of symbols of time in a world without the shared social codes of the former. It consequently proved all too easy for temporal ordering in the unit to be seen as a *planned and limited derivative* of the way that, generally speaking, people gear their expectations and behaviour to those of everyone else.

How does one write about the shared history of care workers, timers and young autists without getting oneself bogged down again in a familiar, non-autistic perspective? When care workers and others had their say, we heard the view that in caring for young people with autism it is essential to distance oneself from what would normally be regarded as involvement. In spite of the limitations attached to it, I have examined the consequences of this conclusion in the last part of my argument. Ideas about what is important in the lives of people with autism were exaggerated and expanded into a framework for writing about life in the unit.[43]

This has shed light on events in the unit and made them more understandable. There are no longer any holes in the social fabric that have to be patched with social conventions. By using things as a *way in* rather than as a passive means in care workers' hands, we can demonstrate how temporal order is in part an effect of actions and trials of strength in a heterogeneous ensemble. Instead of seeing time as a ready-made concept that lodges in the mind of the care worker or language community, boredom, waiting, impatience, abstract concepts of time, communal mealtimes and so on are all described as the local, usually unintended and specific results of network building.

It is not only trivial objects like a kitchen timer that bring about temporal logic - the materiality of the furniture, its position in the living room, the layout of the house and so forth are at the same time dependent on and constitutive of the temporal context. Where the organization of time is concerned, they also weigh in the balance despite their inability to share a language with the people who are *said* to be in charge in the community. As Bruno Latour remarked, 'there are a lot more ways of delegating actions than by speaking. And an ideal community is by no means necessarily a language community.'[44] Authority in questions of time is distributed throughout the practice of running the unit. The construction of a temporal order moreover leaves none of its constituent elements untouched: all the capabilities and roles - including those of the care workers - are redefined on the way.

No one remains unaffected by what happens in the everyday life of the unit - immediately, noticeably, tangibly. (Any more than the autistic residents remain unaffected by what happens - symbolically, meaningfully - in normal human relations).

This relocates the social deficit; the lack is no longer solely in the head of the autist, but must at least also be attributed to the context in which the individual finds himself. The same applies to the quarter from which one can expect solutions to the blocking of the interactions between them. The specific, in part non-linguistic way that temporal order is brought about in this praxis can be seen as an extraordinary achievement on the part of the care workers, but also as a feat by the autistic residents and the things that surround them. Despite the shortage of skills on which one normally relies to give shape to mutual relationships, social life does not grind to a halt. Describing the way care workers, kitchen timers and autistic youngsters succeed in attuning their behaviours and expectations to one another therefore takes more than 'socialization' in a 'conventional order.'

A description of this kind can never be all-encompassing. The possibilities of *talking* about the agency of the non-linguistic entities are, by definition, limited. Nevertheless, actor-network theoreticians Michel Callon and John Law argue that this is precisely what the situation sometimes demands of us:

> Though we cannot, to be sure, *say* very much about it, we do not wish to link a notion of agency to linguistic representation. For signification - or so we have suggested - is more general than talk. It comes in all kinds of forms. And some, though only some, we can imagine. Others, no doubt, we will never know. . . .
>
> To imagine that we can assimilate the Other in any of its forms is hubris. Instead, it seems to me that these Others will ignore us for most of the time. Instead, they

will continue, as they always have, to perform their specific forms of agency to one another. And all that we can do is to say that these performances go on. And then to create appropriately monstrous ways of representing them on those rare occasions when our paths happen to cross and we find, for a moment, that we need to interact with them.[45]

Our paths crossed long ago. And there will always be 'something' that will escape the non-autistic conception of a shared existence with the autistic other.

> *While the others are leaving the table, David places his chair with neat precision along a seam in the carpet. Then he leaves, too.*

# With Lacelike Precision
## The Communication Deficit and Autobiographical Works by Autistic People

> Language sets everyone the same traps;
> it is an immense network of well kept wrong turnings.[1]

'This is Christian. He can see, hear, feel, touch but he cannot speak. He was born with autistic tendencies that cut him off from the world around him.'[2] So runs the advertisement for a new type of monitor produced by electronics giant NEC (see figure 1). 'Until he found this window,' writes NEC, Christian Murphy 'lived with a wall between himself and the world.' This wall is symbolized by a deserted forest path hemmed in by tall trees on both sides. The photograph has been cropped into the shape of an egg. Christian himself seems to emerge from the egg. Thought bubbles escape from the isolation of his world - a golden retriever, a paw print, biscuits and a dog's bowl. They show us what is going on in Christian's head and lead our gaze to the 'window' that makes the suggested insight possible: the monitor on which we read in clear, bold letters, 'This is my puppy Harvey.'

One of Christian's teachers, explains the advertisement, discovered that the eleven-year-old reacted well to pictures, so she created a special keyboard visualizing the story of Christian's new puppy. The mediation of this medium, which made it possible to convert mental images into readable text, gave Christian a means of expressing himself - 'the monitor became his voice.' At the same time, the discovery allowed onlookers insight into Christian's autistic experience.

> With the pictures, he made sentences. With the sentences, he made friends. Christian's monitor is the window between his non-verbal world and the speaking world of his friends. Through it, he teaches them many things.[3]

In the last picture we see Christian standing in the playground surrounded by his friends. From the pictures, by way of language, to a full and accepted member of the playground community - thanks to NEC, goes the message, a channel of communication has been opened up between Christian and the world around him.

This advertisement encapsulates a number of ideas that are typical of discussions about the autistic deficit in the ability to communicate and how to deal with it - the final aspect of the shared existence that I shall consider.[4]

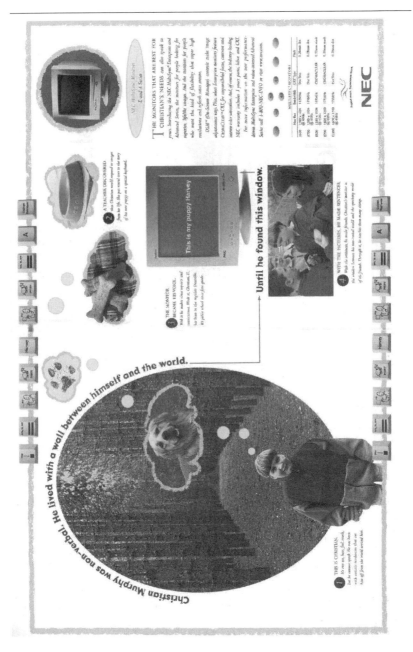

*Figure 1.* Christian Murphy. NEC Advertisement. *WIRED*, July 1997.

To start with, the advertisement expresses feelings of human solidarity and appeals to deeply-rooted ideas about what binds people to one another: it is a striking illustration of the crucial importance that we attach to *reciprocal communication*. In the second place, the advertisement taps into a specific preconception of what lies at the basis of the binding power of language and other means of communication. The words create a *window* between ourselves and the other person - between the verbal, non-autistic world of a group of friends and the mute, closed in on itself world of the autist. Language is a medium for meaningful communication by means of which messages can be exchanged 'about' ourselves and the world to which language 'refers.' If all is well, the words appear *transparent*, so that the person who is inside can 'bring out' what he feels, and the person who is outside can gain 'insight' into what is going on in the other.[5]

It is not only in the advertisement that the primacy of the communicative community and the window metaphor are the leitmotiv; the desire of autistic people to be involved in the community lies behind every effect to develop alternative means of communication for the non-communicative majority. A concept of language that elaborates on the window metaphor moreover underlies the way autists who do have language skills are usually understood. There is a small minority of communicatively able autists who are sometimes regarded as *interpreters* for the inward-turned majority who can express themselves barely if at all. These are often small openings, but fully-fledged autobiographical works have also been published in recent years.[6]

As 'bilingual' individuals, autistic speakers and writers would appear to be perfectly equipped to introduce us to an extraordinary autistic perspective on all sorts of things. What do they have to tell the reader? What can we deduce from their work about the structure of a shared life? What role does this entail for *verbal* players amidst all the silent, material elements that we have so far encountered? At the same time, autobiographical works by people with autism raise pressing questions about the role of the reader. What must readers watch out for as they read so that they really do hear the autistic voice? How does one prevent a non-autistic interpretation from gaining the upper hand after all?

**Listening to the Autistic Voice**

On the lookout for hidden ways by which autists and non-autists sometimes succeed in bridging the gulf between them, it makes sense to listen to what people with autism themselves have to say about it. This search consequently takes a contrary direction. Interactions through communication between people with and without autism are, after all, anything but a matter of course. Even if around half of the autistic population is verbal in one way or another, many of them use language in a way that is not, to our mind, communicative. Jerry, for instance, whom Kanner described as a child, did learn to talk, but without there apparently being any question of meaningful communication.

> At age three he suddenly began talking profusely but did not use speech for communication. His mother attempted to encourage conversation by reading 'alphabet' and 'number' books to him and pointing out letters on street signs, newspapers, etc. Jerry gradually learned the alphabet and a number of words that he would repeat over and over again, but not for communication with others. He also memorized an amazing number of song lyrics, although he did not seem to understand the meaning of the words.[7]

Kanner initially devoted a great deal of time and attention to this sort of verbal behaviour in his autistic patients, particularly their tendency towards echolalia, the 'bald' and literal repetition of what other people say. On the basis of his original study, as we saw earlier, Kanner observed that even in those children who did speak, language did not function as a means of conveying a message to other people. The words, numbers and rhymes they were able to reproduce, he said, 'could hardly have more meaning than sets of nonsense syllables to adults.'[8] Reviewing his findings, Kanner came to the conclusion that as far as the communicative function of language was concerned, there was 'no fundamental difference' between the children who did speak and those who did not.

Kanner subsequently qualified this position by acknowledging the existence of private references in autistic linguistic usage. While autists may have problems with the symbolic referential function of language, the echolalic use of language often actually does have meaning. Usually, though, this can only be recognized by someone who has shared with the child experiences to which the utterance is linked. 'Lack of access to the source shuts out any comprehension, and the baffled listener, to whom the remark means nothing, may too readily assume that it has no meaning at all.'[9] Paul's habit of saying 'Don't throw the dog off the balcony,' for example, proved to be associated with situations that were *like* the circumstances in which he had once heard this said (when he threw a toy dog out of a hotel window). Every time he had an urge to throw something, he used the phrase to call himself to order.

Self-directive language is one of the more functional forms of echolalia that Schuler and Prizant identify.[10] The echolalic behaviours that the authors describe cover a continuum which runs from directionless and completely automatic repetition on the one hand to intentional, meaningful utterances on the other. These communicational and cognitive dimensions reveal that echolalia is not a useless and meaningless activity that can simply be dismissed as 'parroting.' But despite their re-evaluation of what, for many autists, is the highest that can be attained in terms of language, the gulf between this and the flexible and creative language skills of non-autists is unbridgeable - too wide at any rate to explain the appearance of complete autobiographical works by autistic authors.

It would seem to be an internal contradiction - the idea that an autist could write an autobiography. The communication disorder is a key part of the syndrome.[11] Autistic people seem to lack the skills and motives to achieve shared understanding with others. Above all, the social function of language is disrupted. To learn to use language as such, one must have an idea of the *purpose* of communication, and this is something that is usually absent in people with autism. As Clara Park explained about her daughter Elly:

> If it's all one to you whether mama comes or not, you aren't likely to call her. If you don't want teddy enough to reach out for him with your own hand, you will hardly ask for him with a word. But even when she did begin to acknowledge desires - she was reaching two and a half - she did not communicate them by speech. She had other methods. If the object was near, she would take your hand and use it as a tool . . . Language, for Elly, was so non-functional that I often felt that what was inexplicable was not why she didn't have more words but why she had as many as she did . . . Each of Elly's words started in the public domain. Yet it was as if as soon as she acquired it, it became her own and nobody else's. Words are channels of communication, but Elly's words were things-in-themselves that led to nowhere and nobody.[12]

Over and above this, autists are not considered cognitively capable of reflecting their own or others' states of mind because they are said to lack the theory of mind this requires. In the case of autism, introspection and retrospection definitely seem to be much too big a stretch. Individuals who do appear capable of this can probably not be described as autistic.

This lands us in the middle of a debate about the question as to whether the 'classical' autism first described by Kanner does or does not differ essentially from Asperger's syndrome.[13] Wing places people of the Asperger's type together with cognitively high-functioning autists at the milder end of the autistic spectrum. People with Asperger's can be identified by, among other things, good grammatical and intellectual skills. Obviously, as Wing acknowledges, there is great diversity within the spectrum, and language skills make a lot of difference. Making a distinction can therefore also be useful, asserts Wing, to indicate the range of behaviours in which the underlying disorder may be expressed. But she maintains that in essence it is the same fundamental disorder in everyone on the spectrum that blocks their participation in reciprocal social interactions.[14]

Sacks's view of the mutual relationships between different forms of expression is a natural extension of this idea.

> The ultimate difference, perhaps, is this: people with Asperger's syndrome can tell us of their experiences, their inner feelings and states, whereas those with classical autism cannot. With classical autism, there is no window, and we can only infer. With Asperger's syndrome there is self-consciousness and at least some power to introspect and report.[15]

In recent years, their supposed access to a world behind the silence has meant that autistic people with good communications skills have enjoyed considerable sympathetic interest from the public and professionals alike. This fits well in the focus on including the patient perspective, those suffering from chronic conditions and people with a functional impairment as a critical supplement to a medical perspective. In disability studies in particular, every effort is being made to engage the active input of people with a disability in the research *about* their disability and what it means to be living with it.[16] At the same time it has to be acknowledged that this is not evident in the case of cognitive handicaps. Traditional research that asks for the viewpoint or the perception of the person involved assumes a cognitively and verbally able subject, and this means that the inclination to silence - found, for example, in non-speaking psychogeriatric patients - is ruled out in advance.[17]

Great excitement consequently greeted the appearance of the first autobiographical writings by people with autism, which seemed to demonstrate that language really could act as a shared window. In view of the way the speakers in question present themselves, this would appear to be incontrovertible. It is sometimes expressed quite literally: 'as an autist I serve other autists as their proper spokesman,'[18] wrote Birger Sellin in *I Don't Want to Be Inside Me Anymore: Messages from an Autistic Mind.* Who are we, mindful of the disability studies maxim 'nothing about us without us,' to cast doubt on such a cry from the heart issuing from what Sellin calls the 'autistic dungeon'?[19]

Kees Momma, with his Dutch work *En toen verscheen een regenboog; hoe ik mijn autistische leven ervaar* [And Then There Was a Rainbow; How I Experience My Autistic Life], also seems to offer an unusual, autistic perspective on a shared existence. Let us turn to what he has to tell us.

## A Look Through the Window

At the end of his autobiography, Kees Momma (whom we briefly encountered in chapter 4) looks back on the series of events he recorded in the story of his life. To go by the subtitle and the usual way of reading, we can regard Momma's book as a 'report' of his experiences as an autist. It is the account of Momma's desire for a 'flawless' order and of the way this order was repeatedly violated.

> The deep background of all the incidents summed up can be explained as follows. I do not want to be overwhelmed by the pain. I must mount a counter-attack. Pain and sudden noise cause a sensation as if an attack is being committed on my perfectionistically appointed realm of thought. Things that are precious to me, such as drawings and model aeroplanes, are stored in this realm. Deep in my brain they keep me constantly occupied and as a result I have a sort of feeling of pride, because these works came into being so flawlessly. I often let these wonderful images roam through my imagination when I'm going for a walk.[20]

Let us look for a moment at the 'works' of which Momma speaks, starting with the things that so fascinated him as a child, only later arriving, by way of model-making and drawings, at an order that we would normally call *linguistic*.

### Things

What Kees Momma tells us about his earliest childhood - unlike the rest of the book, this part is written in the third person, as if it is about someone else's life - is that he could be completely absorbed in the world of things. For him, as an autistic child, objects embodied a perfect, regular order. Everything else was out of reach.

> The fact that everything had to be perfect down to the tiniest detail, a mindset that is part and parcel of autism, would continue to play a major role for many, many years. Now, what were those objects? The toy cars that belonged to him and his brothers, for instance. The little doors and the bonnet that could be opened and closed were fascinating. He was also fascinated by an old electric razor with two flaps that could be opened by twisting a knob. . . . Kitchen equipment, such as a hand mixer with a handle you could turn to make the two beaters rotate, was another favourite. All these objects that did interesting things fitted

into that inner dream world. He still knew nothing at all
about the real outside world. That was a vague, unknown
and strange place that he could not get to, but could just
see, superficially.[21]

By 'real outside world' Momma is referring to the world of his
parents, brothers, grandma and grandpa. It is the same world that Gunilla
Gerland, whom we also met before, struggled with. She, for instance, could
not understand what the meaning of 'parents' was; might she be able to
exchange them? 'I just didn't know I ought to belong to them, or that I ought
to love them.'[22] It is also the world Temple Grandin longed for, 'but as a
child, the 'people world' was too stimulating to my senses,'[23] as she
describes it in her autobiography.

Although Momma says he was not insensible to the care and
attention of the people around him, the reader finds out very little about them.
What fascinated Momma most was the ingenious mechanism of the revolving
doors in the bus, the way lift doors closed hermetically, the way tights and
stockings 'delicately' enclosed legs and feet, the operation of the doors on his
toy buses. He opened and closed them incessantly until they broke. But as
soon as something stuck or broke it had to vanish from sight. One broken bus
after another disappeared down the drain in the back yard.[24]

Through Momma's earliest memories the reader remains close to
things in their flawless state. As such they embody a concrete, tangible,
predictable order. Momma recounts how he could lose himself utterly in this
material order; the verbal, meaningful world of people-among-themselves
had little to say to him. This does not alter the fact that, as he grew up,
Momma began to be more aware of the people around him. 'But I still had
difficulty in communicating.'[25]

### Making Models

A subsequent step in which we can follow Momma brings us to the
first in a long series of works where the mechanical regularity of things is
pursued through other means. It was not so much about creating a symbolic
representation, but far more about achieving an exact repetition of the desired
mechanism, an expansion in time and space using whatever came to hand.
The doors of the toy bus, for instance, were given carefully measured paper
draught excluder strips.

Although the doors worked fine, the bus was still not
perfect. Paper draught excluder strips had to be fitted to the
door openings, because I discovered that when the doors
were closed, there were long cracks between them. That did

not match the reality. If they were to work flawlessly, they had to shut without cracks. [26]

Momma's book contains countless examples of such simulations.

> My Lego mechanisms had to work ever more perfectly. I wanted to copy everything I saw in reality. Usually diggers that were working in the neighbourhood. I began by staring mesmerized at one of these tractors with its grabs and levers. Then I would start tinkering. Over and over again I discovered new mechanisms and movements in the trucks and these had to be copied exactly so with Lego. But it didn't always work, because Lego had its limitations and the structures were anything but stable. Everything fell apart and I felt thoroughly wretched. [27]

A baby-sitter took him to see buildings in the city. He was blown away by them and became completely enthralled by the perfectly closing sliding doors in the lift.

> At home I played out these fantastic experiences with my bricks. These wooden blocks in different colours were fabulous for me, because there was nothing else I could use that simulated the working of the lift doors so realistically. Unlike the Lego constructions, which always failed, it could never go wrong with the bricks.[28]

Momma developed a passion for metal scale models of aeroplanes and started to collect them. His fascination with buildings, meanwhile, expanded to include the geometric regularity of blocks of flats. He began to build skyscrapers on a small scale, drawing floors and lifts on them. But the scale models he made had to be more and more perfect, contain more and more lifelike details. What had begun with Lego and toy bricks gradually mutated into carved wood and eventually even into models of castles with refined antique interiors.

> I started with a skyscraper I designed myself. Then a Roman Catholic church, and the absolute showpiece is the Byzantine palace in the style of Ravenna, a building complex with a polygonal chapel in the middle. It is possible to take a look inside, where you can see drawings of religious subjects and geometric decorations. In order to show the interiors to other people, I constructed the roofs

and walls so that they could be taken off without too much
difficulty. I still have the models, although I don't look at
them so much anymore. I hope I can keep them for many
years to come.[29]

Two strategies can thus be seen in the way Momma works on a
flawless order. One seeks an extension of order in tiny details; the other looks
for it in the direction of large numbers, in repetition. Both are manifestations
of a craving for more of the same. And, in principle, there is no end to either
approach. Both refining and collecting prove ideal ways of putting things in
order, in accordance with a regularity that provides Momma with a better
grasp than all the conventional rules put together.

Strikingly, Momma does not create this order just for himself. The
maker/collector wants to show his possessions to other people. The roof and
walls can easily be opened; it is possible to see inside. And thus this seamless
order of things, this house that can be hermetically sealed, does not rule out
the possibility of finding an opening to social interaction.

### Drawings

Alongside his three-dimensional models, Momma made his first
drawings as a child, taking a seemingly clear step further towards symbolic
representation. All the same, the transition from the thing itself to an image of
the thing was not without problems. Breathlessly, Momma looked at the
antique clocks he saw hanging on the wall on a visit to some people in an old
folks' home. When he got home he tried to draw a clock like it, but because
he had not yet had enough practice his attempt was unsuccessful, so he made
do with a picture that was evidently closer to the original.

> We did have an encyclopedia with pictures of clocks on
> one of the pages. I copied that page a lot. Once I cut the
> illustrations out and stuck them on paper because I wasn't
> happy with my drawings. That way I had good clocks after
> all. But the clock mania got worse.[30]

Skilled as he was in drawing clocks, Momma obviously found it
hard to relinquish the concrete reality and imagine something else in its place,
something that would be good enough to withstand the comparison and could
pass for more of the same. But once something did stand for the things
themselves, then *that* became the place which, for Momma, had to be the
locus of the action. As well as a symbolic representation in the hands of the
maker, a reference to the ordered reality beyond it, this picture became a
world in itself in which the maker could lose himself entirely - a process to
which, in principle, there was no end.

The feeling of satisfaction with the things I cut out of my parents' books did not last long. They had to be bigger, more realistic, more beautiful. The absolute perfection of my mental world assumed huge proportions. I started to draw them again, but this time much bigger. I needed at least six sheets of paper for my big clocks. I wanted one of these things hanging on the wall like the neighbours had. At one point the wallpaper in my room was covered with stuck-on clocks.[31]

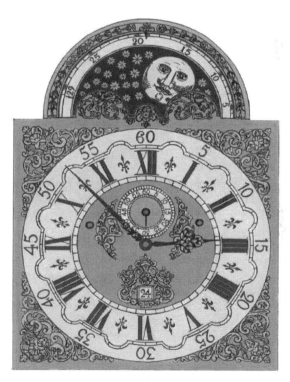

*Figure 2*. Clock dial with moon phase disc. Poster paint on paper.
Kees Momma, July 1999.

The order he sought thus had to be as lifelike and representative as possible, but as soon as it seemed that this might succeed, Momma lost himself on the spot in a desire for repetition. In no time, the newly-acquired playroom began to turn into a *store* room.

Even when he gradually learnt to accept a difference in size between original and image, it proved impossible to curb his craving for perfection. Instead of seeking flawless order in larger and larger clocks, he now looked for it in the details - getting as close as possible to concrete reality, with the precision of a Swiss watchmaker. And again in the collection, in the complete world called an 'album.'

> I carried on drawing clocks. Fortunately I got more and more skilled at it in time. I didn't need giant specimens any more. I stuck my proud timepieces, which now had normal, small-scale dimensions again, in an album.[32]

Gradually Momma's preferences and collecting mania broadened to embrace lavishly ornamented mansions, Jugendstil houses and antique furniture, castles and Oriental architecture with its infinite details. For his drawings of the interior of a Gothic cathedral, a Burmese temple complex and the interior decorations of his models, he says that he used the 'finest pens,'[33] which made it possible 'to work out the drawings with lacelike precision.'[34] Kees Momma became an extremely accomplished artist; the drawing of the clock with the phases of the moon (figure 2) is by him.

### How Should We Read an Autist's Autobiography?

There we have a number of initial impressions of Momma's autistic existence. It is the story of Momma's need for a concrete, thing-related order and of his difficulty of freeing himself from such an order once he had found it. Once he had achieved the desired perfection on paper or elsewhere, he was not really able to make that leap back. He was unable, as the non-autistic norm has it, to shuttle flexibly between reality and image, between original and representation, between the outside world and himself - a first-hand description that confirms the picture of the autistic disorder already outlined, particularly the difficulty in attributing meaning, the inability to rise above the details of the physical world and the tendency towards perseveration.[35]

All the same, there is a problematic side to Momma's story. Properties that are regarded as typically autistic only seem to apply to a time and place 'outside,' as Momma describes it in his book, not to the process of writing itself. All the attention appears to be focused on a tangible, visible, ideally extra-verbal world. Invisible as such in the life that Momma describes, language plays an implicit, not an explicit role, as a medium with which it is possible, in an unproblematic way, to refer to a world outside himself (to a deep, autistic past, for instance). This creates a gulf between form and content; between the difficulty about which Momma speaks and the seeming ease with which, as a transparent 'window' on the reality of the time, he uses words to describe these events. Is the difficulty Momma refers to a thing of the past, then? Does he no longer get lost in the world of things?

*Learning to Write*

The initial answer to this question would seem to be yes. Momma is apparently one of the minority of autistic people who has learnt to communicate and in this respect has 'outgrown' his autism. As he developed into a competent speaker, so the explanation would go in this case, a window of communication opened for Momma, and this enabled him to *transcend* the concrete reality of the past. This accords with the way Momma himself explains his linguistic skill. 'Thanks to the excellent teaching method and the relaxed approach to dealing with other people, I got a lot better at having conversations and making sentences.'[36] The linguistic ability he has acquired may explain the gulf between then and now, form and content, rigidity and flexibility.

There we have a customary interpretation that is found in a great deal of the literature on autobiographical works by autists. Although authors are not blind to the epistemological pitfalls that lurk here, they usually welcome writings of this kind as a unique opportunity to obtain a more or less unmediated insight into the inner life of autistic people. Just take, for instance, the way Jerry's story was received:

> One of the elusive yet intriguing questions that occurs to almost anyone who deals with autistic children is an overwhelming curiosity about what they are experiencing or thinking. Since such children are rarely able to describe their internal states, I attempted to get Jerry to reconstruct his memories of childhood in order to obtain a glimpse, however slight, of what it had been like to be an autistic child.[37]

The foreword to Grandin's autobiography is also very revealing in this regard. Rimland, who wrote it, praises Grandin's ability to convey her deepest emotions and fears. The window she opens from the inside in her book, he says, grants her readers 'an insight into autism that very few have been able to achieve.'[38]

Although Volkmar and Cohen have their doubts as to whether Tony actually still meets the criteria for autism, his 'first-person account' of adaptation strategies can 'contribute to our understanding of the core problems and experience of infantile autism.'[39] And according to Cesaroni and Garber, too, we can generalize from the experiences of the two people they followed. 'Insights into Jim and Albert's experiences can assist in the reconstruction of the world of other autistic children and adults who are not as communicative.'[40]

The primacy of the communicative community and the influence of the window metaphor are easily detected in this material, and it is this that concerns me. On the one hand the autistic author evidently has enough normal qualities to be able to communicate with non-autists. The unproblematic attribution of competencies to which Cesaroni and Garber's generic use of terms like 'report,' 'speculate,' 'theorize' and 'interpret' points is clearly grafted on to the traditional form of representational thinking that is summarized in the window metaphor. On the other, however, the author or speaker is assumed to be (or to have been) so autistic that it is *this* into which he or she provides insight.

One consequence of this approach is that language itself is shielded from the otherness of autism: while the autistic author writes *about* his desire for an external material order, his lucid command of language seems to have escaped that same limitation. In the course of his life, the autistic author has increasingly come to resemble us, at least in so far as his communications skills are concerned. From the developmental perspective that is implicit here, this is put forward as a question of growth and progress, 'a story of struggle and overcoming' in which autism is the negative and every utterance is regarded as a new waypoint 'on a path towards an undefined state of normalcy and acceptance.'[41] Momma's book is thus hailed as an extraordinary achievement that has brought him closer to the non-autistic ideal.

### Learning to Read

In her examination of the autobiographical work of people with Asperger's syndrome, however, Francesca Happé questions the way these writings are usually read.[42] She rejects, in particular, the naïve empiricist bias of existing analyses, which often assume that such sources provide a pure insight into the author's life - in other words uncoloured by his handicap. She would therefore contest the suggestion that the difficulty of which Kees Momma speaks is a thing of the past.

Happé believes that to avoid empirical pitfalls one must approach these writings cautiously, with a preconceived idea of the limitations that are characteristic of autistic people - deficits that must also impact on them when they write. Here she focuses not just on what authors write, but on *how* they write it. Such an awareness of questions of *style* creates an additional chance of bringing to light autistic symptoms that one might overlook were one to concentrate solely on the content.

Abstracting the content from these accounts, without considering style or possible limitations in the writer's insight, not only discards valuable data, but must lead to questionable conclusions. What are we to make, for example, of an autistic person's comment that his mental processes or sensations are radically different from other people's when he is likely to have severely impaired insight into other minds? Is it not probable too, that an autistic adult will have peculiarly unreliable memories from a childhood without self-awareness? While these remain open questions, we must be careful in how we use the contents of autistic autobiographies.[43]

Her yardstick enables us to carry out an analysis of variance. On the one hand a number of typical autistic form characteristics can be identified in autobiographical sources. Happé points, among other things, to a tendency to perseveration in which the same formulations are repeated. She also notes the unprepared introduction of new subjects and abrupt changes of subject that may indicate the author's inability to put himself in the reader's place. There is often, she finds, a degree of insensitivity to social and moral conventions, witness the naïve (for example, extraordinarily frank) way that subjects are tackled. On the other hand, information can be found that has to be regarded as exceptional on the grounds of the autist's assumed handicaps. In such cases it is important to check whether there might be an external explanation (for instance echoing other people, the hand of a co-author) before deciding to relate the content of an utterance to the author's capabilities.

We thus see how Happé calls into question the transparency of the window that autistic authors are said to open. But for her, too, the question of the extent to which language provides insight remains the yardstick by which the practical value of these writings has to be measured. We are still hearing an echo of the window metaphor. It all turns on the question as to whether the text does or does not reliably represent that to which, all being well, it refers: the perceptions and vicissitudes of the autist. Admittedly, alertness to the stylistic aspect of a text can prevent a naïve interpretation of the content, but the tendency to see language as a 'sign' of something that is *elsewhere* is something that is evidently hard to resist. As soon as language itself and its specific form enter the picture, the focus is on what it says 'about' the social-cognitive deficits of the autist that are expressed in it. Even if its semantic content is placed between brackets, language enters the picture as a sign of what lies *behind and beyond* the words. The form serves a higher ideal.

### *Learning to Stammer*[44]

The idea of language as a more or less transparent window that enables communication between competent linguistic subjects is revealed to be the background against which discussions about the work of autistic

authors take place as a matter of course, 'judging these writers by normal
rather than handicapped standards.'[45] Having first asked what lies behind the
window that autistic authors have opened, Happé wonders whether the
window is clear enough to be able to see anything, and, if not, what this says
about the author's limitations. They both, though, know what is 'normal':
language is a medium for meaningful communication. And thus, in reading
autobiographical writings by autistic people, despite all our good intentions to
watch our words, we bring in a deeply-rooted idea about the essence of
language through the back door. Evidently we tend to interpret something
that *resembles* our language as being just that; the very fact that we find it
almost impossible to refrain from *interpreting* texts underlines this.[46]

    What precedes our interpretations? Any enquiry into autism needs to
take autistic 'presence' as a starting point, argues Stuart Murray. Such
presence is what *goes before* all our talking and thinking about autism, and
resists and escapes our efforts to capture autism in narrative forms, scientific
and popular alike. In his analysis of life narratives like those of Temple
Grandin and Donna Williams, Murray is therefore concerned not solely with
opening a window on their autistic lives, but also with the specifically autistic
form of subjectivity that may be expressed in them. Autistic individuals who
speak up themselves can make their presence felt in a way that holds a
promise of autistic agency, of the autistic taking the 'narrative foreground,'
and possibly, in a critical way, having 'some say in the definition of terms
through which he or she is seen.'[47]

    We see a prime example of just such a radical, contrary expression
of autistic subjectivity in the eight-and-a-half-minute video entitled 'In my
Language' that Amanda Baggs posted on YouTube in January 2007. Murray
discusses how the video

> ... opens with a succession of humming and other noises
> produced by Baggs and her interaction with what she terms
> 'assorted objects' - a hoop around a doorknob, hands
> rubbed across surfaces, the flapping of a piece of paper. All
> these sounds are, in Baggs' voiced words ... that open the
> second part of the video, part of her 'native language,' her
> daily sense of her articulated self. 'It is about being in a
> constant conversation with every aspect of my
> environment, reacting physically to all parts of my
> surroundings,' Baggs says of her communication ... As she
> neatly observes in the 'translation' of her actions she offers
> the majority audience in the video's second section, it is an
> irony that this complex set of reactions to the multiple
> elements of her surroundings is characterized by many as
> evidence of her being in a world of her own. ... Here, the

assertion of the normativity of Baggs' world is, at heart, a
statement about rights, a demand that her life is seen and
comprehended on her own terms.[48]

Baggs bases 'her articulation of what autistic subjectivity might be'
in her own 'pleasures, preferences and modes of communication,'[49] notes
Murray. These aspects are usually lacking in the public image because the
emphasis is placed on the tragic deficit of autism

> . . . as a terrible and cruel absence of so much that makes
> being human the most familiar wonder we know. The idea
> that anything associated with this could in any way contain
> pleasure seems too perverse, too contradictory. Yet in many
> ways autism centres on an idea of pleasure. The pleasure of
> the straight line of toys, of the endlessly repeated video, of
> that bit of wallpaper - all these are common to those who
> have associations with autism.[50]

While autistic survival and communication strategies may leap out
at us from the screen, Murray is concerned above all with *reading* Baggs's
translation, the content of her layered video message. Baggs, it is true, seeks
her own voice in tactile and physical conversations with her environment,
rather than in linguistic material, although the sounds she makes come close
to it. Where Murray focuses on the life narratives of Grandin and Williams,
in particular on their performance as *writers*, language itself also enters the
picture as material in which 'autistic difference' can be expressed. But
Murray's narrative approach nonetheless remains sensitive, above all, to the
critical potential of their *substantive* message: what do these sources have to
tell us about an autistic form of subjectivity?[51]

We may question whether this does sufficient justice to the specific
input of autistic language users in a shared existence. Are we not forgetting at
such a moment to give weight in our considerations to the *cost* and *effort* that
attaches to autism in our language concept? And on the other hand, in our
notion of language as the most flexible form of representation - as meaning
which has liberated itself from things, which as the conveyor of meaning and
human freedom is compared to and placed above an invalidating autistic
craving for mechanical repetition - do we not lose for the language itself (and
for the autists who have to make do with it) everything *valuable* that an autist
encounters in the world of things, the *pleasure* that he finds in form, details
and repetition?

Kees Momma also talks about his preoccupation with the material
quality of life without this (involuntary) preference for things having been
taken into account, so far, at the level of language. But suppose we take the

autistic author's message literally and try to pass on the costs and benefits that autism entails *to the language itself*. Suppose we decide to reverse the roles and instead of letting language say something *about* the nature of things we invoke the weight of things to overturn familiar concepts of language. Suppose we try to *meet* the autistic desire for a concrete foothold by gradually extracting words from their meaningful context and closing the gap between significance and matter 'from below' (instead of wondering whether and, if so, how the autist has learnt to transcend this reality). Suppose we take the autistic penchant for repetition seriously by staying with the words themselves a little longer, rather than side-tracking time and again to what lies 'behind' the words.[52]

In all this, the autistic author always acts as a guide. Not because, as we have until now tended to say, he opens a window 'from the inside,' but because he is better equipped than non-autistic users of language to resist the temptation to look for a meaning behind every utterance. If we follow in the footsteps of Momma and others, we will not find ourselves straying outside the boundaries of language for a single moment. Nevertheless, processing a text in terms of 'interpretation' and 'meaning' falls short. The fact that we *can* read his text does not mean that we have to leave it at that. There is more going on in language than meaning alone, as Bernlef's actor discovered when he had to express silence with nothing but a scrap of monologue to hand. If we are to do justice to the heterogeneous characteristic of autobiographical work by an autistic author and follow him wherever he may go, we will have to put language to the test at least in terms of its material, structural properties. There is something to be learnt here - by non-autists, not autists. Something different, to be sure.

### Fitting Words
#### *Weather Forecast*
If there is one phenomenon (at least in the Netherlands, where Momma lives) that can be both regular and fickle, can be experienced in person and with which people are inundated in the form of newspaper reports and television items, it is the weather. For years, as we have seen, Momma was fascinated by it. He joined a club for amateur meteorologists and became a loyal reader of the club magazine. It ran stories about exceptional weather phenomena and he saw his own articles, drawings and observations published in it. The weather was not just important because of what Momma saw and read. His efforts to control the elements found a marvellous counterpoint in his fascination with gliding. With the same passion and determination as on paper, which we saw earlier, he has since tried to tame the elements *in fact*.[53]

The author began his battle with the elements on a discursive level, by working on paper on a written account of clouds and meteorological patterns. Later, when he took up gliding, Momma's work took on a more concrete character. But is the difference between the two as great as seems to be suggested here? Note, firstly, that Momma's study of the weather is a *hybrid*: it refers to a physical meteorological order outside, but at the same time it does not. As he did when he drew antique clocks and interiors, in pursuing his hobby Momma creates a self-contained world, a space in which the distinction between image and physical reality makes way for a series of new patterns. Secondly, in this workshop for cloudy skies and statistical calculations, linguistic tools also appear to be available. Take, for example, the moment when order is disrupted.

> Where I'm currently having a problem is in processing unpleasant news items in the paper or on television, such as crime, violence, pollution and forecasts of bad weather. The information about these sorts of events and facts comes across *so* hard that it sometimes makes me feel hopeless. When something I've read in the paper bothers me, I talk to my parents about it. They try to explain that everything is all right and that I mustn't take it so hard.[54]

Momma recounts how it became increasingly difficult for him to handle unpleasant news reports, with forecasts of bad weather and signs that supposedly pointed to 'a possibly imminent greenhouse effect'[55] causing him particular concern. To cope with these atmospheric upsets - leaving open the question as to what caused the most disquiet, the 'outside' event or the report 'about it' - the author talked to his parents; in all respects a normal way of talking about what was causing Kees concern; the conversation reassured him to some extent.

But Momma's linguistic ability extends beyond this. The idea of language as a medium that refers to a world outside itself proves too narrow for a proper understanding of the possibilities that language opens up for him (and perhaps others, too). I am referring here to aspects of language that fall outside a meaningful framework, so that we can all too easily overlook them. Writing itself - at least in the past, before talking to his parents became more important - was also a very concrete activity for Momma.

> For a long time I scrawled comments all over pages in the paper, expressing my displeasure at the negative articles in them. I also crossed out lines in the weather column with a thick black pen. Although other people who hadn't read the paper yet were definitely not happy about it, it nevertheless gave me some satisfaction.[56]

In his scrawling Momma demonstrates something of the use of language as an ordering mechanism that is both *local* and *referential* - as an aid in controlling the world, indeed, but not a world 'outside' per se. The actual action is not necessarily elsewhere but in any event on the spot, in the written text, *on* the printed sheet. In his editing of the weather column Momma moreover uses language as a means of ordering that is at the same time *symbolic* and *material*. He emerges as a competent user of language, certainly, but not in the familiar sense of the term. It is just as much a literal sort of ordering: make it invisible, obliterate it, cross it out, erase it, write over it. With all his might he tries to make the text 'close without gaps,' just as he used to do with his wooden bricks and the doors of the toy bus. Perhaps not as concrete as gliding, but less symbolically charged than speaking is said to be, Momma's pen scratches out the transparent window of language.

*Seamless Fit*

Let us divert briefly to another autistic author, Gunilla Gerland. Her book, like Momma's, tells of her life as an outsider among what she herself calls 'real people.' It is often a harrowing account. Gerland, too, enables the reader to step back from non-autistic preconceptions and shows us the role that language can play in interactions between autistic people and non-autists. She describes herself as exceptionally gifted linguistically and reflects, much more explicitly than Momma, on the role language plays in her relationship with her surroundings. The battle with the meaning function of language she recounts can illustrate this insight.

> There was something strange about their language. I would say exactly what I meant, but then it would become something else. The older I grew, the more often I had the feeling that when I said exactly what I meant, loud and clear, other people seemed to hear something else. And when I heard exactly what they said, it turned out that they had meant something else. I always said exactly what I meant, neither more nor less.[57]

The result of all the failed communication is that the meaning function of the words recedes into the background and their material value comes to the fore.

> But talk about things I couldn't visualize never stuck in my head - it would just fly away and settle somewhere else. The words possibly stuck, but only as words, interesting in their structure or flavour. They might have exciting colours

or contain pleasant sounds, but if I couldn't visualize them they meant nothing.[58]

To Gerland words have their own structure and taste, a stimulating colour or pleasurable sound - an aspect that is in danger of being overlooked if we only measure her achievements in language against the (non-autistic) referential yardstick. This is not to say that meaningful communication could not contribute to the purpose of Gerland's life. In her endeavour to put the world in order, Gerland really does need meaningful context. She seeks a connection that fits perfectly, a one-to-one relationship which links the linguistic order and the world of things to one another such that transport back and forth between the two becomes possible.

> I used to write labels for various things. I wanted everything to be orderly, clear and separate. This was not some way of keeping an inner chaos under control, but an attempt to arrange the external world according to the same system as my inner world, a way of establishing a slightly better accord between me and everything else. Inside me were already closed compartments with labels attached for events, rooms and worlds. Like a computer, these did indeed have a great many ramifications and sub-departments, but the cross-connections were few. Clearly, the worlds outside me would be easier to relate to if I was able to sort them out in a similar way.[59]

In view of her handicap, it is impossible to overestimate Gerland's achievement, like Momma's. Writing itself is the outcome of a long struggle to express herself in words, to grasp the symbolic meaning of language. But again, an evaluation of her work in referential terms can only come up short. In Gerland's craving for an order without any leeway or overlap we can hear echoes of Momma's desire for closure without gaps.

> My mother and I were now left to ourselves in the daytime, totally without any common language. She had some kind of vague, indistinct language, filled with 'in a minute,' 'maybe' and 'later,' and mine was concrete and exact. I mostly didn't grasp what she meant, and she almost never understood that I meant just what I said. This resulted in my sometimes having violent outbursts of temper and throwing things about. When I didn't have these outbursts, I would go and sit behind furniture or get under beds. I would pick at the material with my nails, liking the feel of

the rough surface. I also liked being in small cramped
spaces where it was quiet and calm, especially when I fitted
exactly into the space. I wanted to put on a space, put on a
sort of cave, like a garment - it felt safe when it was
cramped. There were to be no gaps between things, and
when I fitted into something exactly, a calm came over
me.[60]

This desire for seamless closure applies as much to language as it
does to the world of things. In a single-minded fashion, making a stand
against the laxness that non-autistic speakers permit themselves, Gerland
sought an anchor in absolutely correct spelling. The flawless result she
achieved here was not, however, appreciated at school, where pupils were
expected to make at least a few mistakes, for there to be some *play* in the
application of the rules of spelling. So as to seem more like a 'real' person,
she decided to start making mistakes on purpose, something that in itself
required precision.

I was almost a dictionary. Having once seen a word in
writing, the spelling was stored inside me and I plucked it
out whenever I needed it. That talent was not appreciated at
school. The teacher thought I was cheating when I got them
all right in spelling tests. She talked to me in a kind of
understanding, smarmy voice. . . . A great many long gooey
words. Words that said I may be angry now, but I'm a kind
person really. . . . I didn't understand what she wanted, but
so as to please her and be left in peace I started deliberately
making spelling mistakes. I used my talent for language to
calculate which mistakes would be the most likely.[61]

The connection Gerland establishes between the words themselves
and between words and things is not so much of a symbolic order, or at least
not only that. A symbol - 'something that stands for, represents or denotes
something else, not by exact resemblance, but by vague suggestion or by
some accidental or conventional relation'[62] - is too evanescent for the
seamless connection the autistic author is exploring: too one-sided to allow
for her linguistic proficiency. Her search for a space that fitted perfectly,
without any gaps, where she 'wanted it to touch on all sides equally, from all
directions,'[63] is almost tangibly evident in Gerland's use of language. There
is no play here, no gap that has to be bridged. When she speaks of her 'need
for new words that could be discovered and investigated, that would then slip
softly into place in my mind,'[64] she is exploring a region where the meaning
and the material quality of words *merge seamlessly* one into the other.

Words aroused my curiosity and a kind of hunger. I always had any amount of space for new ones. 'Vendetta,' 'dilettante.' ... I revelled in them. ... Although language, words and rhythm were the essentials, what really captivated me were intimations of rejection and suffering - then I could decipher them.[65]

### Street Names

Back to Kees Momma who, although he is less explicit about it than Gerland, does reveal very clearly what it means to speak a language but be an anything but ordinary user of language. In the following example, language is no longer a tool that Momma can use to bring order to things. Language itself proves to be part of the flawless order that fascinates him.

Every Tuesday my grandmother came to collect me from school. I went shopping with her in Ursulaland, a shopping street in Mariahoeve. I thought that was such a strange name for a street and I wondered why it was called that. The estate of tower blocks turned out to have a whole network of streets with girls' names ending in *land*. There was also a housing estate which had streets with names ending in *horst*. With *horst*, instead of a girl's name it was a jewel, for instance Diamanthorst. My grandmother and I explored all the *lands* and *horsts* in Mariahoeve and I loved it. As with the numbers, collecting the *lands* and *horsts* had become a hobby. Once I got all the special street names in this modern neighbourhood, I'd have another wonderful collection in which I could let my imagination roam.[66]

Momma's street plan is a hybrid creation: we recognize words (street names) and things (signs and the precious stones and streets to which the names refer), but Momma himself makes virtually no distinction between them. The room in which he used to work on building up his collection of antique interiors and clouds is now given over to a heterogeneous collection of streets/gemstones/names/signs in which there is no pride of place set aside for meaningful symbols.

My interest in antique objects and architecture seemed to wane for a while and make way for precious stones and long street signs. As well as how many *horsts* there were, I wanted to know what the jewels they had used in the street names looked like.[67]

Momma consulted a variety of sources to find out more about the object of his collection.

> I also had pop-up fairy story books. Books with brightly-coloured pictures that could move, and one of these books had a magnificent print of a large treasure-chamber full of precious stones. Exactly the same precious stones as there were in Mariahoeve. And it was then that I really started to get into the world of fairy tales and jewels.[68]

In Momma's work, fairy tales and jewels, symbolic and physical properties are forged together in what, seen from a dualistic point of view, is an inappropriate way. And just as soon as Momma does seem to make a distinction, for instance by wondering why a street is called by that name, he still goes ahead and links the - in non-autistic eyes - wrong things together. Just as, in our perception, he makes the same mistake in reverse when he thinks that he really can find the gems in his fairy-tale book 'in Mariahoeve.'

It does not bother Momma himself in the slightest. On the contrary, the self-contained world of meteorological data and the album of antique clocks have meanwhile made way for a veritable treasure-chamber: a room full of *horsts*, *lands* and gems. Rather than a solely symbolic representation in the hands of the author - in other words, a window on or allusion to a concrete reality beyond - the streets/gemstones/names/signs form a world of its own in which the maker can lose himself utterly. By adding new gems to his collection. 'I wanted coloured plastic beads in the shape of cut gems. I started to string them into chains and bracelets and so it became a complete treasure.'[69] And by adding letters and words.

> Once I knew the names of all the *horsts* and *lands*, I found all the ordinary street names interesting too. I started to count the number of letters in these names. Where I lived there were many that had a lot of letters in them. Like speedometers and tower blocks, these signs, with their attractive, regular structure, looked very harmonious. I started to copy them, but with made-up names.[70]

Street by street, stone by stone, letter by letter, word by word. Verbal or silent, symbolic or material, in Momma's desire for flawless order the properties of language and things are threaded together with little ado (if only because paragraphs in which he searches for jewels and paragraphs in which he collects streets and names constantly alternate). Momma is what could be called truly 'bilingual.' He finds appropriate words. Not so much because he uses language to report about a world outside, but because in the process of writing he develops a series of activities and builds up a world in his text that encompasses both linguistic and material representation.[71]

Contrary to what non-autistic usage assumes, Momma's language does not stand above and outside reality. In fact, language is part of a heterogeneous series within which various connections can be made - paths that he can wander endlessly, just like his other collections. This calls to mind Wittgenstein's comments about the labyrinth that language is - 'an immense network of well-kept wrong turnings' that 'sets everyone the same traps.'[72] But unlike ordinary 'competent' members of the language community, autists, by virtue of their materially oriented linguistic ability, are able to find their way through this maze unexpectedly well. Where meanings and matter can be held together by a street grid, Momma defines a new locus of action, a *passage* where autists and non-autists can cross;[73] an interface where the increased tension between concrete and linguistic extremes begins to dissolve by way of *linguistic manoeuvres*, which aim to steer a middle course between meaning and matter.

### Letters

Momma's craving for perfection and control down to the tiniest detail takes shape, lastly, in his interest in letters. Language tends to tip over increasingly to the material side when he starts to value letters not so much for their role in meaningful communication as for their aesthetic quality, as calligraphy.

> This developed into more than a hobby. Beautiful lettering and illuminated capitals had always excited me. When I saw on television that even in this day and age there were people who did this calligraphy for a living, it decided me to take a course myself.[74]

Clara Park noted a similar form of pleasure in her daughter, who 'liked letters, as she liked shapes and colours.'[75] She goes on to describe how she built on this liking for sound, colour and form to reinforce her daughter's perception of language.

> The more meaningless a convention, the more purely formal, the better Elly liked it. She liked punctuation. She liked her letter set, but she liked it far less when I used it to spell the words she knew from cards. She never used it this way herself; she preferred to make arbitrary arrangements, or to mix the letters up together and sift them through her fingers. She was fascinated by a book of different type

fonts; predictably, she learned the word 'serif' at once, and had I wished I would have had no difficulty teaching her 'black letter' and 'Gothic.' Spontaneously, long before handwriting was introduced in school, she tried to turn her capitals into cursive by supplying florid connections, saying 'handwriting' as she worked.[76]

But even without didactic lessons, the object character of language is valuable. According to Momma, the added value of the written word lies in the 'expertise of the human hand.' This is work that demands the utmost concentration and must be screened from the chaotic outside world (although the paradox is that his calligraphic work actually generated social contacts for Momma). 'It requires a steady hand, because a text may not swing, dance or wobble; this is why a calligrapher has to be properly equipped, must not be under stress and must guard against interruptions from outside.'[77]

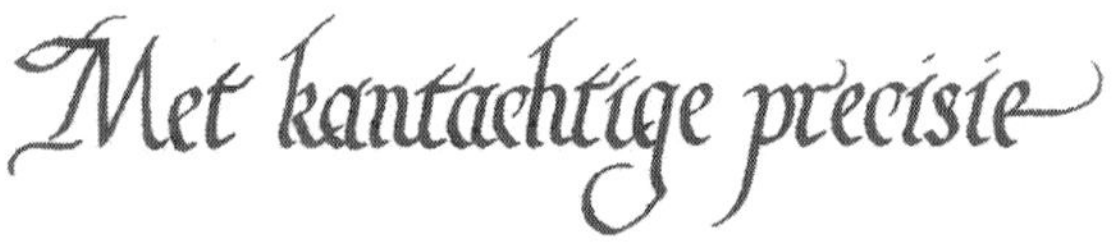

*Figure 3.* 'With lacelike precision,' calligraphy, Kees Momma, July 1999.

The flawless order Momma craves assumes concrete form when he learns to polish and refine his letters (see figure 3). In his calligraphic work Momma literally reveals a no man's land between language and concrete reality; it is the language itself that acquires a heterogeneous connotation in Momma's hands. He is at home in the linguistic no man's land between meaningful and concrete extremes - because of his deficit, not in spite of it.

**Exploring the Wasteland**

A deficit in communications skills lies at the heart of the autistic syndrome. In so far as language plays any role at all in interactions between autistic people and non-autists, it often seems to be confined to one-way traffic. This why I have devoted considerable attention to the key role of non-verbal elements in dealings between autistic and non-autistic people. What is easily overlooked, though, is that recognition of the importance of non-verbal structures in the lives of autists and in living with them is not to say that language and speakers of language no longer have a part to play. On the other hand, we must never lose sight of the fact that linguistic reserves can be tapped in a variety of ways.

As I have shown, the material quality of life also plays an important role in autobiographies by people with autism. We usually tend to look solely at the negative side of this and regard it as an achievement if the author has managed to shed the burden of things. To an extent this battle continues, however, even though the silence has been broken. Writing in reaction to Birger Sellin's book, the Dutch literary critic Jacq Vogelaar says of the autistic struggle to escape from the desire for repetition and find self-expression, 'writing itself is often a continuation of the struggle between the inner and the outer world.' He then goes on to quote Sellin:

> I cannot discover why I have to live so walled in/ in my head I can think inherently clearly and I can feel too/ but when in this outside-the-box world I try breathtakingly to convert the so-called simplest actions into deeds I can't do it/ agitation overcomes me fear and idiotic panic reduce me almost to despair.[78]

This is no 'cured autist,' says Vogelaar, but someone conducting a public struggle in his writing.

To some extent, though, the liking for things is actually an advantage rather than an obstacle. In Momma's book, too, the delight sometimes leaps off the page. His possessions have to look pristine and, like the 'slightly rough or gently ribbed surface' of the cover of a book, 'must feel stimulating to the hand.'[79] His work, therefore, can equally well be read as an ode to the *pleasure* that an autist derives from the visual and tactile properties of things. However, as soon as we come to the *language* Momma uses to talk about his collected work and his collecting, there is often silence. Language itself does not appear to be part of any collection. Nowhere does the needle stick. Writing seems to be pallid, unruffled 'writing about' the tangible, visible things outside - a transparent window for meaning entirely according to the rules of normal usage.

As soon as autists have linguistic abilities that resemble ours, all the precautions intended to avoid an asymmetrical reading are in danger of being jettisoned without hesitation. Not so much because, as David Goode remarks, we are inclined to think that communication is essentially verbal as, conversely, because we make the mistake of thinking that language is always a conveyor of meaning.[80] Time and again we allow ourselves to be taken in by the transparent gloss of words, so that we tend to evaluate the extraordinary performance of autistic authors in *ordinary* terms. What we forget at that moment is to take into account the costs and benefits autism carries with it in language itself and our dealings with it.

As Ian Hacking argues, autistic autobiographers have to 'retool linguistic materials made in an age-long community' and are trying to 'fit' words of non-autistic origin to their own experiences. Thus they are 'creating ways in which to express experiences.'[81] By doing so, these authors play a very different role from the therapies and other regimes that seek to help autistic people better grasp non-autistic behaviour. These autobiographies (and other autism narratives), argues Hacking, 'teach many of us how to compensate in the other. That is, they suggest what to infer from autistic behaviour which on the face of it means nothing to us.'[82] Here I have confined myself to what autistic authors teach us about the value of their linguistic habits.

Language is full of well-trodden paths that tempt language users to repeat non-autistic steps. On the basis of autobiographical works by autistic people I have tried to stretch the distance to familiar interpretations a little further. I have tried to *accommodate* the autistic desire for a material grasp by loosening language bit by bit from its meaningful context. I have tried to liberate not the patient, but in the first place ourselves and our concept of language from non-autistic clichés. The unusual manner of reading that was needed to bring this about, and which I explored in the footsteps of Momma and Gerland, shares with the authors a fascination with sound, texture and taste, with the material form and the collection value of words. It is a way of reading that does not examine the text and its content purely and simply in terms of its meaning, but at the very least also tries to treat the text as a sliding scale, as neither symbolic nor purely material reality.

My reading thus implies criticism of the preoccupation with meaningful communication that dominates much of the debate surrounding linguistic utterances by autists. Which is not to say that meaningful communication could not contribute to the meaning of an autist's life nor that they could not enrich interactions on the interface. What I am concerned with is that a conclusion like this cannot be extended with impunity to what is good and worth aspiring to for autists (and non-autists) in general. The very struggle for the emancipation of the autist's voice, from which the generous interpretation appears to stem, sells that same autist short. Recognition of what the autist has to say requires an effort that runs counter to many of our habits. For is it not *our* preoccupation with the development of the verbal subject, with representation and meaningful content, that leads us to assume automatically that all blessings come, so to speak, 'from above'?[83]

This is not a plea to fill autists, for lack of anything better, with self-contained, meaningless strings of words. What I am saying is that we should question the supposed worthlessness of what is said to be meaningless.[84] Clinging on to the familiar concept of language means that language as a reserve on which it may be possible to draw in a shared life is only relevant to the few autists who have something approaching normal linguistic ability, and only in so far as they do. But the fascination of all those who repeat words, who have a bond with language that most certainly exists but cannot easily be understood as meaningful, is soon lost sight of because of the non-autistic preoccupation with meaning.

We must question the familiar, non-autistic notion of what it means to learn to share a language. Autistic authors prove to be ideal guides in the verbal no man's land between symbolic and material extremes. Their work embraces language from which the meaning has already partially tumbled; language that you can hold like a thing, collect, draw, colour and refine; language you can use to build a safe haven; language you can show other people; language crammed full of letters and words, each with its own sound colour, texture and taste; words that you can attach flawlessly to things; words on which you can chew endlessly.[85] As Kees Momma likes to do, given the chance:

> It was all so recognizable to me. That talking to yourself, repeating the same word - I do that too, when I'm on my own and a word feels good in my mouth. Sometimes I have to tell myself 'Kees, you're being really autistic again.'[86]

It is precisely because of their 'deficit' that autistic authors are able to enrich the language with new possibilities: to bring about an expansion rather than a curtailment of the locus of action; to make the fallow ground that they still often command on their own habitable for non-autists too.

# Autistic Company

It was a hot summer when I did the fieldwork for my research. We went for a walk in the park almost every day - at the end of the afternoon, when it started to get cooler. There were playing fields in the park, flower beds, bushes and a patch of woodland criss-crossed by paths. If we had time we would go a bit further, through the gate at the far side and out of the park, where we knew all the routes like the backs of our hands. We walked beside fields of ripening wheat, along dusty country lanes, past cows in the meadow - Robert usually trailing behind the rest of the group, David way ahead. Others, like Tim and Bart, preferred to stay closer.

I did an awful lot of walking that summer and - mindful of Sartre's observations in the park - often asked myself how I should deal with it in my research. Not that it wasn't a pleasant pastime. On the contrary, it was an activity that the residents and care workers (and I) usually really enjoyed. The problem was just that it all seemed so *ordinary*. That was, of course, to be expected; after all I had worked as a professional care worker with mentally handicapped autistic youngsters for almost three years. So before I embarked on fieldwork I had resolved to be wary of anything that appeared to be a matter of course.

Their everyday nature aside, I suspected that it ought to be possible to infer from these walks something about the shared existence of autistic and non-autistic people that I wanted to write about. To my mind that meant that this would be encompassed during the walk: on the one hand, in situations like this autistic people are evidently just part of the lives of the non-autistic around them; on the other people with autism are so different from other people in crucial areas that we can ask ourselves in what respects there is any question of 'interaction' here. The familiar character of the community of people among themselves, I felt, should also be up for discussion on this occasion.

We will return to this question of opening things up for discussion later, but first let us look at the question as to exactly what is at issue for non-autistic people in their dealings with people with autism. What is understood, according to the accepted non-autistic frames of reference, as 'typical of' and 'familiar to' people? Which norm is at stake here? A great deal has already been written about this, but almost by definition it happened between the lines - these were after all assumptions that largely precede common sense. Let us now try to make a number of aspects rather more explicit, starting with what is usually understood in terms of the *outcome* of normal child development.

*People Among Themselves*
In a number of respects people with autism are so different from other people that being human is threatened to its core. 'Autism as a subject touches on the deepest questions of ontology, for it involves a radical deviation in the development of brain and mind.'[1] Autism is therefore regarded as a disorder *par excellence*, which in its departure from the norm can provide insight into the essential preconditions for normal social-cognitive development. From this comparison it is possible to draw up the inventory of what is understood by 'normal development.' As we read in the *Handbook of Autism and Pervasive Developmental Disorders*:

> Indeed, autism has served as a paradigmatic disorder for theory testing and for research on the essential preconditions for normal social-cognitive maturation - expression and recognition of emotions, intersubjectivity, sharing a focus of interest with other people, the meaning and uses of language, forming first attachments and falling in love, empathy, the nuanced understanding of the mind of others - indeed, the whole set of competencies and motivations that allow a child to become a family member and social being.[2]

The whole set of abilities and drives that enable a person to develop as a member of a family to a member of the extended family of people among themselves - this is where the biological twist of fate impacts on autistic children (and the people closest to them). Conversely, the non-autist appears as someone who does have the necessary competencies and motivations. The complex interaction of empathic competencies, intersubjectivity, social recognition, the meaningful use of language and so forth, is ultimately expressed in what is regarded as an essential human quality: social and emotional connection. If we compare this with an autistic child, whose development into a social being is seriously disrupted, we see that the child who is predisposed towards these social-cognitive competencies usually develops into someone who *feels at home in the community of people among themselves*.

Not, of course, that we have to go to any particular trouble for this. Development into a competent member of the social community generally happens almost of its own accord - at least so runs a second assumption relating to the non-autistic self-image. This matter-of-course way in which normal maturity would usually be reached, stands in stark contrast to the laboriousness of the learning process in autistic people. As Wing observed, 'it is precisely this curiosity and interest in new experiences, and the recognition of and desire to communicate with other human beings that seem to be lacking in autistic children.'[3] Because they show virtually no personal initiative, have no interest in discovering the world and are not curious, Wing argues, autistic children do not pick much up in their contacts with other people. If the child does learn something, it happens mechanically, not because he sees the point of it. 'Most bewildering to an autistic child,' as Wing noted, 'are the social rules that a non-autistic child learns so easily from experience, usually without having to be specifically taught.'[4]

*Naturally and without effort* - this is the conclusion we tend to draw, this is how normal development proceeds. And again attention is focused on what is considered to be the core of human existence: joining in effortlessly with the social traffic. According to this view, children master the various competencies needed to take part in this game of life as a matter of course: as soon as they are ready, when circumstances invite them to do so, in dealings with one another and the world, almost *inadvertently*, usually heedless of any concerted efforts to teach them something formally. An essentialist way of saying that as a rule people learn without effort to deal with the symbolic order that develops between them, is that they *naturally feel at home* in the company of other people.

People with autism lack this self-evident involvement with the other; at best we can impose it on them from outside. This brings special responsibilities for care workers in its wake, because it means deciding what a 'meaningful life' is for another person. This leads on to a third aspect of the norm that we are trying to bring out into the open here: the *ideal* that people persist in keeping in mind, even when the preconditions for normal development are not present. Cohen and Volkmar defend a number of normative choices that are made, usually implicitly, in the care for autistic children.[5] They stand by the ideal of the fullest possible participation of the individual in family life and in society, whereby individual independence must be safeguarded as far as possible, and where, as far as possible, a productive contribution to society is required. They regard it as desirable for a child to be brought up by his parents at home with his brothers and sisters. And should placing him in a care facility prove inevitable, Baron-Cohen and Bolton believe that 'such homes are ideally indistinguishable from and as much a part of the local community as possible.'[6]

A brief look at the ideals that are held in high esteem in the care of people with autism confirms the non-autistic self-image we outlined before. Here again, the endeavour to get them to take part in the community of people among themselves proves to be a guiding principle. As the natural extension of these ideals care workers concentrate on eliminating behavioural problems and encouraging social and communications skills and imagination. Despite the fact that the normal route to this end is broken up and although it is in precisely these three areas that one runs up against the singularity of the autistic 'other,' the ideal of living that they aim for does not undergo any fundamental changes compared with what one would normally want for people. The persistence of this attitude reveals how crucial the *characteristics of our society* are deemed to be in terms of what it means to 'live as a person':

> What counts as happiness for ordinary people is probably the same for people with autism. Only I think that the dimension in which that happiness is attained is a different one. So what the approach boils down to is that you have to adapt as much as possible so that they can discover order in what was previously chaos. But the intention has to be that this adaptation is only a springboard to allow them to get used to, shall we say, more flexibility. Not because it's so important for them to be more like us, but because thanks to that flexibility they can enjoy life more. After all, being locked up inside their brains, in that rigidity, is indeed very limiting.[7]

'What does it mean to perceive, relate to, know about, even *be* a 'person'?' asked Peter Hobson, as I quoted before.[8] What I did not say then, however, was that we usually think that we more or less know the answer. In our efforts to provide people with autism with a roof over their heads - whether we take this literally (by championing the expansion of day care) or figuratively (as in teaching social skills) - we assume that we ourselves are reasonably well housed. We are gregarious by nature; thanks to our social cognition we have distanced ourselves from the world of things, and we feel at home in the meaningful world of people among themselves. The house is spick and span, the table is laid and we all shove up a bit so that the autistic guest can pull up a chair and join us.

It is the self-evident nature of this assumption that has been posited as a problem in this study. The image of the non-autistic self as a social being has in part been articulated in contrast with an autistic existence. Yet in the dealings between autistic and non-autistic people, the tenability of this (ideal) image is also frequently tested and put into perspective. What happens when people are confronted with a fellow human being to whom social reciprocity is anything but self-evident? How do we keep things sociable in such exceptional circumstances? Does our desire for community hold up? And, if it does, in what form?

### A Walk Through the Park

For an answer to these questions let us go back to the walk and the shared existence of autistic and non-autistic people that I hoped to discover. How did this walk differ from the normal activities in the park? A tried and tested method of exposing the underlying order of a situation is to find out where the familiar pattern breaks down. In this case it was with Rick, a resident with serious behavioural problems for whom going for a walk was anything but ordinary. When everyone else set off, Rick often stayed behind. Sometimes a care worker took Rick out on his own. One could see in him to an extreme degree something that people on the autistic spectrum often have to contend with - the great uncertainty that going for a walk involves. How are you supposed to do that; how *do* you go for a walk?

It must be maddening for people with autism - that tendency of the ordinary walker to take short-cuts and turn into another path for no particular reason, to stop now and then and look at what is going on, to avoid dogs running around off the lead, to take account of the speed of other members of the group, meanwhile deciding how long the outing should last. And then to turn for home satisfied, as if they could already depend on getting home, without ever having arrived anywhere. 'Just going for a little walk' brings the latent tension between an autistic and a non-autistic existence to a head.

So as to be able to go for a walk together nonetheless, a compromise sometimes has to be formulated. The walk follows a familiar pattern in order to accommodate the autistic resistance to change. On the basis of a non-autistic idea of what a meaningful occupation is, the care workers try to broaden the margins little by little. (And just hope that other walkers keep their dogs on the lead.)

> It is probably important to a person with autism that you plan the walk to take in certain contact or orientation points, with the last point being that you always come back again. Rick, for instance, will go for a walk, but it has to be the route he knows, so we try to broaden it out so that he knows more routes. By going for a walk and saying, look, it's fine, and now we're going to walk down this way and that's fine too.[9]

Viewed in this light, a walk probably sums up the shared existence of autistic and non-autistic people in a nutshell. The walk is a compromise between an intrinsically meaningful activity (just going for a little walk) and an externalized answer expressed in terms of 'how' (walk from A to B) to the question as to *why* we want to move. The walk generated the beginnings of an answer to the first question in my study - concerning the nature of the interactions between people with autism and those without. But what, meanwhile, was the status of my second question concerning the terms in which the dealings between them can be described? Was this also the tailor-made description I had in mind?

Despite the practical gain that emerges from this example we do not seem to have got much further *conceptually* with a redefinition of going for a walk in terms of time-space coordinates. After all our wanderings, we seem to be right back where we started, with stereotypical images like that of the autist-machine, which chiefly suggests distance from a (no less caricaturish) world of people among themselves. As if going for a walk were an endlessly flexible activity for us! This would seem to be an untenable contradiction - not just in the interaction between autistic and non-autistic people, but also in normal everyday life. The autistic walker is not a robot or dummy; the 'footpath' signpost often leads non-autistic walkers, too, along surfaced roads and pavements. As a framework for my conclusions, a dualistic concept of walking seems too static. (And, as we have seen before, the metaphor of 'a sort of animal' would offer little consolation either, if only because animals are usually not supposed to go for little walks like people do.)

What is missing from this description is, firstly, an impression of the *work* an autistic person and his carer have to do together in order to be able to go for a walk. This work can build a bridge between autistic and non-autistic contributions to a shared existence. Ordinary children learn when they play, children with autism learn when they 'work,' says Peeters.[10] He is referring here to the specific, demarcated nature of the activities with which autistic people learn to cope in social situations and from which they can also derive pleasure. A walk provides someone with autism with the opportunity to learn. His carers, however, are equally involved in a learning process during the walk - not only because skills that do not develop spontaneously have to be specifically learned, but also because it takes effort to step back from a non-autistic life. One has to *learn to value* autistic company - even if it is just so as to be able to go for a walk together.

Not that we could abandon the search for routes that are accessible to both just as easily, a second aspect that has thus far not been sufficiently explored. An autistic person is not like other people, and this means that expectations have to be put into perspective. At the same time we want them to belong with us; it is inconceivable that autistic people should not belong with us, be with us at home. Although living together takes effort, we do not send them off alone into the forest. Even when the care workers say that Rick might be better off 'on his own in a little cabin on the heath where nothing happens,' they are still thinking in terms of a place 'where he can walk' and 'two people to look after him.'[11] *We do our utmost to make them part of our company*. Recalling Park's claim of self-defence:

> Confronted with a tiny child's refusal of life, all existential hesitations evaporate. We had no choice. We would use every stratagem we could invent to assail her fortress, to beguile, entice, seduce her into the human condition.[12]

An autistic child is above all a child whom we treat like any other: a child we desperately want to conform to social expectations, however much that runs up against obstacles; a child that in many respects is like us and with whom we want to communicate; a child we want to give the same enjoyable life we wish for ourselves. For people with autism, in their turn, the fact that their social and emotional development has been disrupted does not mean that they do not want contact with those around them or could not derive pleasure from it. Their 'lack of understanding of the subtle rules of social interaction and communication does not necessarily indicate an absence of feeling or of a desire for a relationship.'[13] A *desire* for one another's companionship is thus an indispensable motive for a shared life.

The matter-of-course way we see ourselves as sociable beings has been sufficiently aired. This book has been about the steps that have to be taken when this self-evidence is lacking, when it is a matter of making people part of our company who are not 'by nature' part of the community of people among themselves. What sort of *work* do we have to do if social relationships remain largely incomprehensible to one of the parties? What effort do we have to put into living together if the linguistic, meaningful world of people among themselves has for the most part to be suspended? How do we learn to value this shared life? I shall bring the main players in this book briefly back on to the stage, starting by recalling the preparatory conceptual work.

### Conceptual Work

Speaking exclusively in terms of people and things, we saw, gets in the way of a good understanding of the interactions between autistic and non-autistic people. As a metaphor for what goes on there, the human-thing dualism suggests a gulf that does not necessarily exist in practice. So as not to lose sight of this practice, we must problematize the conceptual framework itself. At the same time no one can get around these terms. After all, the distinction between people and things also functions as an unproblematic background against which the otherness of the autist stands out and as a tool that enables people to live and to cope with this difference. If we want to discuss the shared existence of autistic and non-autistic people, we must try to clear conceptual barriers out of the way without detracting from the everyday reality of the human-thing distinction.

Taking J. Bernlef's novella *Vallende ster* as our starting point, we explored ways of putting some distance, little by little, between us and familiar oppositions, without pretending that our non-autistic origins can be wiped out. Layer by layer, the author built up time-space frameworks between which the reader could travel back and forth. In this structure, the difference between a linguistic, meaningful world of people among themselves and a concrete world of things beyond it functioned as a model for what we could imagine by non-autistic and autistic worlds. If we cannot detach ourselves from it anyway, ran my interpretation, we can at least make non-autistic *default* values more useful. By maintaining people-thing dualism as a background, exaggerating and idealizing, we have in our hands a yardstick for defining a 'midpoint' between diverse 'places.'

Bernlef mobilized a variety of means of transport for the journey between these two locations - a meaningful world of people among themselves and an autistic world constructed along mechanical lines. By filling the exemplary vacuum with new, unexpected actors and activities, he created scope for bringing to the reader's attention that which cannot easily be conceived in terms of the people-thing distinction.

The same vocabulary and similar means of transport were then used to bring situations outside the novella within reach. The explorations of a shared life began in familiar regions before roaming through an unknown area that lay between meaningful and material extremes. The purpose of organizing the text in this specific way was to enable readers to experience new impressions and offer them the opportunity to adjust prevailing ideas about themselves and the nature of the community of people among themselves.

This may make it sound as though the transport to other characters, places and times was effortless, but in practice it often proved to be a long-drawn-out business. Every attempt to circumvent dualistic terms and put distance between ourselves and some of the self-evident aspects of the non-autistic life showed the well-nigh impossible nature of the whole undertaking. By speaking about 'us' and 'them,' we were happy to use a conventional distinction that only proved to be problematic as the book progressed. And not only that. From the outset every indication of a 'midpoint' between meaning and matter was related to what appeared to be the midpoint from the non-autistic perspective. Although we may have avoided some digressions, there are no guarantees that the terrain we have reconnoitred here also marks a shared life with non-autists from the viewpoint of the autistic person.

It proves extraordinarily difficult to develop a vocabulary that does not immediately reduce the examples of a shared existence to humanistic or mechanistic clichés. What E. A. Burtt observed in 1932 applies here, too: we are tied hand and foot to a modern, dualistic world view.

> The cosmology underlying our mental processes is but three centuries old - a mere infant in the history of thought - and yet we cling to it with the same embarrassed zeal with which a young father fondles his new-born baby. Like him, we are ignorant enough of its precise nature; like him, we nevertheless take it piously to be ours and allow it a subtly pervasive and unhindered control over our thinking.[14]

This study is, in short, an endeavour to get away from the sort of stereotypical images that I outlined in the introduction, knowing that I cannot free myself of them altogether. Because I cannot resolve this duality, I have tried to make this tension tangible. In so doing, I am confronting the reader of this book with my own non-autistic struggles to distance myself as an author from a vocabulary that is grafted on to a world view that makes a distinction between people and things. During attempts to clear away conceptual barriers, this tension recalled the everyday reality of the human-thing distinction. It proves virtually impossible to avoid the pitfalls Wittgenstein describes:

> Language sets everyone the same traps; it is an immense network of well-kept wrong turnings. And hence we see one person after another walking down the same paths and we know in advance the point at which they will branch off, at which they will walk straight on without noticing the turning, etc., etc. So what I should do is erect signposts at all junctions where there are wrong turnings, to help people past the danger points. [15]

Within the possibilities of the language game we grew up with and with all its limitations, we can perhaps avoid a few well-trodden paths. I have tried to do this in the preceding chapters by using textual resources to organize a form of transport to unknown characters, places and times. The preparatory conceptual work for which Bernlef's literary imagination provided inspiration has thus been adequately outlined. Time once again to follow the paths of other figures who were introduced here and to take stock of what we can infer, from their reconnaissances, about the nature of a shared life and the terms in which we can think of a role in such a shared life for imagination, socialization and communication.

### Imagination

One of the first places where the differences between people with and without autism came to light was the cognitive psychologist's laboratory. The reports of what researchers found there suggested that there is a conspicuous difference between autistic and average abilities in social imagination and conceptualization. Whereas children normally develop into mind-readers as a matter of course, autistic subjects, these studies suggested, are barely, if at all, able to recognize the inner states of other people; they can at most deduce it by logic. The way such exceptions were accounted for, however, remained within the dualistic bounds: a person with autism succeeds at best in camouflaging the empathic deficit by means of mechanical calculations; the real scope of the non-autistic imagination remains beyond his reach. In practice, moreover, tapping into cognitive reserves often proves to be a step too far. And yet there are all sorts of situations in which autistic and non-autistic people live together that cannot be attributed to cognitive feats. The imagination also has a place there, albeit in a different way from the one we are accustomed to.

From the empirical situations described we can draw conclusions about the specific *nature* of a shared life. Extra efforts have to be made to find a place for imagination in a shared existence. 'A lot of hard 'work' has to go into 'leisure time.''[16] To a degree, this job of organizing leisure time can be taken over by things. Practices in which things play a part alongside people have more to offer the imagination in a shared existence than a 'theory of mind' that makes a strict distinction between the roles of people and things. Various examples demonstrated that, instead of calling on cognitive reserves, compensation for a shortage of shared ideas could be found in places *other* than the human mind. They make a shared existence conceivable in concrete terms (visible, tangible) without having to abandon the desire to have the autistic person share in a certain measure of freedom.

In response to these explorations, it is also possible to make an evaluation of the *vocabulary* in which we usually speak about the role of imagination in human relationships. The established dualistic frameworks play a dual role in the work of the cognitive psychologist: in the experimental setting where cognitive differences between people with autism and people without are investigated, the people-thing distinction is both *assumed* and *intensified*. The cognitive psychologist's research into autism does more than generate insights into the abnormalities of the autistic mind; it is also a mirror in which the familiar features of a non-autistic self-image can be examined. The dualistic framework is constitutive for our knowledge of the cognitive differences between autistic and non-autistic minds; it provides something to hold on to in training people with autism and allows for exceptions to be explained.

But this vocabulary comes at a price. Because social imagination and understanding are purely mental affairs when seen in this light, they block the view of alternative forms of imagination that depend on their physical presence rather than their strength of mind. This creates friction because it is precisely such extra-mental forms of social imagination that seem to suit the possibilities and preferences of many people with autism. A dualist framing also overlooks the fact that alternative locations of imaginative activities are (to a certain extent) also accessible to the non-autistic. This does, though, require adapting the non-autistic self-image that is imprisoned in a conceptual straitjacket which values the mind above the body and a theory of mind above mechanical thinking, and in which things have a negative and stultifying connotation. It took not just an empirical but also a conceptual detour to value the imaginative value of things and bodies and take the sting out of the supposed *conflict* with human qualities that are held to be essential and assumptions about the nature of the community of people among themselves.

*Socialization*

Another location in which we explored a shared existence was the residential centre for mentally handicapped autistic boys. In order to rescue something of the normal sociability of life, care workers saw to it that other, less obvious elements were involved in mealtimes. This is not to say that standing back from familiar companionable interactions came easily to them. Compared with the sociability which, in the final analysis, this is all about, the constraint of the kitchen timer creates a decidedly desolate impression. The timer, at least in terms of the care workers, is at best a tool in their hands; it is they who, with the best of intentions, actually say what happens at the table. And yet there are also situations where, in time, young residents and care workers learn to gear their actions to one another, without having to make an a priori distinction between humanistic ideals in the distance and material aids within reach - precisely the sort of dualistic distinction we wanted to get away from little by little. Such situations only became apparent, however, if one took seriously, more even than the care workers themselves, the delegation of authority to the world of things and shifted the narrative centre of gravity from their story to the resources being talked about.

From a more detailed exploration of these object-centred forms of sociability, we can again draw conclusions about the specific nature of a shared existence. Care workers, who are usually assumed to delegate tasks in a well thought-out way, manage to go along with the socializing power of local and heterogeneous elements. Things, on the other hand, do not just play a passive, instrumental role, they also have an interactive effect. In the processes of social integration and segregation they help to determine what people do and do not do.[17] This means that holes do not open up in the social fabric even when familiar socialization mechanisms are lacking. Unexpected things and activities often take their place - a seam in the carpet where the chair fits precisely, a step in the grass, a fork and a plate of food. These have a socializing tendency that cannot be reduced to stimulus response relations or good intentions.

On the basis of this sociological microcosm of the meal and other temporal ordering processes, it is also possible to evaluate the current way of speaking about a shared existence. By pointing to the special nature of meaningful human actions, established dualistic frameworks provide a framework for understanding the autistic socialization deficit and directing pedagogically justified attempts to compensate for this deficit 'by the back door.' Dualism moreover provides a conceptual framework within which the involvement of 'objectifying' means can be defended normatively against, among other things, moral doubts about a 'dehumanizing' approach to the other.

Again, though, there are disadvantages to the use of the familiar vocabulary. The notion that social embedding can also be derived from elements other than things which function as an extension of ideas lodged in the minds of care workers and the linguistic community vanishes from sight. This is a problem because forms of socialization that are less heavily charged with interpretations and social conventions appear to chime better with what moves many *autistic* people. A dualist framing, moreover, ignores the fact that that these alternative sources are also accessible (in part) to the non-autistic people around them. However, in order that this potential for a shared life can be utilized, it again requires adjustment of the non-autistic self-image that regards the symbolic side of social relations as being of another and higher order than the physical setting in which they take place. It took an empirical *and* conceptual detour to be able to assess the socializing value of the material order and to mitigate the presumed *conflict* with what are deemed to be unshakable competence requirements for taking part in the community of people among themselves.

### Communication

Thanks to the autobiographical work of autistic people, the reader was in the privileged position of being able to distance himself from some of the self-evident aspects of a non-autistic existence. When familiar ideas about what you need to survive as a person in the company of others come up for discussion, the autistic author takes the work out of the reader's hands. At first sight, however, there appears to be little to learn about a possible alternative role for the language itself. The author appears, as a competent member of the language community, to have a medium for communication 'about' his autistic existence, without any more words having to be wasted on the issue. And in so far as that does happen, in discussions about the value of autobiographical work by people on the autism spectrum, the parties to the discussions usually elaborate on a well-worn pattern: the value of the work is measured in terms of the (epistemological) question as to whether this is a reliable representation and, if so, what is revealed in it. And here we are - back again at a familiar dualistic world view (with a linguistic subject on the one hand and an object outside it on the other) from which we gradually tried to get free. All the same, there is something to be learnt from the work of autistic authors.

By shifting the narrative focus to the material properties of the text itself, it is possible to shed further light on the specific nature of a shared existence. What it *means* to be a competent speaker of language is seen in a different light after re-reading 'auti-biographical' work. We are indeed constantly wrong-footed by the language, even down to our ideas about the nature of language itself. Not only does normal (non-autistic) linguistic competence prove to make no more than a modest contribution to the community of autistic and non-autistic people, it also appears that it is anything but ordinary users of language who point us towards alternative ways. Where Kees Momma leads the way and exerts himself to bring order to the labyrinth of streets/names/signs, he interprets Wittgenstein's task of signposting the path through the maze of well-worn linguistic trails like no one else. He works on the path *literally*, in the language itself, at the level of the text, of the words and letters, the sounds and forms.

On the basis of this reading it is also possible to produce an evaluation of the terms that are usually used in speaking of (the importance of communication in) a shared existence. The familiar vocabulary that makes a distinction between a linguistic subject and a world beyond it is constitutive of our understanding of meaningful communication. It provides a framework for understanding many autistic people's failure in terms of communication and for appreciating the extraordinary achievement by the autistic author.

At the same time the consequence of the non-autistic tendency towards interpretation is that language as a source which can be drawn on in a shared existence is only relevant to the few who can come close to a non-autistic ideal of the meaningful use of language. The thing that people with autism have with language but which does not satisfy a standard for meaningful use - a liking for the taste of words, for the curl on the *r*, for the sound of 'round' - is in danger of being ignored. Time and again we allow ourselves to be taken in by the transparent gloss of words. A less dualistic relationship with the language is also open (to a limited extent) to the non-autistic. However, this does again call for an adjustment of the non-autistic self-image that is dominated by a dualism in which the mind has become the seat of everything we find important about language, and form is wholly subservient to content. An empirical and conceptual detour was required - a detour which, no less than anywhere else, also proved to be a material one - to liberate language from a non-autistic preoccupation with meaning and to reduce the supposed *tension* with the symbolic function of language considered essential in the community of people among themselves.

### A Motley Crew

In our dealings with autistic people it emerges that we are not the people we often think we are. I have specified in three ways the idea that we are by nature gregarious. I have focused attention on pronouncements relating to the outcome of normal development, the way it is usually achieved, and the ideal image we persist in keeping in mind, even when it is clear that the conditions for normal development have not been met. Let us, finally, look at these three one more time to see which traces a shared existence has left here.

If we want to talk about the *outcome* of a shared life of autistic and non-autistic people, terms such as 'community of people among themselves' fall short. Dealings with autistic people make us realize that it is essential to involve other elements in that community in order to give substance to living together. The nature of these relationships is not easily described in purely interpretative terms. It requires a sociality concept that is heterogeneous enough to discount the diverse interactions that take place here. Perhaps we can regard a shared existence, to borrow a metaphor from science and technology studies, as a 'seamless web.'[18] Not so much because the transition between the constituent elements of companionship is ambiguous and every distinction is a matter of convention, but because autistic and non-autistic people, words and things, pictures, ideas, colours, shapes also fit together *physically*. Mutual adaptation requires not so much mental flexibility as for those involved to try to mesh together and be present for one another flawlessly, seamlessly.

Expanding the circle of socially relevant players takes more than a simple addition sum; it is about exploiting the possibilities and experimenting with the properties of the material that is to hand. The abilities needed to join this motley crew encompass both more and less than the social-cognitive abilities that are usually regarded as essential. An irregularity in the pattern of expectation can be resolved according to the convention of the linguistic community by means of words, gestures, symbols. But things can also create a meaningful situation, act as an incentive through which those concerned can respond to one another and to their environment. It is this multiformity of stimuli that coordinate action which guarantees the unfolding of a shared life.

In terms of the *way in which* one develops into a competent member of this community, secondly, there is a paradoxical conclusion to be drawn. On the one hand it appears that, in contrast to what is usually supposed, there is no self-evident or spontaneous development that results in the formation of a community. On the contrary, the interaction between autistic and non-autistic people suggests that 'living together' can more accurately be understood as a laborious learning process. We knew that this is true of people with autism. 'Work' enables them to survive in society, to discover a certain regularity in and to derive pleasure from social relationships. But a shared existence also requires non-autistic people to develop skills that are not within easy reach. Non-autistics also have to make an effort and learn to appreciate alternative options, if for no other reason than to get away from the idea that sociality is a purely symbolic affair - something that is supposedly brought about with careless ease by people among themselves through meaningful communication.

A shared existence does not come naturally to us. On the other hand a great deal of effort ultimately goes into *transferring* work to other members of the company. Whereas the non-autistic will tend to delegate his work to words, texts, subtle gestures and facial expressions, it seems that it is precisely the explicit, tangible, visible forms of order that are more readily accessible to the person with autism. If he is to be able to share in this, the non-autistic will have to make more effort and it is from the *autist* that he will learn things about a shared life: from centre to periphery, from subject to object, from internal to external control, from autonomous to heteronomous ordering, the autistic person reminds us of the possibility of building on the socializing influence of other elements.[19] Conversely, it seems to be very difficult for the autistic person to create a form of subjectivity that does not get lost in the world of things. In that regard the non-autistic has the advantage, and there are things to be learnt from him.

These findings suggest that in this company it is more about the question as to how to live with differences, rather than a one-sided effort to make up the autistic deficit. This brings us, thirdly and finally, to the *ideal* that people continue to cherish and to the normative nature of the work done in a shared existence. What is usually regarded as happiness is probably the same for autistic people, albeit that this happiness, according to Peeters, has in part to be sought in 'another dimension': the aim for development towards the non-autistic ideal is tempered by the realization that it 'stops somewhere' and that 'ordinary forms of meaningfulness are not accessible to them.'[20] Conversely, it has to be said that to some extent the non-autistic similarly has no access to what it is that gives content to the life of a person with autism. What is usually regarded as meaningful is at the same time aiming too high and yet too limited to do justice to what moves this company at all its levels.

The ideals of a 'meaningful life' originating in the familiar non-autistic context are reiterated in the interactions between autistic and non-autistic people. Social, communicative and imaginative competences are still always important ingredients of what it means to live as a human being. Social recognition, however, is no longer solely focused on the recognition of people, but on the socializing contributions that the different members of this motley crew have to offer. Communication is no longer focused on the exchange of messages that shore up the social-emotional traffic, but extends to the maintenance of a whole series of relationships - ranging from meaningful connections to physical connections - that the members of this heterogeneous company maintain among themselves. Social imagination and understanding, finally, no longer give priority to the ability to put oneself in another person's mental experience; it is much more about setting out narratives and other (extra-mental) means of transport that enable us to travel to other characters, places and times within this company and to make a shared form of life conceivable.

*Shower, Teeth and Bed*

What is absent in the relations between autistic and non-autistic people, Ian Hacking argues, is 'a kind of immediate understanding' of the other person's inner life from the look in their eyes, their face, their bodily movements and gestures - an instant 'seeing' that Wolfgang Köhler, in his 1929 *Gestalt Psychology*, considered 'the common property and practice of mankind.'[21] It is precisely these common ways of understanding, Hacking counters, that are '*not* familiar, automatic, immediate or instinctive for most autistic people.'[22] This lack of fluency, however, must not be attributed unilaterally to the autistic side of the relationship. 'Conversely, ordinary people cannot see what an autistic boy is doing when, to take a banal example, he is furiously flapping his hands.'[23] Whereas mutual understanding usually does not require any inferences, what is going on in this autistic boy can, at best, only be inferred. Employing Wittgenstein's phrasing, Hacking concludes from this that 'neurotypicals and severely autistic people do not initially share a form of life because the bedrock is lacking, and so an artificial platform must be constructed.'[24]

I started my book discussing the origins and effects of some popular metaphors of autism. In Hacking's opinion, the popularity of the metaphor of the 'alien' in fiction and factual writing on autism can be explained by the absence of the phenomena that Köhler identified. In order to better appreciate what we may nevertheless share in life and to normalize the discourse between autists and neurotypicals, says Hacking, we need to come up with better terms. Our ordinary language for the understanding of inner experiences falls short, though:

> there has been a language for the intentions, desires and emotions of other people for the whole of history. It was, however, crafted by and for neurotypicals. We are only just beginning to adapt that language to autistic life.[25]

Life-writing, internet blogs and the like may provide a more level playing field for exchange than ordinary communicative situations, because they do not depend on Köhler's phenomena. However, as we have seen, alternative grounds for a shared form of life take shape outside the language community as well. In this book we have visited some of these artificial platforms in the making that revolve around concrete qualities of the world.

Where people with and without autism come in contact with one another, the singular character of the community of people among themselves is a matter of constant discussion. Certainly this is a relatively rare situation with a strange logic of its own. At the same time the shared existence of autistic and non-autistic people displays familiar features. The desire for company, for instance, remains strong even under these extreme circumstances. We *want* autistic people as our companions. But the way that companionship is shaped is often reduced to a stereotypical non-autistic conception of living together. This has proved only partly tenable.

A non-autistic concept of society, in which the mind has become the yardstick for everything we find important in one another's company (empathy, interpretation, communication) and autistic people by definition occupy a marginal position, gets in the way of a proper understanding of a shared existence. It is only by applying a correction to the dualistic vocabulary which is normally at our disposal, that it becomes clear how in practice problems of rapport are often solved in unexpected ways. Admittedly, more and better concepts can do nothing to alter the fact that significant differences between the two will *continue* to exist in practice. But this does not mean to say that the conceptual detour we have taken here makes no difference and that we might just as well have stayed at home. Whereas social deficits and social abilities normally split along the autistic/not autistic dividing line, here they are redistributed among those involved. This sheds a different light on the nature and workings of the community of people among themselves.

In his essay, 'Walker Evans: archeoloog van de oppervlakte' [Walker Evans; Archaeologist of the Surface], J. Bernlef describes a photograph by Evans. Amidst the scattered things in the poverty-stricken interior Evans photographed, a child sits forlornly. 'There is a very good reason why the boy looks so rootless. He does not know what living in a home is. This interior is as changeable and accidental as driftwood washed up on the beach.'[26] Living seems to be the sole preserve of those who have the means to do it. 'Only the well-to-do, within the walls of their house, can force life outside the door to come to a standstill, can domesticate in an interior an order which, however precarious it may be, still gives a sense of duration and hence of safety,'[27] writes Bernlef.

It is tempting to see in this description a metaphor for the contrast between the comfort of the life of a non-autistic and the reality of the rootless existence of the autistic person. The former imagines himself to be safely housed; for the latter, recalling the metaphor in *Vallende ster*, the door to the outside world stands wide open and the draughts whistle through the house. But even if the resources are limited, as they are in the dealings between people with autism and non-autistic people, 'nevertheless no human being ever wholly abandons himself to chaos. Even after a disastrous flood, he takes his hastily grabbed household goods and makes a place, a nest, a sort of interior in the empty hall of an abandoned factory'[28] to protect himself from the elements.

In the interaction between autistic and non-autistic people, the mutual rapport between people is put to the test and placed under a magnifying glass. We are indeed gregarious beings, we can infer from this, but of an unusual species. This presents an interesting perspective on the question as to what work normally remains concealed, what exactly is involved, when non-autistic people make companions of *one another*.

And that walk? It took us along bumpy paths, beside fields of ripening wheat, past cows in the meadow - Robert usually trailing behind the rest of the group, David way ahead. Tim and Bart usually stayed closer, and Rick sometimes went off on his own with one of the care workers. Travelling is work and walking makes you thirsty. So when we got home, we had some lemonade. And then it was time for showers, teeth and bed.

# Notes

## Introduction

[1] F. Happé, *Autism: An Introduction to Psychological Theory*, Harvard University Press, Cambridge, MA, 1995, p. 112.

[2] To paraphrase the title of one of the earliest publications on autism in a popular ladies' magazine in the Netherlands. See: J. Bromet, 'Kinderen die van onze wereld niets begrijpen,' *Margriet*, Vol. 39, 12 June, 1976, p. 70.

[3] American Psychiatric Association, *Diagnostic and Statistical Manual of Mental Disorders*, 4th rev. text edn, Author, Washington DC, 2000, pp. 69-85. Estimates vary according to the criteria that are used in defining the syndrome. See chapter 2 on the epidemiology.

[4] American Psychiatric Association, op. cit., p. 75.

[5] U. Frith, *Autism: Explaining the Enigma*, 2nd edn, Blackwell Publishers, Malden MA/Oxford UK, 2003. The developmental psychologist Frith says that myths, legends and fairy tales reveal that there have probably always been children living in the public consciousness whom today we would call autistic, with features that are independent of socio-cultural influences. For a brief discussion on constructivist alternatives for such a realist history of autism, see chapter 2.

[6] Source: W. R. Albury, 'From Changeling to Space Alien: Popular Culture and the "Otherness" of the Autistic Person,' *Building Bridges: Proceedings of the 1995 National Autism Conference*, Autistic Children's Association of Queensland, Brisbane, 1995, pp. 1-6. For the comparison, see e.g. C. C. Park, *The Siege: The First Eight Years of an Autistic Child, With an Epilogue, Fifteen Years Later*, Little, Brown and Company, Boston and Toronto, 1982.

[7] See: J.-M. G. Itard, 'The Wild Boy of Aveyron' (1801/1807), in L. Malson, *Wolf Children and the Problem of Human Nature*, Monthly Review Press, New York, 1972.

[8] L. Kanner, 'Autistic Disturbances of Affective Contact,' *The Nervous Child: Quarterly Journal of Psychopathology*, Vol. 2, 1943, p. 249.

[9] L. Wing, 'Review of H. Lane, The Wild Boy of Aveyron,' *Journal of Autism and Developmental Disorders*, Vol. 8, No. 1, 1978, p. 121.

[10] Albury, op. cit.

[11] O. Sacks, *The Man Who Mistook His Wife for a Hat*, Simon and Schuster, New York, 1985, p. 220.

[12] Ibid., p. 218.

[13] 'Multiverse' is a term that Sacks borrowed from William James to indicate that the worldview of autistic people, lacking any concept of meaningful connections, cannot be called a *universe*. According to this view, an autistic person sees the world in fragments.

[14] Ibid., p. 221.

[15] See: A. F. Bance, 'The Kaspar Hauser Legend and its Literary Survival,' *German Life and Letters*, Vol. 28, No. 3, 1975, pp. 199-210 and RD Theisz, 'Kaspar Hauser im zwanstigsten Jahrhundert: der Aussenseiter und die Gesellschaft,' *The German Quarterly*, Vol. 49, No. 2, 1976, pp. 168-180.

[16] The analogy with Sacks's interest in the abilities of José and other autistic artists is evident. See also Sacks's description of Stephen Wiltshire, in whose drawings he sees great similarities to José's work, in: O Sacks, *An Anthropologist on Mars: Seven Paradoxical Tales*, Alfred A. Knopf, New York, 1995. Still, Frith (op. cit.) comes to the conclusion that Hauser was probably not really autistic, because in her view he did not display the characteristic autistic aloneness, the inability to engage with other people.

[17] Theisz, op. cit.. Sacks (op. cit., 1985) also makes the connection between moral purity and autism, after he has rejected a symbolic explanation for José's drawing and concludes: 'Back to the safe, Edenic, prelapsarian Mother Nature' (p. 214). This idea is exemplified in the opening sentence of Rousseau's *Emile*: 'tout est bien, sortant des mains de l'auteur des choses: tout dégénère entre les mains de l'homme' ('everything is well, leaving the hands of the author of things: everything degenerates in man's hands') (cited in: Bance, op. cit., p. 202). This idea of the social origin of evil did not, however, go unchallenged (B. Rang, ''When the Social Environment of a Child Approaches Zero,' *Comenius*, Vol. 27, No. 3, 1987, pp. 316-343). Rousseau's concept is opposed by Jean-Marc Itard for one, who held a more culturally optimistic view. In the 1802 foreword to his essay on the 'savage' of Aveyron, Itard therefore stressed the moralizing character of human society, which for that reason bore the responsibility for civilizing the wild child. 'MAN can find only in the bosom of society the eminent station that was destined for him in nature, and would be, without the aid of civilization, one of the most feeble and least intelligent of animals' (Itard in Malson, op. cit., p. 91).

[18] I. A. van Berckelaer-Onnes, 'Leven naar de letter,' *Tijdschrift voor Orthopedagogiek*, Vol. 31, No. 9, 1992, p. 423. This and other quotes from originally Dutch sources are translated into English by Lynne Richards. Cf. also Haddon's *The Curious Incident of the Dog in the Night-Time*, in which Christopher differentiates as strictly between right and wrong as between the different colours that he associates with these values and cannot stand being mixed up. Take f.i. his reaction when the police ask him whether he killed the dog. The answer is no. But, does Christopher speak the truth? He says he always does: it is not so much a moral *choice*; he simply is incapable of lying.

[19] U. Frith, 'Autism,' *Scientific American*, Vol. 268, June 1993, p. 84. Frith (op. cit., 2003, chapter 1) therefore considers that myths concerned with

autism are important for two reasons. We can sometimes glean surprising insights from early attempts to understand autism, like those which, according to Frith, occur in myths. But we must also be aware of the limitations of myths so that traditional wisdom can be replaced by the system and rigour of scientific knowledge, which is also envisaged in Frith's work.

[20] Albury, op. cit., p. 3.

[21] With a percentage of approximately 15% with an IQ in the normal or above-normal cohort, and a percentage of approximately 70% with an IQ lower than 70, the majority of the autistic population has an *additional* mental impairment. This does not alter the fact that there is an unbalanced development profile within the limited abilities. Aside from the IQ score, some 10% of the autistic population possess exceptional talents, also measured against the non-autistic norm. Conversely, around 50% of the population with exceptional talents in a particular area are autistic (Frith, op. cit., 2003). These talented exceptions used to be described as 'idiot savants'; nowadays people prefer the term 'savant syndrome.'

[22] D. A. Treffert, *Extraordinary People: Understanding Idiot Savants*, Harper and Row, New York [etc.], 1989.

[23] Sacks, op. cit., 1995, p. 241.

[24] S. Murray, *Representing Autism: Culture, Narrative, Fascination*, Liverpool University Press, Liverpool, 2008, p. 99.

[25] Frith, op. cit., 2003, p. 24.

[26] Haddon, op. cit.. For a comparative discussion of the detective and comic, and their bond with the autistic person, see chapter 3 and: R Hendriks, 'De autist, de komiek en de detective,' *Wetenschappelijk Tijdschrift Autisme*, Vol. 5, No. 2, 2006, pp. 60-70.

[27] Sacks, op. cit., 1995, p. 275.

[28] J. Sinclair, 'Bridging the Gaps: An Inside-Out View of Autism (Or, Do You Know What I Don't Know?),' in E. Schopler and G. B. Mesibov (eds), *High-Functioning Individuals With Autism*, Plenum Press, New York and London, 1992, p. 302.

[29] 'Living by the letter' is the opposite title of Van Berckelaer's oration on her inauguration as professor of remedial assistance for children with serious developmental disorders, particularly autistic children, at the University of Leiden, the Netherlands. See: Van Berckelaer-Onnes, op. cit..

[30] Frith, op. cit., 2003, pp. 27-28.

[31] S. Turkle, *The Second Self: Computers and the Human Spirit*, Simon and Schuster, New York, 1984.

[32] Frith, op. cit., 2003, pp. 26-27. But see chapter 5 on the relationship between autism and humour.

[33] Ibid., p. 27.

[34] J.-P. Sartre, *L'être et le néant: essai d'ontologie phénomenologique*, Galimard, Paris, 1943, pp. 298 ff.

[35] L. W. Nauta, *Jean-Paul Sartre*, Het Wereldvenster, Baarn, 1966, p. 48.

[36] H. E. Barnes, 'Sartre's Ontology: The Revealing and Making of Being' in C Howells (ed), *The Cambridge Companion to Sartre*, Cambridge University Press, Cambridge [etc.], 1992, p. 13.

[37] The 'nihilating function of the consciousness' is how Sartre describes this. The jargon in *Being and Nothingness* here relates to the contrast between being as a whole, which has no other consciousness and coincides wholly with itself or is *en-soi* (in-itself), and the consciousness of something that exists as the consciousness of not being this something or is *pour-soi* (for-itself). Sartre also identifies the relationship to the other, the *pour-autrui* (for-others), which we look at in more detail in the main text.

[38] Nauta, op. cit., p. 45.

[39] Ibid., p. 86.

[40] S. Shapin, *The Scientific Revolution*, The University of Chicago Press, Chicago and London, 1998, p. 159.

[41] Sartre's philosophy itself is an attempt to nuance this dualism. The consciousness in Sartre is not located somewhere in the human being, but is an intentional consciousness that is anchored in the world (the consciousness of not being 'something'). The knowing man thus appears as someone who stands in the centre of the world, who acts, observes, et cetera, and hence, according to Nauta (op. cit.), pure rationalism as in Descartes is avoided. Yet, an essentially human quality is preserved with the concept of 'freedom.'

[42] L. Wittgenstein, *Philosophical Investigations*, 3rd edn, Basil Blackwell, Oxford UK/ Cambridge MA, 1994, p. 126e/§ 420.

[43] J. Searle, *Mind, Language, and Society: Doing Philosophy in the Real World*, Weidenfeld and Nicolson, London, 1999.

[44] L. Wing, *Autistic Children: A Guide for Parents*, Constable, London, 1971, p.113.

[45] The fact that the author has skipped the doll-part, keeping the 'passively' in later editions of her book (see e.g. L. Wing, *The Autistic Spectrum: A Guide for Parents and Professionals*, Constable, London, 1996, p. 135) does not mean that it is no longer an issue, but precisely confirms the problematic and sensitive character of a comparison of people with things.

[46] Happé, op. cit., p. 111.

[47] Murray, op. cit., p. 5.

[48] Albury, op. cit.

[49] Park, op. cit., p. 13.

[50] Sacks, op. cit., 1985, p. 220.

[51] Dyson is talking about Jessy Park, whom features as Elly in her mother's work. See: F. Dyson in: W. Kayzer, *A Glorious Accident*, Freeman, New York, 1997, p. 138.

[52] R. P. Hobson, 'Social Perception in High-Level Autism' in Schopler and Mesibov, op. cit., p. 164.

[53] R. Barnes quoted in D. Birkett, 'See It My Way,' *The Guardian*, 23 November, 2002, p. 33. Cf. Murray, op. cit., p. 109, who points at the erasing effects of the portrait.

[54] See: S. Sontag, *Illness as a Metaphor and Aids and Its Metaphors*, Anchor, Doubleday [etc.], 1990. And: M. Somers, 'The Narrative Constitution of Identity: A Relational and Network Approach,' *Theory and Society*, Vol. 23, No. 5, 1994, pp. 605-649.

[55] I. Hacking, 'Autistic Autobiography,' *Philosophical Transactions of the Royal Society Biological Sciences*, nr. 364, 2009, p. 1467.

[56] Albury, op. cit., p. 4. The use of an all-embracing metaphor also brushes out individual differences so that the autistic population is presented as being more coherent than it is. Next, the use of static metaphors conceals the fact that, even for a person with autism, development is possible. If these metaphors are taken literally, there is a risk of overlooking personal stories and studies in which it is clear that the non-metaphorical reality is more complex than suggested, and that the deficits do not necessarily imply the absence of a *desire* for contact.

[57] Murray, op. cit., xvi. On the other hand, we may turn to existing narrative forms to banish our fears, 'we seek to blunt its difference, precisely because of the worries we sense such differences might contain' (pp. 211-212).

[58] Ibid., p. 99.

[59] L. J. Davis (ed), *The Disability Studies Reader*, Routledge, London and New York, 1997.

[60] O. Sacks, *Seeing Voices: A Journey Into the World of the Deaf*, University of California Press, Berkeley, 1989.

[61] Murray, op. cit., xvi.

[62] Sinclair, op. cit., p. 302. Sinclair is the founder of ANI-L, Autism Network International - an electronic communications network for autistic people and their relatives. ANI-L provides an electronic forum where autism is the norm. For years Sinclair has been trying to achieve the emancipation of the world of autistic people as a separate culture rather than a medically-defined departure from the neurologically typical (or non-autistic) norm.

[63] Sinclair adds that it is essential to radically overhaul the familiar concept of culture, rather than conclude that autistic people do not have a culture: 'It takes more work to communicate with someone whose native language isn't the same as yours . . . You're going to have to learn to back up to levels more

basic than you've probably thought about before, to translate, and to check to make sure your translations are understood. You're going to have to give up the certainty that comes of being on your own familiar territory, of knowing you're in charge, and let your child teach you a little of her language, guide you a little way into his world.' (J. Sinclair, 'Don't Mourn for Us,' *Our Voice: Newsletter of Autism Network International*, Vol. 1, No. 3, 1993.

[64] See, for the origin of this characterization: A. Mol, *The Body Multiple: Ontology in Medical Practice*, Duke University Press, Durham, 2002. Mol asks how people manage to integrate illness and the knowledge of illness in their lives, how they succeed making initially alien medical events an ordinary part of life. Mol thus raises the problem of the distinction between the domain of illness claimed by sociologists (the perception of being ill, to which research into disabilities is often confined) and the domain of the disease (the knowledge of a physical disorder), which is left to the doctors.

[65] L. A. Sass, J. Parnas, J. Whiting, 'Mind, Self and Psychopathology: Reflections on Philosophy, Theory and the Study of Mental Illness,' *Theory and Psychology*, Vol. 10, No. 1, 2000, pp. 87-98.

[66] See: S. Baron-Cohen, H. Tager-Flusberg and D. J. Cohen, *Understanding Other Minds: Perspectives From Developmental Cognitive Neurosciences*, 2nd edn, Oxford University Press, Oxford [etc.], 2000. See also chapters 2 and 4.

[67] As Baron-Cohen and Bolton argue: 'In line with the current thinking in the field of disability, we have taken seriously the issue of avoiding terms that may be offensive. In particular, we follow the recent practice of labelling the disability, rather than the person, and agree that this is both more accurate and more humane. This book is therefore about 'children with autism,' and not 'autistic children' or 'autistics.' (S. Baron-Cohen and P. Bolton, *Autism: The Facts*, Oxford University Press, Oxford [etc.], 1993, v.)

**Given Reality**

[1] O. Sacks, *An Anthropologist on Mars: Seven Paradoxical Tales,* Alfred A. Knopf, New York, 1995, p. 246.

[2] U. Frith, *Autism: Explaining the Enigma*, 2nd edn, Blackwell Publishers, Malden MA/Oxford UK, 2003, p. 34.

[3] M. Nadesan, *Constructing Autism: Unravelling the 'Truth' and Understanding the Social*, Routledge, London and New York, 2005, p. 2. One might wonder, for instance, how an autistic person would survive in a world where formal structures like railway timetables, measurements and clocks occupied a less prominent place. How did the autistic mind develop compared with the normal psyche during the history of the development of

the modern individual? What difference did various institutional approaches make?

[4] I. Hacking, *The Social Construction of* What? Harvard University Press, Cambridge, MA/London, England, 1999, esp. pp. 100-124. For another non-essentialist, historicizing view of the origin and development of a psychiatric condition, in this case anorexia nervosa, see: S. van 't Hof, *Anorexia Nervosa, The Historical and Cultural Specificity: Fallacious Theories and Tenacious Facts*, Swets and Zeitlinger, Lisse, 1994. Van 't Hof describes how the modern form of starvation could come about as a meaningful diagnostic category in the course of the nineteenth century, when the possibility that individual mental suffering could be expressed physically actually became conceivable. This is not such a strange comparison when one thinks that anorexia nervosa may perhaps be a female variant of a continuum of empathic disorders to which ('male') autism has been said to belong. See: C. Gillberg, 'Autism and Autistic-Like Conditions: Subclasses Among Disorders of Empathy,' *Journal of Child Psychology and Psychiatry*, Vol. 33, No. 5, 1992, pp. 813-842.

[5] Paedologisch Instituut Nijmegen, *Verslag over de jaren 1937-1938*, Author, Nijmegen, 1938, p. 40.

[6] Paedologisch Instituut Nijmegen, *Verslag over de jaren 1939-1940*, Author, Nijmegen, 1940, p. 39.

[7] The Nijmegen children were said to have stood out because of a stereotyped form of repetitive behaviour and a deficit of automatic behaviour regulation, a lack of vital contact with their environment, generally delayed development, among other things of the communication functions, and, in comparison, a remarkable superiority in conceiving and controlling form, great resistance to change, a discrepancy between a good memory and a lack of independent insight, and anxiety prompted by uncertainty.

[8] L. Kanner, 'Autistic Disturbances of Affective Contact,' *The Nervous Child: Quarterly Journal of Psychopathology*, Vol. 2, 1943, p. 217 *et passim*. Emphases in the original.

[9] These children also did not experience the deterioration usual in schizophrenia, but actually improved, so that over time their aloneness was overcome to varying degrees: 'One might perhaps put it this way: While the schizophrenic tries to solve his problem by stepping out of a world of which he has been a part and with which he has been in touch, our children gradually *compromise* by extending cautious feelers into a world in which they have been total strangers from the beginning.' See: Ibid., p. 249.

[10] Ibid., p. 250.

[11] L. Eisenberg and L. Kanner, 'Early Infantile Autism, 1943-1955,' *American Journal of Orthopsychiatry*, Vol. 26, 1956, p. 557.

[12] Ibid., p. 558.

[13] M. Rutter, 'Diagnosis and Definition of Childhood Autism,' *Journal of Autism and Childhood Schizophrenia*, Vol. 8, No. 2, 1978, pp. 139-161.

[14] When he used the term 'autism' at the beginning of the twentieth century, Bleuler was referring to a *withdrawal* from social reality and an escape into a fantasy world typical of schizophrenia, whereas the children concerned here seemed to be conspicuous for their *lack* of imagination and inability to *develop* meaningful relationships (see: Rutter, op. cit.). The hallucinations typical of schizophrenia also proved to be absent here. The term 'autism' was therefore also burdened with a connotation that did insufficient justice to the nature of the disorder as it was presented by Kanner.

[15] The study looked at sixty-three children 'for [each of] whom an unequivocal diagnosis of child psychosis, schizophrenic syndrome of childhood, infantile autism, or any symptoms of these had been agreed by all Maudsley Hospital consultant psychiatrists who had seen the child.' (M. Rutter, M. and L. Lockyer, 'A Five to Fifteen Year Follow-Up Study of Infantile Psychosis: I. Description of Sample,' *British Journal of Psychiatry*, Vol. 113, No. 504, 1967, p. 1169) This group was compared with a non-psychotic control group, matched for age, sex and IQ, who did, however, have other mental disorders and behavioural problems. Criteria customary at the time were used in the selection of the psychotic group. Another selection criterion was that the children had not yet reached puberty, so that the chance of selecting better-known forms of schizophrenia, which peaked in adolescence, was slight. The groups were tested for the presence and severity of 34 characteristics that were then seen as indicative of 'infantile psychosis.'

[16] Disintegrating conditions later in childhood (which first come to light after the third year), in contrast, are admittedly reminiscent of autism, but these children differ in their behaviour and in that they are suffering from demonstrable, structural, progressive brain conditions (Rutter, op. cit.).

[17] According to the multiple rationale behind the classification: a reflection of and at the same time a means of increasing knowledge, an aid in early diagnosis and in clinical interventions and a rhetorical tool for use in securing public funds (cf. National Society for Autistic Children, 'Definition of the Syndrome of Autism,' *Journal of Autism and Childhood Schizophrenia*, Vol. 8, No. 2, 1978, pp. 162-167). For the pragmatic and other aspects of classification, see: F. R. Volkmar, A. Klin and D. J. Cohen, 'Diagnosis and Classification of Autism and Related Conditions: Consensus and Issues' in D. J. Cohen and F. R. Volkmar (eds), *Handbook of Autism and Pervasive Developmental Disorders*, 2nd edn, John Wiley and Sons, New York [etc.], 1997, pp. 5-40.

[18] At an IQ of below 50, neurological disorders are more frequent, epilepsy is more likely to set in puberty, the affective disorder is more severe and deeper, and there are more stereotypical behaviours and self-mutilating tendencies (I. A. van Berckelaer-Onnes and H. van Engeland, *Kinderen en autisme: onderkenning, behandeling en begeleiding*, (2nd edn, Boom, Meppel and Amsterdam, 1992). Abnormalities in social or communicative behaviours must therefore always be viewed in relation to the developmental age.

[19] Rutter, op. cit., p. 156.

[20] This shift in orientation was expressed in the change in the name of the *Journal of Autism and Childhood Schizophrenia* founded by Kanner in 1971: since its ninth volume (1979) it has been called the *Journal of Autism and Developmental Disorders*. For the motivation behind this change in scope and title, see the editorial by: E. Schopler, M. Rutter and S. Chess, 'Change of Journal Scope and Title,' *Journal of Autism and Developmental Disorders*, Vol. 9, No. 1, 1979, pp. 1-10.

[21] See: L. Wing and J. Gould, 'Systematic Recording of Behaviors and Skills of Retarded and Psychotic Children,' *Journal of Autism and Childhood Schizophrenia*, Vol. 8, No. 1, 1978, pp. 79-97. And: L. Wing and J. Gould, 'Severe Impairments of Social Interaction and Associated Abnormalities in Children: Epidemiology and Classification,' *Journal of Autism and Developmental Disorders*, Vol. 9, No. 1, 1979, pp. 11-29.

[22] It should be noted that over time, influenced by new insights, there has been a shift in the way Wing defines the 'triad of impairments' (later: the triad of *social* impairments). In 1988, Wing refers to an impairment in *social* recognition, *social* communication and *social* imagination and understanding. (See: L. Wing, 'The Continuum of Autistic Characteristics,' in E. Schopler and G. B. Mesibov (eds), *Diagnosis and Assessment in Autism*, Plenum Press, New York and London, 1988, pp. 91-110). Abnormal language alone, in 1979 still one of the necessary criteria (together with, among other things, motor and sensory abnormalities), is no longer regarded as essential: in terms of language what remains as the core of the autistic disorder is the impairment in social use.

[23] In 1981 Wing was the first author to introduce the term Asperger's syndrome to the English-speaking world. In his 1944 book Asperger described four children between the ages of 6 and 11, who represented a larger group of patients with manifest difficulties in social integration, despite apparently normal intelligence and verbal skill (For an annotated English translation, see: U. Frith (ed), *Autism and Asperger Syndrome*, Cambridge University Press, Cambridge [etc.], 1991). The defining social problem existed alongside a number of associated characteristics: difficulties with non-verbal communication, idiosyncratic use of language, egocentric

preoccupation that gets in the way of social integration, an intellectual rather than an intuitive approach to emotional matters, physical clumsiness and poor kinaesthesis, and behavioural problems (such as aggression and social maladjustment). Asperger reported that the disorder was not recognizable in early childhood and occurred almost exclusively in boys, and that similar traits were always found in the family. Source: A. Klin and F. R. Volkmar, 'Asperger's Syndrome' in Cohen and Volkmar, op. cit., pp. 94-122.

[24] Frith, op. cit., 1991.

[25] L. Wing, 'The Relationship between Asperger's Syndrome and Kanner's Autism' in Frith, op. cit., 1991, pp. 93-121. Klin and Volkmar, op. cit., provide an overview of studies in which the supposed distinction is argued, but they also point to the lack of generally accepted diagnostic guidelines. There is, though, agreement about a provisional working definition - in *DSM-IV-TR* Asperger's syndrome is defined according to the following criteria: a qualitative impairment in social interaction; restricted repetitive and stereotyped patterns of behaviour, interests, and activities; the disturbance causes clinically significant impairment in social, occupational, or other important areas of functioning; there is no clinically significant general delay in language; there is no clinically significant delay in cognitive development or in the development of age-appropriate self-help skills, adaptive behaviour (other than in social interaction), and curiosity about the environment in childhood; and criteria are not met for another specific Pervasive Developmental Disorder or Schizophrenia (American Psychiatric Association, *DSM-IV-TR*, p. 84). Asperger himself acknowledged that there were similarities between the two groups, but was nonetheless convinced that the children he had described belonged in an essentially different category from Kanner's (F. Happé, *Autism: An Introduction to Psychological Theory*, Harvard University Press, Cambridge, MA, 1995). 'Whether Asperger's Disorder will remain a distinct category or will be reintegrated in the spectrum of autism remains to be seen,' was the more cautious formulation of: Volkmar, Klin and Cohen, op. cit., p. 28.

[26] Wing, op. cit., 1988, p. 92.

[27] Frith, op. cit., 2003, p. 60.

[28] Wing, however, points out that her spectrum is still slightly broader on the one hand than the *DSM-IV* system, since it includes 'the most subtle manifestations of the triad' (L. Wing, 'Syndromes of Autism and Atypical Development' in Cohen and Volkmar, op. cit., p. 153) and on the other narrower than the WHO's ICD-10 classification, because that includes a category that does not require any deficit in socialization, whereas this is considered essential for the autistic spectrum.

[29] I. Kok and P. Koedoot, *Hulpverlening bij autisme in Nederland*, Trimbos-instituut, Utrecht, 1998.

[30] American Psychiatric Association, *Diagnostic and Statistical Manual of Mental Disorders*, 4th rev. text edn, Author, Washington DC, 2000, pp. 69-85. Autism - described as 'infantile autism' - appeared for the first time as a separate diagnostic category in the *DSM-III* (1980); Rutter's 1978 definition was influential here. In this version, however, there was a striking lack of developmental perspective and an exclusive focus on a language (rather than communication) disorder (Volkmar, Klin and Cohen, op. cit.). There was a response to this criticism in the successor *DSM-IIIR* (1987), under the heading 'autistic disorder': it left scope to take into account changes that could occur over the years and in a person's individual development. *DSM-IIIR* drew on Wing and Gould's broader 1979 definition and dropped the early onset requirement. After empirical testing, another correction was made in *DSM-IV*: it specified an age limit of three years and gave proportionally greater weight to the impaired socialization function. PDD-NOS (PDD Not Otherwise Specified) offers a diagnostic refuge within the category for a great many children (including those with 'atypical' autism) whose condition cannot be taken into account for various categories because they only partly satisfy the required criteria. The criteria for PDD-NOS were tightened up in the revised *DSM-IV-TR*: in order to merit the diagnosis there has to be an impairment in more than one area, instead of the erroneously stated requirement that there needed to be an impairment in just one of the areas (social interaction, communication, stereotypical behaviours).

[31] M. Rutter and E. Schopler (eds), *Autism: A Reappraisal of Concepts and Treatment*, Plenum Press, New York and London, 1978, p. 16.

[32] Cohen and Volkmar, op. cit., p. 2.

[33] American Psychiatric Association, op. cit., p. 73.

[34] For Asperger's syndrome alone, Gillberg and Gillberg in 1989 reported even higher (albeit less reliable) results: 10 to 26 per 10,000 children of normal intelligence. Klin and Volkmar, op. cit., in 1997 report a minimal prevalence of Asperger's Syndrome in 3.6 per 1,000 children in the 7-16 year-old age group, rising to 7.1 per 1,000 children if suspect cases are added! If future research confirms these figures it would mean that Asperger's syndrome is a much more common disorder than the relatively rare autistic disorder.

[35] Frith, op. cit., 2003, p. 59. Cf. S. Chakrabarti and E. Fombonne, 'Pervasive Developmental Disorders in Preschool Children,' *JAMA*, Vol. 285, No. 24, 2001, pp. 3093-3099.

[36] R. R. Grinker, *Unstrange Minds: Remapping the World of Autism*, Basic Books Inc, New York, 2008, p. 11. Grinker's realism seems to rule out the

possible effect of cultural changes on the way autistic symptoms manifest themselves. For a critique, see the work of Ian Hacking discussed before.

[37] Ibid., p. 5.

[38] Of the group of 63 children Rutter and Lockyer examined, 40% had an IQ below 50, and 30% an IQ between 50 and 70. Half of the 30% with an IQ of more than 70 achieved a normal score. Of the children with the triad in the Camberwell Study (which showed a bias towards low IQs because these were children known to the social, health and/or educational services), only 3% could be placed in the normal range (IQ 70+), 14% displayed mild mental retardation (IQ 50-70), 42% had an IQ between 20 and 50 (severe to moderate), and 41% were very severely mentally retarded children (with an IQ < 20). See: Frith, op. cit., 2003.

[39] See also: N. O'Connor and B. Hermelin, 'Low Intelligence and Special Abilities. Annotation,' *Journal of Child Psychology and Psychiatry*, Vol. 29, No. 4, 1988, pp. 391-396. Treffert, going on a study by Rimland, even refers to a figure of 9.8% with special skills (D. A. Treffert, *Extraordinary People: Understanding 'Idiot Savants,'* Harper and Row, New York [etc.], 1989. Conversely, a maximum of 50% of the population with what is nowadays known as savant syndrome are autistic (Frith, op. cit., 2003). There are no adequate explanations for the phenomenon. Treffert discusses a number of possible causes, such as an exceptionally well-developed visual memory. Another is that savants are not distracted by the normal (social and communication) worries of human existence, and can (and must) focus on isolated facets of a concrete order.

[40] S. E. Bryson, 'Epidemiology of Autism: Overview and Issues Outstanding,' in Cohen and Volkmar, op. cit., pp. 41-46. It should be noted here that the PDD label may have a sex-specific bias: it is suggested that as a result of compensating skills an underlying defect is less likely to be expressed in social deficits and can come out in other ways in females, whereas *DSM-IV-TR* differentiates chiefly according to social skills or the absence of them. Asperger regarded the syndrome that bears his name as an extreme variant of typical male cognitive capacities.

[41] Eisenberg and Kanner, op. cit.. In order to describe the nature of the social impairment in the autistic syndrome, I can only touch on a few of the main points in the extensive and detailed reports that exist in this field. I derive the structure according to age stages from: Van Berckelaer-Onnes and Van Engeland, op. cit.. In addition to the sources that are specifically referred to, I am drawing on: T Peeters, *Autisme: van begrijpen tot begeleiden*, Hadewijch, Antwerpen and Baarn, 1994; F. Volkmar, A. Carter, J. Grossman and A. Klin, 'Social Development in Autism,' in Cohen and Volkmar, op. cit., pp.

173-194; and: L. Wing, *The Autistic Spectrum: A Guide for Parents and Professionals*, Constable, London, 1996.

[42] Wing, op. cit., 1988, p. 92. Note that in the triad of social impairments Wing includes social recognition, communication and imagination in their social capacity. Here I confine my use of the term socialization chiefly to what she calls 'social recognition.' Communication and imagination are treated separately.

[43] S. Baron-Cohen and P. Bolton, *Autism: The Facts*. Oxford University Press, Oxford, New York, Tokyo, 1993.

[44] Wing and Gould, op. cit., 1979.

[45] I have called upon just a few main points in the literature to describe the nature of the communication impairment. I have taken the information in this section from: Baron-Cohen and Bolton, op. cit.; Van Berckelaer-Onnes and Van Engeland, op. cit.; Kanner, op. cit.; S. van der Kolk-Wolthaar, 'Taalstoornissen bij kinderen met autisme,' *Logopedie en Foniatrie*, Vol. 56, No. 2, pp. 12-16; C. Lord and R. Paul, 'Language and Communication in Autism' in Cohen and Volkmar, op. cit., pp. 195-225; Peeters, op. cit.; D. M. Ricks and L. Wing, 'Language, Communication and the Use of Symbols' in L. Wing (ed), Early Childhood Autism, 2nd edn, Pergamom, Oxford [etc.], 1996, pp. 93-134; H. Tager-Flusberg, 'On the Nature of Linguistic Functioning of Early Infantile Autism, *Journal of Autism and Developmental Disorders*, Vol. 11, No. 1, 1981, pp. 45-56.

[46] In part A of the *DSM-IV-TR* criteria deficits in language and imagination are *both* classified under communication skills. Taking my lead from Wing, op. cit., 1988, I deal with impairments in communication as separate, albeit closely related symptoms. Unlike Wing, I also include language impairment under the heading of communication.

[47] Opinions differ as to what precisely should be understood by 'usable' language. There is often an absence of consistent behaviours, for instance when a child incidentally says a few words or even one or two whole sentences in the 12-18 months period, but then never says another meaningful word. In general such incidental use of words seldom leads to usable communication. Any discussion of usable language raises the question as to how spontaneous the use of language has to be, how frequent and how comprehensible, and the extent to which what has been learned is generalized. In the absence of standardized criteria in these areas, there are various figures for the number of autistic children who never achieve usable language. With all the reservations mentioned, Lord and Paul (op. cit.), report some statistical support for a figure of 50% in whom usable language develops.

[48] The transposition of 'I' and 'you' has always appealed strongly to the imagination. A since discredited psychodynamic interpretation held that the transposition of personal pronouns represents the refusal of the 'I' to become involved in the world. From the point of view of theory of language, however, it is a problem of deixis, of indicating with the aid of language, in which the pragmatics of the relationship between speaker and listener is a factor (Van der Kolk-Wolthaar, op. cit.).

[49] In the APA system impairments in imaginative play and social imitation play are therefore included under the heading of 'communication.' In line with Wing's triad, I treat the impairment in imagination as a separate category. The information, again only in broad outline, is taken from: Van Berckelaer-Onnes and Van Engeland, op. cit.; Lord and Paul, op. cit.; T. Peeters, *Over autisme gesproken*, Dekker and V.d. Vegt, Nijmegen, 1980; Peeters, op. cit., 1994; Volkmar, Carter, Grossman and Klin, op. cit.; L. Wing, J. Gould, S. R. Yeates and L. M. Brierley, 'Symbolic Play in Severely Mentally Retarded and in Autistic Children,' *Journal of Child Psychology and Psychiatry*, Vol. 18, No. 2, 1977, pp. 167-178; Wing and Gould, op. cit., 1979; next to sources that are referred to in the text.

[50] S. B. Wulff, 'The Symbolic and Object Play of Children with Autism: A Review,' *Journal of Autism and Developmental Disorders*, Vol. 15, No. 2, 1985, p. 140.

[51] A comparative study found that none of the autistic children in the group studied displayed imaginative play and 33% played only in a stereotypical way, by simple, constantly repeated manipulation of objects; 87% of the mentally handicapped children showed symbolic play, 2% stereotypical play and only 11% no imaginative play at all. See: Wing, Gould, Yeates and Brierley, op. cit.

[52] Wing, op. cit., 1988, p. 94.

[53] Ricks and Wing, op. cit., p. 107.

[54] Although always present, according to Wing this rigid proclivity for repetition is not diagnostically relevant in itself because it sometimes also occurs in individuals who are not autistic. Wing regards the rigid, repetitive pattern of behaviour rather as an *effect* of the triad of social impairments (Wing, op. cit., 1988). The APA, though, does mark the deficit as an essential characteristic. Essential or not, it is without doubt an important behavioural characteristic. For this section I have used: Van Berckelaer-Onnes and Van Engeland, op. cit.; M. Davies and L. Kommandeur, *Anders dan anderen*, Donker, Rotterdam, 1982; Wing, op. cit., 1988; and Wing and Gould, op. cit., 1979.

[55] Kanner, op. cit., p. 245.

[56] Davies and Kommandeur, op. cit., p. 46.

[57] R. P. Hobson, 'Social Perception in High-Level Autism' in E. Schopler and G. B. Mesibov (eds), *High Functioning Individuals with Autism*, Plenum Press, New York and London, 1992, p. 157.

[58] W. R. Albury, 'Autism: The Experts Still Differ,' *Australian Doctor*, April 2, 1993, pp. 65-66.

[59] Bettelheim, *The Empty Fortress: Infantile Autism and the Birth of the Self*, Free Press, New York, 1967, p. 126.

[60] L. Kanner, Problems of Nosology and Psychodynamics in Early Infantile Autism, *American Journal of Orthopsychiatry*, Vol. 19, 1949, p. 422, p. 425 [Reprinted in: L. Kanner, *Childhood Psychosis: Initial Studies and New Insights*, Winston and Sons, Washington, 1973, p. 58, p. 61].

[61] Eisenberg and Kanner, op. cit., p. 562.

[62] Ibid., p. 561.

[63] Ibid., p. 562.

[64] Ibid., p. 563.

[65] Albury, op. cit.

[66] Eisenberg and Kanner, op. cit., p. 563-564.

[67] Ibid., p. 563.

[68] According to Albury (op. cit.), in 1968 Kanner found himself between two extremes: between Bettelheim, who supported a purely psychodynamic approach and Rimland (on whom more later), who advocated a purely biological explanation. Bettelheim completely lost sight of the message that a biological predisposition can be a factor. But seen from Kanner's position, Rimland's biological approach overlooked equally crucial factors. Rimland was, however, closely involved in the founding of the American parents' association in 1965. Although in terms of substance Kanner was actually closer to Bettelheim than Rimland, the parents' hero, in his address to the American parents' association in 1968 he publicly distanced himself from Bettelheim's psychodynamic theory. Kanner blamed suggestions that he also supported a psychogenic explanation on selective quoting (which was indeed the case). Wisely, however, he did not mention his unchanged psychobiological view, which advocated the integral study of biological, psychological and social factors. This meant that after 1968 Kanner could be embraced as the founding father of autism research.

[69] N. Tinbergen and E. A. Tinbergen, *Autistic Children: New Hope for Cure*, Allen and Unwin, London, 1983, p. 155. Also see: E. A. Tinbergen and N. Tinbergen, *Early Childhood Autism: An Ethological Approach*, Verlag Paul Parey, Berlin and Hamburg, 1972.

[70] Tinbergen and Tinbergen, op. cit., 1983, p. 147. Italics are in the original.

[71] Admittedly, organic brain disorders could by no means always be demonstrated in people with autism, but conversely there was a connection.

Rimland also rebutted the notions of 'nurture' rather than 'nature' being to blame by pointing out that parents with an autistic child often had other, non-autistic children. Autistic children behaved abnormally from the moment they were born. In almost all cases of autism in twins, they were identical, and there was a consistent male/ female ratio. According to Rimland, many, but not all, parents of autistic children fitted the picture described by Kanner of detached and intelligent personalities, but he believed that this could indicate a genetic factor. Finally, Rimland argued that the autistic symptomatology was unique and specific and that there was no sliding scale from normal to impaired. (B. Rimland, *Infantile Autism: The Syndrome and Its Implications for a Neural Theory of Behaviour*, Meredith Publishing Company, New York, 1964)

[72] Tinbergen and Tinbergen, op. cit., 1983, p. 133.

[73] For a review of the pattern of mother blaming that emerged in this debate see: J. T. McDonnell, 'Mothering an Autistic Child: Reclaiming the Voice of the Mother' in B. A. Daly and M. T. Reddy (eds), *Narrating Mothers: Theorizing Maternal Subjectivities*, The University of Tennessee Press, Knoxville, 1991, pp. 58-75.

[74] E. Schopler, C. A. Andrews and K. Strupp, 'Do Autistic Children Come From Upper-Middle-Class Parents?,' *Journal of Autism and Developmental Disorders*, Vol. 9, No. 2, 1979, pp. 139-152. Cf. Frith, op. cit., 2003.

[75] D. Cantwell, L. Baker and M. Rutter, 'Family Factors' in Rutter and Schopler, op. cit., pp. 269-296.

[76] See: Baron-Cohen and Bolton, op. cit.; Frith, op. cit., 2003; Happé, op. cit.

[77] Cf. Frith, op. cit., 2003. Or: 'The capacity for emotional bonding, attachment behaviour, is buried so deep in our brains (in the limbic system) that it appears to be 'protected' from lesser defects of the cerebral system. It is only in autism that these deep structures, which usually safeguard the roots of social conduct, also seem to be affected.' (Peeters, op. cit., 1994, p. 136)

[78] EEG measurements show, among other things, abnormal processing patterns for unknown sounds. Brain scans produce an abundance of confusing and non-specific results. Post-mortem studies have revealed a series of abnormalities in the brains of autistic individuals, particularly in the frontal lobes of the cerebrum (responsible for, among other things, planning and control), in the limbic system (responsible for, among other things, emotional response), in the brain stem and the fourth ventricle, and in the cerebellum (responsible for, among other things, motor coordination). The hippocampus (important to memory function) has a different structure, as does the pineal gland, where sensory and other information is integrated. Autistic persons have enlarged ventricles, and other areas of the brain are also larger; only the frontal lobe is (possibly only relatively) small. The cerebellum is either too

large or too small. Caution is crucial, however, wrote Baron-Cohen and Bolton (op. cit.): it is unclear which defects are specific to autism and which relate to the mental handicap that often accompanies it.

[79] B. Hermelin and N. O'Connor, *Psychological Experiments with Autistic Children*, Pergamon Press, Oxford [etc.], 1970, p. 126.

[80] Ricks and Wing, op. cit., p. 122.

[81] U. Frith, 'Autism,' *Scientific American*, Vol. 268, June, 1993, p. 83. For the Theory of Mind hypothesis, see: S. Baron-Cohen, A. M. Leslie and U. Frith, 'Does the Autistic Child Have a Theory of Mind?,' *Cognition*, Vol. 21, No. 1, 1985, pp. 37-46.

[82] S. Baron-Cohen, *Mindblindness: An Essay on Autism and Theory of Mind*, MIT Press, Cambridge, MA and London, 1995.

[83] Frith, op. cit., 2003.

[84] C. Hughes and J. Russell, 'Autistic Children's Difficulty with Mental Disengagement From an Object: Its Implications for Theories of Autism,' *Developmental Psychology*, Vol. 29, No. 3, 1993, p. 507. Also see: S. Baron-Cohen and J. Swettenham, 'Theory of Mind in Autism: Its Relationship to Executive Function and Central Coherence' in Cohen and Volkmar, op. cit., pp. 880-893.

[85] S. J. Weeks and R. P. Hobson, 'The Salience of Facial Expression for Autistic Children,' *Journal of Child Psychology and Psychiatry*, Vol. 28, No. 1, 1987, pp. 137-151.

[86] Hobson, op. cit., p. 164.

[87] 'While agreeing that autistic subjects fail to acquire a fully developed concept of 'persons' with minds, Hobson disagrees with those who want to diagnose this deficit in intellectualistic or cognitivist terms. He views this deficit as caused and perhaps even constituted largely by failures of affect, or more precisely by 'affective-cognitive-conative' factors' (L. A. Sass, J. Parnas and J. Whiting, 'Mind, Self and Psychopathology: Reflections on Philosophy, Theory and the Study of Mental Illness,' *Theory and Psychology*, Vol. 10, No. 1, 2000, p. 93). Hobson derives his arguments in part from the philosophical work of Merleau-Ponty, Heidegger and Wittgenstein. See: R. P. Hobson, 'Against the Theory of 'Theory of Mind',' *British Journal of Developmental Psychology*, Vol. 9, No. 1, 1991, pp. 33-51.

[88] Psychodynamic theorizing in regard to autism is now almost exclusively referred to by way of a negative point of departure - a seemingly somewhat dutiful exercise for which authors nonetheless found good reasons in the past. According to some (e.g. Wing, op. cit., 1996), psychotherapy can provide helpful support in the event of mental need in people with autism who have mastered language and developed an ability to symbolize. Rather than dismissing psychodynamic theorizing about autism as unscientific, outdated

and immoral, Hobson examines its strengths and weaknesses (R. P. Hobson, 'On Psychoanalytic Approaches to Autism,' *American Journal of Orthopsychiatry*, Vol. 60, No. 3, 1990, pp. 324-336).

[89] There are moreover countless specific therapies for autism doing the rounds to which I could not possibly do justice here, ranging from 'daily life' therapy in which children are immersed in intensive physical and artistic activities as part of a structured regime that provides no scope for retreating back into autism to dolphin therapy. Some of them seem to have favourable effects; others promise the moon, sometimes even a cure, although their claims are not underpinned by any scientific evidence whatsoever (see: Baron-Cohen and Bolton, op. cit.).

[90] C. C. Park, *The Siege: The First Eight Years of an Autistic Child. With an Epilogue, Fifteen Years Later*, Little, Brown and Company, Boston and Toronto, 1982, p. 12.

[91] P. Howlin and M. Rutter, *Treatment of Autistic Children*, John Wiley and Sons, Chichester [etc.], 1987, p. 227.

[92] Baron-Cohen and Bolton, op. cit., p. 68.

[93] I. A. van Berckelaer-Onnes, 'Leven naar de letter,' *Tijdschrift voor Orthopedagogiek*, Vol. 31, No. 9, 1992.

[94] Peeters, op. cit., 1994.

[95] G. J. Nijhof, *Herhaalgedrag bij mensen met autisme en een verstandelijke beperking*, Pons and Looijen, Wageningen, 1999.

[96] Howlin and Rutter, op. cit.; Wing, op. cit., 1996.

[97] L. Wing, *In zichzelf gekeerd: voor ouders en opvoeders van het autistische kind*, 2nd edn, Lemniscaat, Rotterdam, 1981, p. 112.

[98] F. Schrameijer, *Een wankele wereld*, Dr. Leo Kannerhuis, Doorwerth, 2007, pp. 52-53.

[99] Grinker, op. cit., p. 6.

[100] S. Murray, *Representing Autism: Culture, Narrative, Fascination*, Liverpool University Press, Liverpool, 2008, p. 208.

[101] Sacks, op. cit., p. 246. See note 1.

## On Stage

[1] L. Rood, *Het boek Job*, Prometheus, Amsterdam, 1994, p. 23.

[2] S. Murray, *Representing Autism: Culture, Narrative, Fascination*, Liverpool University Press, Liverpool, 2008, p. 7.

[3] J. Bernlef, *Vallende ster*, Querido, Amsterdam, 1989, p. 24. Like other quotes originally in Dutch, excerpts taken from *Vallende ster* are translated into English by L. Richards.

[4] Ibid., p. 40.

[5] Ibid., pp. 40-41.
[6] Ibid., p. 21.
[7] Ibid., p. 81.
[8] Ibid., p. 60.
[9] Ibid., p. 44.
[10] Ibid., pp. 59-60.
[11] Ibid., pp. 31-32.
[12] Ibid., p. 60.
[13] Ibid., p. 12.
[14] Ibid., p. 85.
[15] Ibid., p. 59.
[16] Ibid., p. 27.
[17] Ibid., pp. 32-33.
[18] Ibid., pp. 33.
[19] Ibid., pp. 37-38.
[20] Ibid., p. 37.
[21] Ibid., p. 46.
[22] Ibid., p. 82.
[23] Ibid., p. 47.
[24] Ibid., p. 21.
[25] Ibid., p. 70.
[26] Ibid., p. 9.
[27] Ibid., p. 84.
[28] Ibid., p. 29.
[29] Ibid., p. 80.
[30] Ibid., p. 86.
[31] Ibid., p. 86.
[32] NPS/VARA, Zembla, 'De wereld in fragmenten,' 7 May 1998.
[33] Animals are machines, thought Descartes. Animal behaviour (unlike that of people) could be explained by the same mechanical laws as the movements of automatons - the figures of people and animals that were set up in parks and incorporated in clock towers in his day. 'There was no problem in conceding that the movements of such automatons were produced by wholly mechanical causes - after all, human beings constructed them - and there was, for Descartes, also no problem in construing every aspect of animal bodies in similarly mechanical terms' (S. Shapin, *The Scientific Revolution*, University of Chicago Press, Chicago and London, 1998, pp. 158-59). Also see Noske's overview of debates about the human/animal relationship, in which animals prove to be in a problematic intermediate position. According to Noske it is difficult to get away from the basic dualistic model that determines our thinking about animals. 'We may fail to acknowledge and respect animals'

Otherness. Basically we face a dilemma in that there seems to be no option to imposing upon animals either object status or *human* subject status' (B. Noske, *Humans and Other Animals: Beyond the Boundaries of Anthropology*, Pluto Press, London, 1989, p. 157). For other contributions to this debate, see: M. Lynch and H. M. Collins (eds), 'Humans, Animals, and Machines [Special Issue], *Science, Technology, and Human Values*, Vol. 23, No. 4, 1988.

[34] Bernlef, op. cit., p. 43.

[35] J. Bernlef, 'Twee heren zonder verleden: over Stan Laurel en Oliver Hardy,' *Op het Noorden: essays*, Querido, Amsterdam, 1987, pp. 118-123.

[36] Ibid., p. 122.

[37] A. Mertens, 'Het fonetisch serveersysteem,' *De Groene Amsterdammer*, Vol. 118, 11 May 1994, p. 27.

[38] I have borrowed the ice metaphor from Mertens (op. cit., p. 27), who addresses Bernlef's explorations of a mysterious reality that the latter suspects is under the surface of a thin layer of meanings and interpretations that people have put over it and in which, as a rule, they dare to trust unthinkingly. Until a hole in the ice opens up, through which you fall to end up in a world 'that can no longer be analyzed using words and sentences.' Mertens points in this connection to the influence that Wittgenstein's work had on the literary climate in which Bernlef wrote his first books.

[39] Nauta relates this observation to the sort of act in which a clown has no idea what to do with a thing that is universally regarded as a chair. See: L. W. Nauta, 'Notities,' *Kennis en Methode: Tijdschrift voor Wetenschapsfilosofie en Wetenschapsonderzoek*, Vol. XVIII, No. 1, 1994, p. 66. See also Chapter 4 for the figure of the clown.

[40] Cf. in this context the disturbing effect of photographs of people in a waiting-room situation (such as in the subway) by the American photographer Walker Evans: 'They are being transported to a place where their actions will become purposeful again, but now, for a moment, they have nothing to do. An empty, absent stare. Their personality momentarily drained away,' wrote Bernlef in his essay 'Walker Evans: Archeologist of the Surface.' (See: J. Bernlef, 'Walker Evans: archeoloog van de oppervlakte,' *Op het Noorden: essays*, Querido, Amsterdam, 1987, p. 88).

[41] Bernlef, op. cit., 1989, p. 21.

[42] Given the prominent role of Beckett's plays in *Vallende ster* and the autistic traits often identified in his characters, the association with Beckett is an obvious one. There also appear to be philosophical parallels between *Film* and *Vallende ster*. My interpretation is inspired in part by that of the art historian Wilma Siccama, in her essay on the philosophical point of *Film*. (See: W. Siccama, 'De filosofische clou van een komedie: Samuel Becketts

Film,' in E. Mulder and H. Ester (eds), *De schone waarheid en de steen der dwazen: transartistieke studies*, Ambo, Baarn, 1996, pp. 185-201).

[43] 'L'apparition d'autrui dans le monde correspond donc à un glissement figé de tout l'univers, à une décentration du monde qui mine par en dessous la centralisation que j'opère dans le même temps' (J-P Sartre, *L'être et le néant: essai d'ontologie phénoménologique*, Galimard, Paris, 1943, p. 301). See also Chapter 1.

[44] Bernlef, op. cit., 1989, pp. 59-60.

[45] Ibid., p. 85.

[46] Ibid., p. 43.

[47] Cf. I. Hacking, 'Humans, Aliens and Autism,' *Dædelus*, Summer 2009, p. 56.

[48] Bernlef, op. cit., 1989, pp. 43-44.

[49] G. H. de Vries, 'Wittgensteins afscheid van de epistemologie,' in E. L. G. E. Kuypers (ed), *Wittgenstein in meervoud*, Garant, Leuven and Apeldoorn, 1991, pp. 17-28.

[50] Other members of the subject family point, for instance, to the Cartesian *cogito* or to Kantian transcendental categories of the human intellect. The confidence in the corrective powers of members of the language community reveals a kinship with Wittgenstein's ideas in *Philosophical Investigations* about the relationship between language and world, or at least with an idealistic interpretation of his views (Cf. G de Vries, Ibid., and: GH de Vries, *Zeppelins: over filosofie, technologie en cultuur*, Van Gennep, Amsterdam, 1999). Wittgenstein introduced the concept of 'rule-governed behaviour' as an explanation of what it means to know a word: meaning is rule-governed use. Our interpretations of reality depend on the rules of the 'language game' in which we take part. But rules do not contain the rules for their own application; the correct application (according to this reading) would require an additional explanation. In this context authors usually refer to the community of language-users, to other people who correct our mistakes: without sufficient embedment in the language community our perception loses all its points of reference (cf. Winch's influential reading). It is interesting in this context to read the suggestion that Wittgenstein suffered from Asperger's syndrome put forward by the autism expert Christopher Gillberg (cf. O. Sacks, *An Anthropologist on Mars: Seven Paradoxical Tales*, Alfred A Knopf, New York, 1995, p. 295). An idealistic reading of Wittgenstein, ironically, appeals to typically *non*-autistic pre-conceptions, such as the importance of social conventions. See De Vries (op. cit., 1991, and op. cit., 1999) for a criticism of and an alternative to this idealistic interpretation.

[51] Bernlef, op. cit., 1989, p. 47.

[52] In *Vallende ster*, close to home, a problem that has been put on the agenda in cultural anthropology and elsewhere has been brought to a head. Problems the anthropologist encounters far from home can often be traced back to the supposed untranslatability between diverse world views that meet one another. On the one hand, the anthropologist is seeking communication with and understanding of the other. On the other, this presents him with the dilemma that his wish to 'do justice' to the other can compel the anthropologist to suspend his own pretentions to truth. The danger that the anthropological preoccupation with (avoiding) ethnocentrism brings with it in the most extreme case is total identification with the object of the research, the risk of going native (See: M. Hammersley and P. Atkinson, *Ethnography, Principles in Practice*, 2nd ext. edn, Routledge, London and New York, 1995). In order to avoid an enforced choice between the two extremes, between ethnocentrism and cultural relativism, various attempts have been made to bridge the gulf between anthropologist and 'savage' in a manner other than by way of the ideal of 'truthful representation.'

[53] G. H. de Vries, 'Bewogen bewegers: ironie in het intellectuele bestaan,' in L. Nauta, G. de Vries, H. Harbers, S. Koenis, A. Mol, D. Pels and R. de Wilde (eds), *De rol van de intellectueel: een discussie over distantie en betrokkenheid*, Van Gennep, Amsterdam, 1992, pp. 111-127.

[54] Ibid., p. 125.

[55] Ibid., p. 119.

[56] See Runia on the tension between 'being present on the spot' and 'maintaining an overview' as a problem in historiography, as it is presented in Tolstoy's *War and Peace*. Runia regards Tolstoy's refusal to reduce history to what historians and others project into it as a central aspect of his philosophy of history. The quadrille-like, spontaneous ordering that reigns on the spot is often ground down after the event into chess-like plots, which people are only too happy to believe so as not to have to live with the idea that they are part of a contingent, meaningless series of events. Tolstoy, in contrast, argues in favour of confining oneself to the surface in historiography, to phenomena, and always stresses the mediated character of the way the past is brought into the present. (E. Runia, *De pathologie van de veldslag: geschiedenis en geschiedschrijving in Tolstoj's Oorlog en Vrede*, Meulenhoff, Amsterdam, 1995, chapter 1).

[57] This insight was developed with a view to a symmetrical analysis of so-called science-in-action (See: B. Latour, *Science in Action: How to Follow Scientists and Engineers Through Society*, Harvard University Press, Cambridge MA, 1987. And see: B. Latour, *The Pasteurization of France: War and Peace of Microbes - Irreductions*, trans. A. Sheridan and J. Law, Harvard University Press, Cambridge, MA, 1988a). In order to gain insight

into the dynamic of controversies in which the distinction between the subjective and objective character of claims is created, the description must steer clear of terms that presuppose such a difference. Instead, the significance of claims is seen, in a semiotic way, as an intertextual relational effect. Latour and other actor-network theoreticians (most notably Michel Callon and John Law) have extended this approach to the world beyond the text: during a process of 'network building,' heterogeneous elements are forged into an 'inner world' where the knowing subject and the object of knowledge, the world of people-among-themselves and the world of things, are 'co-produced' as two sides of the same coin as a result of transformations in chains of association. 'Our general symmetry principle is . . . to obtain nature and society as twin results of an . . . activity . . . that [we call] . . . network building, or collective things, or quasi-objects, or trials of force . . . : and others call it skill, forms of life, material practice . . .' (M. Callon and B. Latour, 'Don't Throw the Baby out With the Bath School! - A Reply to Collins and Yearley,' in A. Pickering (ed), *Science as Practice and Culture*, University of Chicago Press, Chicago, 1992, p. 348.

[58] Bernlef, op. cit., 1989, p. 10.

[59] These three forms of delegation - in time, in space and to an actor - form the essential narrative building blocks from which each event is constructed. By means of *shifting out*, the implied author moves the focus from himself in the here and now to another actor who is acting in a different time and at a different location (See: B. Latour, 'A Relativistic Account of Einstein's Relativity,' *Social Studies of Science*, Vol. 18, 1988b, pp. 3-44. And see: B. Latour, 'Pasteur on Lactic Acid Yeast: A Partial Semiotic Analysis,' *Configurations*, Vol. 1, 1992, pp. 129-145). Such a shift of vantage point can be repeated ad infinitum, and a new narrative layer can be added each time.

[60] Bernlef, op. cit., 1989, p. 82.

[61] Ibid., p. 47.

[62] Ibid., p. 75.

[63] Having first had his focus shifted to other actors, places and times, the reader's attention is brought back to the implied author by way of a reverse semiotic shift. This creates in the reader the impression that the delegated actors and the one who sent them off on their adventures coincide and can speak with one and the same voice. 'The result of these two movements is to create characters which play the role of delegates for the main enunciator' (Latour, op. cit., 1988b, p. 6).

[64] Bernlef, op. cit., 1989, p. 46.

[65] As Latour observes, 'the actors (or more exactly actants) which are shifted out in this way need not be human characters; they can be anything' (Latour, op. cit., 1988b, pp. 5-6). The radioactive element (actant) which makes it

possible, at certain intervals (time) to follow fluid flows in the tubules of a hamster's kidney (place) - referring to a study by Latour and Bastide - is just such a 'non-human' delegate, which is sent out as a messenger so that, as an accredited reporter, it can give an account of its journey through the kidney. (See: B. Latour and F. Bastide, 'Writing Science - Fact and Fiction,' in M. Callon, J. Law and A. Rip (eds), *Mapping the Dynamics of Science and Technology: Sociology of Science in the Real World*, Macmillan, Basingstroke, UK and London, 1986, pp. 51-66). Latour (op. cit., 1992) introduced the term 'shifting down' for this delegation to a technical object.

[66] Bernlef, op. cit., 1989, p. 70.

[67] The translation-concept aims to hold the middle ground symmetrically between linguistic and material organization, between linguistic 'translation' and geometric 'shifting.' This concept is painstakingly worked out in: B. Latour, 'The 'Pedofil' of Boa Vista: A Photo-Philosophical Montage,' *Common Knowledge*, Vol. 4, No. 1, 1995, pp. 144–187. Abstraction is not a cognitive affair - so it emerges from a typical piece of translation work undertaken by the soil experts in the article - but a question of putting a clod of earth (still just belonging to the world of things) into a cardboard box. At that moment the earth becomes a symbol, for the box is part of a matrix made up of a number of boxes that assigns coordinates with which further calculations can be done. The actual soil thus becomes a *known* soil, which in turn forms a fertile medium for the next process. The abstract, large ontological gap between the meaningful and the material world is thereby reduced to a series of minuscule cracks between things and symbols which, in practical terms, can be effortlessly bridged by means of hand gestures, with the aid of a ruler, a look, an action.

[68] Bernlef, op. cit., 1989, p. 5.

[69] When we describe a thing as 'intermediary' we conceive of it in the familiar sense of the word, as a passive link, as a carrier of meanings that have been assigned to it by people, in short as a faithful messenger that simply transports information. 'Everything changes if the word mediation fills out a little in order to designate the action of mediators. The meaning is no longer simply transported by the medium but in part constituted, moved, recreated, modified, in short expressed and betrayed.' (B. Latour, 'The Berlin Key or How to Do Words With Things,' in P. M. Graves-Brown (ed), *Matter, Materiality and Modern Culture*, Routledge, London, 2000, p. 19).

[70] This corresponds with what Latour (op. cit., 1987) calls the 'Janus face' of science: after the event, when the network has stabilized and we can speak of ready-made science, there is a 'correspondence' between the subject's pronouncement and a property of the known object; it is then possible to check the reporting against the facts, as the saying goes.

[71] Bernlef, op. cit., 1989, p. 29.

[72] Ibid., p. 10.

[73] Ibid., pp. 79-80. In his analysis of *Vallende ster*, professor of general and Dutch literature Wiel Kusters emphasizes the 'dizzying circular situation' that occurs at the moment Witteman tries to read and reads that he is trying to read (W. Kusters, 'Autisme: over 'Vallende Ster' van J. Bernlef',' *Tijdschrift voor Gezondheidszorg en Ethiek*, Vol. 1, 1991, p. 23). Kusters describes the circle form, which recurs countless times in *Vallende ster* (the circles that Peter, turned in on himself, draws, the way he spins on his axis and so on), as a metaphorical connection between the subject of autism and the (theoretically autonomous) ontological status of literary work.

[74] Bernlef, op. cit., 1989, p. 69.

[75] Ibid., p. 53.

[76] Cf.: 'But aren't we, as audience, interpreting the events on stage? Yes, of course, in a certain sense we are, but that is not the point. On stage, in normal cases, there is no 'interpretative flexibility.' Props speak in a clear voice: 'I'm a crown.' The actors on stage take this for granted, as does the audience captured by the play.' (G. H. de Vries, 'Should We Send Collins and Latour to Dayton, Ohio?,' *EASST Review*, Vol. 14, No. 1, 1995, p. 6)

[77] I take inspiration here from Carlo Ginzburg's history of a specific paradigm that enjoyed growing popularity in life sciences at the end of the nineteenth century that he traces in Conan Doyle's stories about Sherlock Holmes but also in art history and Freudian psychoanalysis. This paradigm held that on closer scrutiny all kinds of data that appeared to be of marginal importance at first sight (appearances, unconscious gestures, mistakes, side issues), could provide a great deal of information about a deeper-seated reality that had been unreachable until then. Ginzburg traces the roots of this so-called evidential or conjectural paradigm to man's primeval knowledge as a hunter, who, thousands of years ago, when following his invisible prey, learned to collect even the smallest and most insignificant traces and to organize empirical facts such that the plot could be read from them. 'The hunter would have been the first 'to tell a story' because he alone was able to read, in the silent, nearly imperceptible tracks left by his prey, a coherent sequence of events.' (C. Ginzburg, 'Clues: Roots of an Evidential Paradigm,' in *Clues, Myths, and the Historical Method*, trans. J. and A. C. Tedeschi, Johns Hopkins University Press. Baltimore, Md. [etc.], 1989, p. 103).

[78] The detective thus provides a fitting role model for the reader when, following in the wake of the messengers I send out in my research, he approaches an autistic existence. 'Detectives and clowns can be called thing-researchers,' writes Nauta (op. cit., p. 66), since they have the same talent for

abandoning the familiar order, following seemingly irrelevant traces, and thus finding out about the world beyond ready-made narratives.

[79] Bernlef himself, reacting to the reception of his bestseller *Out of Mind* as if by definition it gave a realistic picture of dementia (cf. A. Peters, 'Echt gebeurd' als amputatie van de verbeelding: J. Bernlef verdedigt de literatuur tegen modieuze beperkingen,' *De Volkskrant*, 17 April 1998, p. 35), spoke of a 'neurological cocktail' that he had composed intuitively and in which he had sometimes deliberately distorted the truth - in so far as it was known. It then proved that this created an image which apparently appealed to what people imagine by something like the experience of a person with dementia (Bernlef, 2 March 1994). Something similar applies, it seems to me, to *Vallende ster*.

[80] Kusters, op. cit., p. 20.

[81] This expression, borrowed from Bernlef, again refers to the evidential paradigm described by Ginsburg. Bernlef, himself, in his essay on Walker Evans as 'anthropologist of the surface' drew inspiration from Ginzburg's article. Evans's photographs are always about people. That they are so telling, writes Bernlef, is because people themselves so seldom appear in them personally and they do not 'immediately evoke a ready-made story' (Bernlef, op. cit. 'Walker Evans,' p. 82). Fireplaces and sideboards are among the trivial places that Walker Evans photographed - 'all the places where people more or less heedlessly came to make a collection' (p. 82). Precisely because no more than traces of human habitation are found in places like these, they compel the reader to reconstruct an underlying story.

**Body and Mind Shows**

[1] L. Wittgenstein, *Culture and Value: A Selection From the Posthumous Remains*, Basil Blackwell, Oxford, 1998, p. 90e. Cf. 'Es ist *schwer* etwas zu wissen, and zu handeln als wüßte man's nicht.' MS 137 143a: 7.-8.1.1949.

[2] J. T. McDonnell, 'Mothering an Autistic Child: Reclaiming the Voice of the Mother' in B. A. Daly and M. T. Reddy (eds), *Narrating Mothers: Theorizing Maternal Subjectivities*, The University of Tennessee Press, Knoxville, 1991, pp. 58-75.

[3] L. Wing, 'The Continuum of Autistic Characteristics' in E. Schopler and G. B. Mesibov (eds), *Diagnosis and Assessment in Autism*, Plenum Press, New York and London, 1988, pp. 91-110.

[4] S. B. Wulff, 'The Symbolic and Object Play of Children with Autism: A Review,' *Journal of Autism and Developmental Disorders*, Vol. 15, No. 2, 1985, pp. 139-140. Also see: L. Wing and J. Gould, 'Severe Impairments of Social Interaction and Associated Abnormalities in Children: Epidemiology and Classification,' *Journal of Autism and Developmental Disorders*, Vol. 9,

No. 1, 1979, pp. 11-30. And: L. Wing, J. Gould, S. R. Yeates and L. M. Brierley, 'Symbolic Play in Severely Mentally Retarded and in Autistic Children,' *Journal of Child Psychology and Psychiatry*, Vol. 18, No. 2, 1977, pp. 167-178.

[5] J. Bromet, 'Kinderen die van onze wereld niets begrijpen,' *Margriet*, Vol. 39, 12 June, 1976, p. 76.

[6] L. Eisenberg and L. Kanner, 'Early Infantile Autism, 1943-1955,' *American Journal of Orthopsychiatry*, Vol. 26, 1956, p. 559.

[7] S. Baron-Cohen, *Mindblindness: An Essay on Autism and Theory of Mind*, MIT Press, Cambridge, MA and London, 1995, p. 4.

[8] Dyson in: W. Kayzer, *A Glorious Accident: Understanding Our Place in the Cosmic Puzzle*, Freeman, New York, 1997, p. 138. Islets of ability are found in both mentally handicapped and intelligent people with autism, although they are seldom as well developed in the former case as in the latter. All the same, the disharmonious development profile is a striking characteristic of the syndrome.

[9] B. Hermelin and N. O'Connor, *Psychological Experiments with Autistic Children*, Pergamon Press, Oxford [etc.], 1970.

[10] D. M. Ricks and L. Wing, 'Language, Communication and the Use of Symbols' in L. Wing (ed), *Early Childhood Autism*, 2nd edn, Pergamom, Oxford [etc.], 1976, pp. 93-134.

[11] L. Wing, 'Language, Social, and Cognitive Impairments in Autism and Severe Mental Retardation,' *Journal of Autism and Developmental Disorders*, Vol. 11, No. 1, 1981, p. 41.

[12] S. Baron-Cohen, AM Leslie and U Frith, 'Does the Autistic Child Have a 'Theory of Mind'?,' *Cognition*, Vol. 21, No. 1, 1985, pp. 37-46. I certainly do not intend to give an overview here of the formation of cognitive psychological theories on autism to date, nor concern myself with current discussions. I shall confine myself to a few crucial experiments and debates that throw light on assumptions about the nature of imagination and the imagination deficit that are accepted in this field and how these premises determine what can be said about the division of roles between people and things in compensating for the deficit.

[13] Baron-Cohen, Leslie and Frith, op. cit., p. 38.

[14] S. Baron-Cohen and J. Swettenham, 'Theory of Mind in Autism: Its Relationship to Executive Function and Central Coherence,' in D. J. Cohen and F. R. Volkmar (eds), *Handbook of Autism and Pervasive Developmental Disorders*, 2nd edn, John Wiley and Sons, New York [etc.], 1997, pp. 880-893.

[15] G. Gerland, *A Real Person - Life on the Outside*, Souvenir Press, London, 1997, p. 20.

[16] Ibid., p. 64.

[17] Ibid., p. 66.

[18] See: J. R. Bemporad, 'Adult Recollections of a Formerly Autistic Child,' *Journal of Autism and Developmental Disorders*, Vol. 9, No. 2, 1979, p. 192.

[19] McDonnell, op. cit., p. 64.

[20] A. M. Leslie, 'Pretence and Representation: The Origins of 'Theory of Mind',' *Psychological Review*, Vol. 94, 1987, pp. 412-426.

[21] Wing, op. cit., 1988, p. 94.

[22] The mental age is important because the capacity to pass this sort of test is not developed until the fourth year. 'The results for Down's Syndrome and normal subjects were strikingly similar. 23 out of 27 normal children, and 12 out of 14 Down's Syndrome children *passed* the Belief Question on both trials (85% and 86% respectively). By contrast, 16 of the 20 autistic children (80%) *failed* the Belief Question on both trials. . . . All 16 autistic children who failed pointed to where the marble really was, rather than to any of the other possible locations . . .' (Baron-Cohen, Leslie and Frith, op. cit., p. 42).

[23] Ibid., pp. 43-44.

[24] P. Steerneman, *Leren denken over denken en leren begrijpen van emoties*, Leuven and Apeldoorn, Garant, 2004.

[25] Wulff, op. cit., p. 144.

[26] S. Baron-Cohen, 'Are Autistic Children 'Behaviorists'? An Examination of Their Mental-Physical and Appearance-Reality Distinctions,' *Journal of Autism and Developmental Disorders*, Vol. 19, No. 4, 1989, p. 585.

[27] Ibid., p. 538. The author derives these criteria for the distinction between mental and physical entities from: H. Wellman and D. Estes, 'Early Understanding of Mental Entities: A Re-Examination of Childhood Realism,' *Child Development*, Vol. 57, 1986, pp. 910-923. In this source the authors use as additional criteria for the definition of physical entities 'a public existence' and 'a consistent existence.' Compare the articulation of uncertainty regarding the mental/ physical divide here with remarks under note 87.

[28] Baron-Cohen, op. cit., 1989, p. 538.

[29] I write 'tend' because Baron-Cohen ultimately gives a nuanced answer to his initial question: people with autism appear to be able to predict human behaviour not only on the grounds of conditions like 'feeling hungry,' but also on the grounds of 'desires' (for example wanting a biscuit), inner drives that can be understood without having to call on metarepresentation (of the 'beliefs' of other people). This subtle distinction does not alter the thesis that their psychology differs radically from that of normal children: .' . . they may be able to predict people's actions in terms of desires and physical causes, but fail to develop a 'belief-desire psychology' characteristic of even normal 3-

year-olds.' (Ibid., p. 598) 'Common sense mentalistic psychology' is taken from: Steerneman, op. cit., p. 14.

[30] D. Williams, *Nobody, Nowhere: The Extraordinary Autobiography of an Autistic*, Avon Books, New York, 1992, p. 51.

[31] Baron-Cohen, op. cit., 1989, p. 587. No fewer than 84.2% of the normal children and 68.8% of the children with learning disabilities in the control groups mentioned mental activities as against 23.5% of the autistic children. The latter mentioned *physical* activities in 70.5% of the cases.

[32] V. Lewis and J. Boucher, 'Spontaneous, Instructed and Elicited Play in Relatively Able Autistic Children,' *British Journal of Developmental Psychology*, Vol. 6, 1988, pp. 325-339. The authors suspect that autism is the result of a *conative* rather than a cognitive impairment, which is to say that that people with autism do have the potential for symbolic play, but do not do it spontaneously because, for some unknown reason, they lack the motivation and perseverance. *Eliciting* this play is therefore essential and, according to the authors, measures the ability to play symbolically or functionally without calling on the child's conative or generative ability. The criticism is part of a school that is known as the 'executive function' approach, which explains autism on the grounds of an inability to escape mentally from a course once taken within purposeful and strategic behaviour (cf. chapter 2).

[33] S. Baron-Cohen, 'Instructed and Elicited Play in Autism: A Reply to Lewis and Boucher,' *British Journal of Developmental Psychology*, Vol. 8, 1990, p. 207.

[34] Discussions about the reliability and the validity of measuring instruments and about the role of (representations of) people and things are indissolubly linked to the researcher's project. For instance Boucher and Lewis in their turn deny that the measurement results were coloured by the nature of the things or the input of the researcher. (see: J. Boucher and V. Lewis, 'Guessing or Creating? A Reply to Baron-Cohen,' *British Journal of Developmental Psychology*, Vol. 8, 1990, pp. 205-206.) All the autistic children who were tested, they claim, proved capable of original symbolic play that could not possibly have been derived from the researchers' instructions. Doubts have also been raised as to the validity of a method like the Sally-Anne test in distinguishing between representations of mental and physical phenomena. Children up to the age of six often interpret a question about what Sally *thinks* as a question about a physical rather than a mental activity. Moreover, the use of a puppet show as a measuring instrument presupposes that the test subject has a narrative set, such as a concept of shared imagination, at his or her disposal. 'For these reasons it would appear that deception tasks [the alternative they studied] might be purer tests of false belief understanding -'purer' in the sense of being less verbal and less

narrative,' according to: J. Russel, N. Mauthner, S. Sharpe and T. Tidswell, 'The 'Windows Task' as a Measure of Strategic Deception in Preschoolers and Autistic Subjects,' *British Journal of Developmental Psychology*, Vol. 9, 1991, p. 333.

[35] Baron-Cohen, Leslie and Frith, op. cit., p. 43.

[36] S. Holroyd and S. Baron-Cohen, 'Brief Report: How Far Can People With Autism Go in Developing a Theory of Mind?,' *Journal of Autism and Developmental Disorders*, Vol. 23, No. 2, 1993, pp. 379-385.

[37] Baron-Cohen, op. cit., 1995.

[38] Holroyd and Baron-Cohen, op. cit., p. 384.

[39] Wing, op. cit., 1988, p. 95.

[40] O. Sacks, *An Anthropologist on Mars: Seven Paradoxical Tales*, Alfred A. Knopf, New York, 1995, p. 272.

[41] Ibid., p. 270.

[42] T. Grandin, 'My Experiences as an Autistic Child and Review of Selected Literature,' *Journal of Orthomolecular Psychiatry*, Vol. 13, No. 3, 1984, p. 145.

[43] Sacks, op. cit., p. 283.

[44] Ibid., p. 272.

[45] Gerland, op. cit., p. 244.

[46] One could counter on this point that the ability to distinguish is in itself located in a complex calculator and hence is in essence based on a monistic (mechanistic) world image (cf. J. Searle, *The Rediscovery of the Mind*, MIT Press, Cambridge MA and London, 1992). 'We inhabit mental worlds populated by the computational outputs of battalions of evolved, specialized neural automata,' is how it is put in the foreword to Baron-Cohen (op. cit., 1995, xii) by Tooby and Cosmides. Against this it could be adduced that the crucial mind-reading system that Baron-Cohen describes is part of a *social* module. 'Mind reading is by definition a system for use within the social environment,' (Ibid., p. 96) he claims, so that the characteristic that distinguishes people with and without autism is projected back into the sphere of the human subject anyway.

[47] Steerneman, op. cit., p. 21. Steerneman notes that the training presupposes a level of social-cognitive functioning of at least a four-year-old. In the groups studied the calendar ages were also relatively high (the average age in the studies ranged from eight to 26 years; the average IQs were in the 63-89 range). The best results were moreover obtained with socially anxious children and children with a contact disorder related to autism; the training was less successful in children with autistic spectrum disorder.

[48] S. Murray, *Representing Autism: Culture, Narrative, Fascination*, Liverpool University Press, Liverpool, 2008, pp. 83-89.

[49] T. Peeters, in the foreword of the Dutch translation of Gerlands book. See: G. Gerland, *Een echt mens*, Houtekiet, Antwerpen/Baarn, 1998, p. 8.

[50] The familiar concept of imagination (and in subsequent chapters the thinking about socialization and communication), in other words, deserves to be reconsidered. For an inspiring analysis of the topological (i.e. regional) assumptions concealed in ideas about knowledge and in social theorizing, see: A. Mol and J. Law, 'Regions, Networks and Fluids: Anaemia and Social Topology,' *Social Studies of Science*, Vol. 24, No. 4, 1994, pp. 641-671. The authors (following Michel Serres) advocate exploring alternative conceptions of this theoretical space, among other things in fluid terms.

[51] R. Marchant, P. Howlin, W. Yule and M. Rutter, 'Graded Change in the Treatment of the Behaviour of Autistic Children,' *Journal of Child Psychology and Psychiatry*, Vol. 15, No. 3, 1974, p. 223.

[52] Ibid., p. 223.

[53] Ibid., p. 223.

[54] R. J. Gaylord-Ross, T. G. Haring, C. Breen and V. Pitts-Conway, 'The Training and Generalization of Social Interaction Skills With Autistic Youth,' *Journal of Applied Behavior Analysis*, Vol. 17, 1984, p. 230.

[55] Gaylord-Ross, Haring, Breen and Pitts-Conway, op. cit., p. 235.

[56] The script concept, like that developed for technical equipment, could prove useful in this context to encapsulate the way techniques guide people's behaviour in words and meanings, or conversely, to see how the lack of inner scripts in people with autism can be compensated from outside. The 'prescription' of an artefact is, for example, defined as 'what a device allows or forbids from the actors - humans and nonhuman - that it anticipates; it is the morality of a setting both negative (what it prescribes) and positive (what it permits)' (M. Akrich and B. Latour, 'A Summary of a Convenient Vocabulary for the Semiotics of Human and Nonhuman Assemblies,' in W. E. Bijker and J. Law (eds), *Shaping Technology/Building Society: Studies in Socio-Technical Change*, MIT Press, Cambridge, MA and London, 1992, p. 261.) In the case in question, it had to be concluded that the scripts of the objects that were introduced (downward delegation, or *shifting down* to use Latour's term, see chapter 2) did not provide sufficient guidance for the autistic students. Additional written scripts were consequently added to these things.

[57] T. Peeters, Interview, Opleidingsinstituut Autisme, Antwerp, 23 June 1995. For his source of inspiration, see: T. Grandin and M. M. Scariano, *Emergence: Labeled Autistic*, Arena Press, Novato, 1993.

[58] Ibid., p. 246. The addition of the script produced a result, according to Gaylord-Ross et al., but after four months and the discontinuation of the training, most of the social skills proved to have been forgotten. This would

seem to provide support for the interpretation of H. M .Collins, G. H. de Vries and W. E. Bijker, 'Ways of Going On: An Analysis of Skill Applied to Medical Practice,' *Science, Technology, and Human Values*, Vol. 22, No. 3, 1997, pp. 267-285. They claim that the simulation of a form of life can serve to teach 'novices' complex behavioural repertoires that only gradually differ from the simple routines that can be learned from a textbook or a set of formal instructions for use (cf. the skills lab of the medical faculty studied by the authors, where specific - for instance, surgical - skills that could not be learned from a textbook are taught). According to the authors there is, however, a radical difference between learning complex repertoires like these and so-called 'embodied capabilities' that can never be learned in isolation from the natural situation, the social context from which they derive their specific meaning. In Collins's terms this is about the difference between mimeomorphic and polimorphic actions (cf. chapter 5). In my next examples, however, this boundary appears to be less clear than is suggested here.

[59] T. Peeters, *Autisme: van begrijpen tot begeleiden*, Hadewijch, Antwerpen and Baarn, 1994, p. 102.

[60] Ibid., p. 102.

[61] Ibid., p. 102.

[62] Gerland, op. cit., p. 57-58.

[63] Ibid., p. 58.

[64] Ibid., p. 248.

[65] K. Momma, *En toen verscheen een regenboog: hoe ik mijn autistische leven ervaar*, Prometheus, Amsterdam, 1996, p. 112.

[66] Ibid., p. 167.

[67] K. Momma, *Achter de onzichtbare muur: een autist op reis door het leven*, Bert Bakker, Amsterdam, 1999, p. 39.

[68] Ibid., p. 44.

[69] Ibid., p. 41.

[70] Ibid., p. 62.

[71] Ibid., p. 56.

[72] Ibid., p. 59.

[73] A. Lebert, 'Howard Buten: Ohne Worte die richtige Sprache finden,' *Süddeutsche Zeitung Magazin*, 5 July, 1991, p. 13.

[74] Here I am quoting from my personal correspondence with Buten (22 April 1999; 12 January 2000) and a visit to the Adam Shelton Centre, Saint Denis, on 27 May 1999.

[75] Buten, Personal communication, 12 January 2000.

[76] Lebert, op. cit., p. 14.

[77] Ibid., p. 14.

[78] Other disciplines are more qualified than I to answer the question as to the verifiable effects of the alternative approaches to social imagination and concept formation that I am exploring here. I am concerned solely with exploring the conceptual space that is opened up in these unusual interactions.

[79] Lebert, op. cit., p. 13.

[80] Ibid., p. 13.

[81] In the language-games I have contrasted the role of the senses is radically different. The dominant sensory metaphor in the language-game of the cognitive psychologist is sight, which is expressed in the use of terms like observation and insight (cf. also the visual metaphors in the description of the components of the mind-reading mechanism in: Baron-Cohen, op. cit., 1995). Buten, in contrast, moves through space primarily by touch (a meaning that is retained in the word *sense* in English and French, but has been lost in many languages). See: S. van der Geest, 'Zin en zintuig in gezondheid en ziekte: voorbeschouwing op een symposium,' *Medische Antropologie*, Vol. 5, No. 1, 1993, pp. 63-69.

[82] Buten, op. cit., 12 January 2000.

[83] Lebert, op. cit., p. 11, 13.

[84] H. Buten, *Through the Glass Wall: Journeys Into the Closed-Off Worlds of the Autistic*, Bantam Books, New York, 2004, p. 86.

[85] Ibid., p. 99.

[86] Ibid., p. 101. Similarly, miMakkus, a special form of clowning in dementia care, can be understood in terms of developing an embodied form of sensitivity and thus becoming more interesting for the individual with dementia. See: R. Hendriks, 'Tackling Indifference: Clowning, Dementia and the Articulation of a Sensitive Body,' *Medical Anthropology*, forthcoming, 2012. (DOI 10.1080/01459740.2012.674991)

[87] L. Wittgenstein, *On certainty*, Basil Blackwell, Oxford, 1979. If some event or other causes us to doubt, we go and look for evidence: for an explanation, for good reasons, convincing proof, in short for anything that can provide reassurance and reasonable certainty. This quest for evidence takes place, however, against a background of things that are beyond all doubt, which are not based on research but on a familiar way of doing things. People would find it strange if you were suddenly to assert that you 'know for sure' things that they take for granted. A statement about 'knowing' presupposes a reason for doubt. Expressing doubt is therefore related to the situation: it assumes agreement about the context in which it is appropriate to do such a thing. Take the statement 'I know for sure that this is a thing and not a person.' In contrast to our response to the statement 'I know for sure that I have a tenner in my pocket,' in the former case we cannot imagine why

it should be necessary to make such an assertion. It seems to be a meaningless statement because, unlike the case of the ten-pound note, there does not seem to be any good reason for doubt. Why should you say that you *know* something for certain if it is something that you take for granted? (cf. G. H. de Vries, 'Wittgensteins afscheid van de epistemologie,' in E. L. G. E. Kuypers (ed), *Wittgenstein in meervoud*, Garant, Leuven and Apeldoorn, 1991, pp. 17-28. Also see chapter 1 on Searle's default position. In the psychologist's project, however, a debate about what is a person and what is a thing no longer sounds strange to us: because it nibbles away at this constitutive distinction the exact boundary suddenly becomes the subject of fierce discussion and controversy (cf. note 27).

[88] Buten, op. cit., 12 January 2000.

[89] O. Sacks, *A Leg to Stand On*, Duckworth, London, 1984, p. 159. In this book Sacks writes about the certainty of the body that is aware of itself. He describes how an accident temporarily dissociated his body and his mind from his own leg. At that moment he lacked the sense of self - proprioception - telling him that the leg was a part of him. This (unconscious) awareness of self, he writes, is often overlooked but is actually the vital 'sixth sense' which enables the body to know itself and its position in space. (pp. 46-47). What concerns Sacks is that impairments in physical function - in his case an injured leg - display a remarkable similarity to mental perceptions. Such an experience always involves an 'experimentum suitatis' (an experiment with the self).

[90] In the interview by Lebert (op. cit., p. 13) we read: 'Autistic people are clowns . . . or the other way around: the clown is the only way to portray an autistic person, so that people dare to laugh.' In my personal communication with Buten (op. cit., 22 April 1999; op. cit., 12 January 2000), however, he said this interpretation of his words was misleading.

[91] M. M. Bakhtin, 'Forms of Time and Chronotope in the Novel: Notes Toward a Historical Poetics,' in M. Holquist (ed), *The Dialogic Imagination: Four Essays*, University of Texas Press, Austin, 1981, pp. 159-160.

[92] Buten, op. cit., 12 January 2000.

[93] L. W. Nauta, 'Notities,' *Kennis en Methode*, Vol. XVIII, No. 1, 1994, p. 66.

[94] H. Plessner, *Lachen en wenen: een onderzoek naar de grenzen van het menselijk gedrag*, Utrecht, 1965, p. 92.

[95] J. Bernlef, 'Er valt niets te lachen. Over Buster Keaton' in *Ontroeringen: essays*, Querido, Amsterdam, 1990, p. 129, p. 131.

[96] Lebert, op. cit., p. 11.

[97] Buten, op. cit., 22 April 1999.

[98] Buten, op. cit., 12 January 2000.

[99] The Dutch term *voorstelling*, referring to both 'mental image' and 'stage performance,' neatly fits the intended transition of a mentally conceived to an extra-mental sense of imagination.

[100] A question that could be raised from the field of science and technology studies is the extent to which cognitive abilities that are defined in laboratory conditions correspond with the working of human cognition outside the lab, 'cognition in the wild' as it is called in: E. Hutchins, *Cognition in the Wild*, MIT, Cambridge MA and London, 1995. Is the outside world as purely dualistic as laboratory research assumes? It is not, Hutchins shows. However, should we not extend Hutchins' analysis to the laboratory shop-floor itself? See: R. Benschop, *Unassuming Instruments: Tracing the Tachistoscope in Experimental Psychology*, ADNP, Groningen, 2001 for such a move and a re-evaluation of the diversity of lab work. The criticism regarding Hutchins's failure to consider psychological laboratory work itself also, of course, applies to my approach. Aside from the fact that I studied lab 'practice' by way of written material, what concerns me is more what can be said about people and things in the language of cognitive psychology, and not so much what people at the sharp end actually *do*. For research which does justice to the complexity, the theory loading and the practical skill and inventiveness of experimental psychological work itself, particularly where achieving *precision* is concerned: R. Benschop and D. Draaisma, 'In Pursuit of Precision: The Calibration of Minds and Machines in Late Nineteenth-Century Psychology,' *Annals of Science*, Vol. 57, No. 1, 2000, pp. 1-25.

[101] Wittgenstein, op. cit., 1979, p. 71e.

[102] Cf. also that the deficit of a 'theory of mind,' although it can often be very clearly identified, is not a sufficient explanation for autism. 'This can be attributed to the fact that certain children never reach the level of social development at which this skill would normally manifest itself,' according to: I. A. van Berckelaer-Onnes, 'Leven naar de letter,' *Tijdschrift voor Orthopedagogiek*, Vol. 31, No. 9, 1992, p. 417). Cf. also Hobson's criticism of the theory of a 'theory of mind' referred to in chapter 2.

[103] Wittgenstein, op. cit., 1998, p. 36e.

**On Words and Clocks**

[1] M. Daru, 'Technologie aan tafel: de opkomst van de gezelligheids-technologie,' in R. Oldenziel and C. Bouw (eds), *Schoon genoeg: huisvrouwen en huishoudtechnologie in Nederland 1898-1998*, SUN, Nijmegen, 1998, p. 175.

[2] This and subsequent observations were made in a unit for young autistic people at a residential institution for the mentally handicapped in the south of

the Netherlands. The fieldwork was done between June and September 1994. For reasons of privacy, all residents and care workers have been given fictitious names.

[3] At the time I undertook my fieldwork a majority of the staff working in Dutch residential institutions for the mentally handicapped held a special nursing license (*Verpleegkunde-Z*) or were doing their in-service training (with extended internships in different units) to become licensed. However, rather than calling themselves 'nurses' the common and less 'medically charged' way of referring to their job was *groepsleider*. This term would translate somewhere between personal support worker (PSW) or care worker, and I shall use the latter throughout this chapter.

[4] This view derives from, among other things, Winch's idealistic reading of the late Wittgenstein (see note 50, chapter 3).

[5] See L. Wing, 'Manifestations of Social Problems in High-Functioning Autistic People,' in E. Schopler and G. B. Mesibov (eds), *High-Functioning Individuals with Autism*, Plenum Press, New York and London, 1992, p. 131.

[6] L. Wing, *The Autistic Spectrum: A Guide for Parents and Professionals*, Constable, London, 1996, p. 88.

[7] As H. M. Collins puts it in 'Dissecting Surgery: Forms of Life Depersonalized,' *Social Studies of Science*, Vol. 24, No. 2, 1994a, p. 316: 'What one is trying to do as a sociologist is (among other things) to discover the range of ways of experiencing the world that are generally available to actors in particular cultural locations in particular societies. The best way of doing this is to come to share the form of life of the actors, and to find out at first hand if this is how actors might reasonably see things.'

[8] All quotes, unless otherwise stated, originate from (partly informal) interviews I had with the care workers and members of the (advisory) autism team, and from my field notes. The everyday language in the quotes has been corrected here and there to promote readability.

[9] L. de Jaegher, *Structuur en zichtbaar maken van verbanden bij de behandeing van autistische personen*, Introductory folder, 21 February, 1989.

[10] The vagueness of the concept of *gezelligheid* does not mean that no meaningful structure can be detected in it, at least by competent members of the language community. On the contrary, it is extremely important to be *tactful* in this situation. Georg Simmel considers it the ideal playground of necessarily tactful and self-restrained social intercourse, which would explain why people with autism cannot see the point of remarks referring to it: 'Von den soziologische Kategorien her betrachtend, bezeichne ich also die Geselligkeit als die Spielform der Vergesellschaftung und als - mutatis mutandis - zu deren inhaltsbestimmter Konkretheit sich verhaltend wie das Kunstwerk zur Realität.' For this interpretation of the concept of *Geselligkeit*

see G. Simmel, 'Die Geselligkeit,' *Grundfragen der Soziologie (Individuum und Gesellschaft)*, Walter de Gruyter, Berlin and New York, 1984, p. 53.

[11] The ability to draw on recollections is not the same as the mechanical memory, which is often very well-developed in autists: this relates to memories that are mobilized in order to do something new with them or are seen in a different light as a result of current happenings.

[12] Wing, op. cit., 1996, p. 89.

[13] Socialization technology at the dinner table in the form of a fondue or raclette - which, says Daru (op. cit., p. 175) is about 'prolonging time: sitting at the table, enjoying the companionship' - also plays an important regulatory part in non-autistic people's lives. The same thing applies to objects like watches, the electronic signalling system indicating the time until the next bus arrives, and the like. For the moment, therefore, focusing on the role of material objects does not indicate any fundamental distinction, but refers only to a relative difference between autistic and non-autistic people's needs.

[14] De Jaegher, op. cit., p. 3.

[15] G. B. Mesibov, 'Treatment Issues with High-Functioning Adolescents and Adults with Autism,' in E. Schopler and G. B. Mesibov (eds), *High-Functioning Individuals with Autism*, Plenum Press, New York and London, p. 151. TEACCH stands for Treatment and Education of Autistic and related Communication handicapped CHildren. The TEACCH-department of the University of North Carolina in Chapel Hill provides services to children with autism and their families as well as staff training and consultation for classrooms, group homes and other services.

[16] L. Wing, *Autistic Children: A Guide for Parents*, Constable, London, 1971, p. 114.

[17] Wing, op. cit., 1996, p. 93.

[18] G. Simmel, 'Sociologie van de maaltijd,' in J. M. M. de Valk (Keuze en Inleiding), *Brug en deur: een bloemlezing uit de essays*, Kok Agora, Kampen, 1990, p. 70.

[19] Wing, op. cit., 1996, p. 125. Wing's engagement with the daily experience of raising a child with autism was allowed more room in the 1971 version, where she refers to families who find every mealtime 'a nightmare' because their child 'insists on eating his food in snatches while running round the room' (Wing, op. cit., 1971, p. 91).

[20] T. Peeters, *Autisme: van begrijpen tot begeleiden*, Hadewijch, Antwerp and Baarn, 1994, p. 63.

[21] L. Wittgenstein, *Culture and Value: A Selection from the Posthumous Remains*, Basil Blackwell, Oxford, 1998, p. 40e.

[22] A. O. Hirschman, *Crossing Boundaries: Selected Writings*, Zone Books, New York, 1998.

[23] Wing, op. cit., 1996, p. 91.

[24] As a rule, the history of humans and machines (formal structures and routines included) is particularly associated with the unbounded extension of mindlessness and the suppression of human creativity. Harry Collins provides a surprising reversal of such assumptions. His theory of action was originally developed in debating problems in human-machine interactions, with a special focus on artificial intelligence (H. M. Collins, *Artificial Experts: Social Knowledge and Intelligent Machines*, MIT Press, Cambridge, MA and London, 1990). In order to learn how to react appropriately to the continuously changing circumstances of social life, one has to be brought up by people who correct our mistakes. The only way for people to become familiar with the subtle rules of the social community is by going through a process of socialization in the language community. This is how people learn to carry out what Collins calls *polimorphic* action (H. M. Collins and M. Kusch, *The Shape of Actions: What Humans and Machines Can Do*, MIT Press, Cambridge, MA and London, 1998). Machines, however, are not raised by people the way children are. Thus, one would not expect machines to be part of society, except maybe as the 'strangest of strangers.' Yet, machines and people sometimes mingle very well. How can this be? According to Collins, the boundary between humans and machines disappears for a certain class of acts only. For the non-socialized to be able to mix with the socialized in a more or less trouble-free way, the socialized *simulate* the behaviour of the non-socialized. They try to restrict themselves to what Collins calls *mimeomorphic action* (the term 'machine-like action' may also be used). Rather than refer to 'mind-numbing' human/machine relations, therefore, Collins postulates the creative (polimorphic) achievement by people who learn to behave (mimeomorphic) according to the model of things. Collins's thesis helps us to re-evaluate the efforts of the care workers along similar lines. For an examination of this point see: R. Hendriks, 'Egg Timers, Human Values, and the Care of Autistic Youths,' *Science, Technology, and Human Values*, Vol. 23, No. 4, 1998, pp. 399-424. For a digression into the subject of autism see also: H. M. Collins, 'Socialness and the Undersocialized Conception of Society,' *Science, Technology, and Human Values*, Vol. 23, No. 4, 1998, pp. 494-516.

[25] Peeters, op. cit., 1994, p. 106.

[26] This may appear to be a personal argument against the conditioning of young autists in favour of a more humanistic approach towards them. To be sure, I do find it unpleasant to compare people with autism to machines, but that is not the position I want to champion here. The argument is that it is care workers *themselves* who cannot bear to reduce autists to machines.

[27] T. Peeters, *Uit zichzelf gekeerd: leerprocesen in de hulpverlening aan kinderen met autisme en verwante communicatiestoornissen*, Dekker and Van de Vegt, Nijmegen, 1984, pp. 33-34.

[28] T. Peeters, Interview, Opleidingsinstituut Autisme, Antwerp, 23 June, 1995.

[29] L. Rood, *Het boek Job*, Prometheus, Amsterdam, 1994, p. 25.

[30] Ibid., p. 26. The extent to which professional staff really live with residents consequently has to be put into perspective. 'You eat together, certainly,' said one of the care workers, 'but at night you go back to your own home. If they had to choose, everyone who works here would choose their private life. This really is work.'

[31] S. Murray, *Representing Autism: Culture, Narrative, Fascination*, Liverpool University Press, Liverpool, 2008, p. 49.

[32] In Collins's terms, too, there is always tension between the conviviality of the social community and what unfolds around the kitchen timer. At best the timer provides a quasi-translation of the polimorphic actions that are beyond David's ken - 'quasi' because, according to Collins, concepts like *conviviality* are supposed to be of a socialized, open-ended nature, and thus irreducible to formal rules.

[33] In its logocentrism and anthropocentrism, such a point of view mirrors the deeply rooted presumption that language speakers, members of the interpretative community, are primarily responsible for the way social order is accomplished. See for a critique on the logocentric bias in mainstream social theory: M. Callon and J. Law, 'Agency and the Hybrid *Collectif*,' *South Atlantic Quarterly*, Vol. 94, No. 2, 1995, pp. 481-507.

[34] Distance with respect to the interpretations of non-autistic members of the community being studied is not easily achieved by a researcher who is to a certain extent familiar with the language and skills of the care workers. But even if I had been a complete stranger to their practice, I would still have been a fellow member of the interpretative community. The researcher and care workers suffer the same handicap: they are all 'too ordinary.'

[35] Actor-network theory (see chapter 3) provides some excellent examples of stylistic experiments with a naturalized use of, among other things, the vocabulary of nature ('forces'), which aims to describe heterogeneous processes of ordering in a less logocentric and anthropocentric, and hence more symmetrical way.

[36] Stefan Hirschauer explores a comparable style in his analyses of a cultural practice like surgery in S. Hirschauer, 'The Manufacture of Bodies in Surgery,' *Social Studies of Science*, Vol. 21, No. 2, 1991, pp. 279-319. Stories of surgeons could be used to gain an inside out access to the surgical form of life, as Collins (op. cit., 1994a, p. 316) has pointed out. Hirschauer

takes a different stance. Instead of considering (self-) representations of surgeons as a representation of what they believe and intend, he takes them literally: 'realizing that there were no persons in surgeons' descriptions of an operation, I took them at their words. The consequence of this hyper-realist reading was that I described an operation as an encounter of two bodies, consistently applying the surgeons' perspective to themselves. While surgeons look in the body for the anatomic images which have been made of it, I was looking in surgical practice for the descriptions surgeons made of it.' For this argument, see: S. Hirschauer, 'Towards a Methodology of Investigations into the Strangeness of One's Own Culture: A Response to Collins,' *Social Studies of Science*, Vol. 24, No. 1, 1994, p. 342). A literal, hyper-realist reading of texts on autism may be a good candidate for simulating an 'autistic world,' and not only because of the *content* of these accounts: 'autism' may also resonate in a *method* of 'taking things literally,' as literal understanding is considered typical of an autistic cognitive style.

[37] To paraphrase Annemarie Mol. Cf. A. Mol, 'Decisions No One Decides About: Anaemia in Practice,' Paper Presentation for Ethics in the Clinic. An International Conference on Normative and Sociological Aspects of Clinical Decision Making. Rijksuniversiteit Limburg, 1993.

[38] By the observer who is familiar with the ordinary concept of 'boredom' as well as with the alienating vocabulary in which it is conceptualized here. Mol and Law make this point with regard to topological ordering. They note that a description of spatial arrangements as a *network* effect presupposes a regional topology: displacement in space is only *displacement* if it is seen from a regional point of view. See A. Mol and J. Law, 'Regions, Networks and Fluids: Anaemia and Social Topology,' *Social Studies of Science*, Vol. 24, No. 4, 1994, p. 649. In the same way, an analysis of the production of temporal order as a network effect presupposes familiarity with symbolic conceptions of time, if only because this provides some bearings in order to recognize change and stability in the progress and order of events. These strange forms of time are distortions of familiar concepts.

[39] Power differences, like any other differences, can be regarded as the outcome of network building. I will not treat these effects at length here. This undoubtedly does not do justice to this complicated matter and may paint a rosy picture of the distribution of right of speech in matters of time. However, because of the point of this chapter - to question familiar (logocentric, interactionist) conceptualizations of ordering power - I believe that this imbalance is justified. See also: A. Mol and J. Mesman, 'Neonatal Food and the Politics of Theory: Some Questions of Method,' *Social Studies of Science*, Vol. 26, No. 1, 1996, pp. 419-444.

[40] A qualified view holds that repetitive behaviour fulfils all sorts of functions for autistic people and that it is unwise to deprive them of survival mechanisms like these. In everyday practice in the community the care workers, who have learned from experience, implicitly take this into account by providing frequent scope for repetitive behaviours and reading them for their communicative value.

[41] See chapter 3 for the concept of 'mediation' and the difference between mediators and intermediaries. For the concept of 'interactive materialism' that is implied here, see: H. Harbers and S. Koenis (eds), 'De bindkracht der dingen,' *KandM*, Vol. XXIII, No. 1, 1999. And: H. Harbers and A. Mol (eds), 'De aard der dingen,' *Kennis en Methode*, Vol. XVIII, No. 1, 1994.

[42] Simmel, op. cit., p. 73.

[43] Such a hyper-realistic magnification of 'what a handicap means' might be used as a heuristic device to think about (coping with) handicapped lives in general. An exaggeration of an 'autistic world' of this kind need not be restricted to texts. In a faculty building at the University of Groningen, the Netherlands there is a lift with a mechanism for wheelchair users, which holds the door open for about 15 seconds to allow them time to enter and exit. Able-bodied people using the lift unexpectedly find themselves in a *material magnification* of the 'handicapped' situation.

[44] B. Latour, 'De antropologisering van het wereldbeeld - een persoonlijk verslag,' *Krisis*, Vol. 15, No. 58, 1995, pp. 33-34. A variant on the theme of delegating action to a non-linguistic prosthesis could be heard several years ago in the VARA radio programme 'Spijkers met koppen' (18 February 1998), when the designer Erik Nap unveiled a special range of clothing for people with autism. As well as a pair of trousers with legs that could be zipped together so that the wearer could restrain his physical panic reactions himself, Nap presented a seaman's jersey with an extra large collar that could be completely zipped up, which meant that the wearer could easily shut himself off as soon as social stimuli got too much for him.

[45] See Callon and Law, op. cit., pp. 503-504.

**With Lacelike Precision**

[1] L. Wittgenstein, *Culture and Value: A Selection From the Posthumous Remains*, Basil Blackwell, Oxford, 1998, p. 25e.

[2] NEC, 'Christian Murphy' [Advertisement], *WIRED*, July 1997.

[3] Ibid.

[4] I do not, therefore, quote this advertisement to denounce the commercial exploitation of autistic people that one might see here. Nor am I concerned with testing the sweeping claims against the reality, although the suggestion

that Murphy could learn to use abstract information like the term 'golden retriever' through the keyboard seems hard to explain if he could previously neither read nor write; it is more likely that visual cues can support reciprocal communication.

[5] This referential concept of language may perhaps come across as naïve, particularly since it has long been rejected in the philosophy of language, in Wittgenstein's notion of 'language games' (note 49, chapter 3). I am, however - again - concerned with everyday notions, where this idea still persists.

[6] For an inventory that listed fifty-four autobiographical texts in English, published by autistic authors between 1985 and 2004, see I. Rose, 'Autistic Autobiography - Introducing the Field,' October, 2005, <http://www.cwru. edu/affil/sce/Texts_2005/Autism%20and%20Representation%20Rose.doc>. Last accessed 16 June 2010.

[7] J. R. Bemporad, 'Adult Recollections of a Formerly Autistic Child,' *Journal of Autism and Developmental Disorders*, Vol. 9, No. 2, 1979, p. 180.

[8] L. Kanner, 'Autistic Disturbances of Affective Contact,' *The Nervous Child: Quarterly Journal of Psychopathology*, Vol. 2, 1943, p. 243.

[9] L. Kanner, 'Irrelevant and Metaphorical Language in Early Infantile Autism,' *The American Journal of Psychiatry*, Vol. 103, No. 2, 1946, p. 243.

[10] A. Schuler and B. Prizant, 'Echolalia,' in E. Schopler and G. Mesibov (eds), *Communication Problems in Autism*, Plenum Press, New York and London, 1985, pp. 163-184.

[11] Schopler and Mesibov, op. cit.

[12] C. C. Park, *The Siege: The First Eight Years of an Autistic Child. With an Epilogue, Fifteen Years Later*, Little, Brown and Company, Boston and Toronto, 1982, pp. 74-75.

[13] See note 25, chapter 2 for studies in which the supposed difference is substantiated but which also point to the lack of generally accepted diagnostic guidelines.

[14] L. Wing, 'The Relationship Between Asperger's Syndrome and Kanner's Autism,' in U. Frith (ed), *Autism and Asperger Syndrome*, Cambridge University Press, Cambridge [etc.], 1991, pp. 93-121. Cf.: L. Wing, 'The Continuum of Autistic Characteristics,' in E. Schopler and G. B. Mesibov (eds), *Diagnosis and Assessment in Autism*, Plenum Press, New York and London, 1988, pp. 91-110.

[15] O. Sacks, *An Anthropologist on Mars: Seven Paradoxical Tales*, Alfred A. Knopf, New York, 1995, p. 247.

[16] L. J. Davis (ed), *The Disability Studies Reader*, Routledge, London and New York, 1997.

[17] J. Pols, *Good Care: Enacting a Complex Ideal in Long-Term Psychiatry*, Trimbos Instituut, Utrecht, 2004. According to Murray, autism, like other cognitive disabilities, is virtually invisible within disability studies, although in his view this is caused mainly by the focus on visible, physical, functional limitations. See Murray, *Representing Autism*, pp. 8-9.

[18] B. Sellin, *I Don't Want to Be Inside Me Anymore: Messages from an Autistic Mind*, Basic Books, New York, 1995, p. 141.

[19] The work of the young German, Birger Sellin, which aroused widespread interest, supposedly came about with the aid of facilitated communication (FC). FC involves training non-verbal people to use auxiliary communication resources such as a word processor, where a trusted person (the facilitator) physically supports the elbow or hand of the user in indicating and typing letters and words. In the early nineteen-nineties Douglas Biklen in the US claimed to have achieved remarkable successes using this approach. See D. Biklen, *Communication Unbound: How Facilitated Communication Is Challenging Traditional Views of Autism and Ability/Disability*, Teachers College Press, New York [etc.], 1993. Other researchers wiped the floor with the 'anecdotal evidence' presented and the claims made by the FC school. The successes that had been claimed could not be replicated, they said, in controlled experiments where the influence of the facilitator was removed. See e.g. the critical review by M. Prior and R. Cummins, 'Questions about Facilitated Communication and Autism,' *Journal of Autism and Developmental Disorders*, Vol. 22, No. 3, 1992, pp. 331-338. An editorial, moreover, talks of the 'emotional blackmailing' of parents and teachers because proponents of the method blame any failure on the absence of a bond of trust. (Editorial Commentary, *Journal of Autism and Developmental Disorders*, Vol. 22, No. 3, 1994, pp. 337-338). Although scepticism is appropriate here, a portrait of Sellin on Dutch television (KRO, Sporen, 'Als een loden last: een roep uit de wereld van een autist,' 6 May, 1994) nevertheless made an overwhelming impression.

[20] K. Momma, *En toen verscheen een regenboog: hoe ik mijn autistische leven ervaar*, Prometheus, Amsterdam, 1996, p. 175.

[21] Ibid. p. 8.

[22] G. Gerland, *A Real Person - Life on the Outside*, Souvenir Press, London, 1997, p. 14.

[23] T. Grandin and M. M. Scariano, *Emergence: Labeled Autistic*, Arena Press, Novato, 1993, p. 25.

[24] The use of an agency from the surroundings to compensate for a lack of internal control over the world is a characteristic of many autistic people, as is the subsequent difficulty they encounter in extracting themselves from a

structure like this and striking out in a different direction. (Ann de Roeck, Interview, Antwerp, 7 August, 1997).

[25] Momma, op. cit., p. 32.

[26] Ibid., pp. 16-17.

[27] Ibid., pp. 46-47.

[28] Ibid., p. 66.

[29] Ibid., p. 156.

[30] Ibid., p. 73.

[31] Ibid., p. 73.

[32] Ibid., pp. 73-74.

[33] Ibid., p. 156.

[34] Ibid., p. 158.

[35] For a definition of perseveration in terms of executive functioning, see C. Hughes and J. Russell, 'Autistic Children's Difficulty with Mental Disengagement From an Object: Its Implications for Theories of Autism,' *Developmental Psychology*, Vol. 29, No. 3, 1993, pp. 498-510.

[36] Momma, op. cit., p. 91.

[37] Bemporad, op. cit., p. 192.

[38] B. Rimland in Grandin and Scariano, op. cit., pp. 7-8.

[39] F. D. Volkmar and D. J. Cohen, 'The Experience of Infantile Autism: A First Person Account by Tony W.,' *Journal of Autism and Developmental Disorders*, Vol. 15, No. 1, 1985, p. 54.

[40] L. Cesaroni and M. Garber, 'Exploring the Experience of Autism Through Firsthand Accounts,' *Journal of Autism and Developmental Disorders*, Vol. 21, No. 3, 1991, p. 312. What is interesting is what Jim and Albert have to say about the auditory, visual and tactile sensations that the sound of a word brings about. Cesaroni and Garber refer here to Luria's mnemonist, who similarly appeared to see, taste and feel things in response to the sound of a word. Cf. also D. Tammet, *Born on a Blue Day: a Memoir of Asperger's and an Extraordinary Mind*, Hodder and Stoughton, London, 2006.

[41] S. Murray, *Representing Autism, Representing Autism: Culture, Narrative, Fascination*, Liverpool University Press, Liverpool, 2008, pp. 8-9.

[42] F. G. Happé, 'The Autobiographical Writings of Three Asperger Syndrome Adults: Problems of Interpretation and Implications for Theory,' in U. Frith (ed), *Autism and Asperger Syndrome*, Cambridge University Press, Cambridge [etc.], 1991, pp. 207-242. Happé initially uses the terms Asperger's syndrome and high-functioning autism interchangeably for autistic individuals with fluent language and normal intelligence. In the end she comes to the conclusion that we probably can and should make a distinction between autists with relatively good social and communications skills connected through the capacity for meta-representation on the one hand

(for which group the label Asperger's syndrome appears to be usable), and a group with a high IQ but low scores on verbal and social skills.

[43] Ibid., pp. 222-223.

[44] In this allusion to the object character of linguistic usage there resonates a remark Wittgenstein made in regard to the inadequacy of familiar language to express what he saw in music, architecture and pictures: 'I never more than half succeed in expressing what I want to express. Indeed not even so much, but perhaps only one tenth. That must mean something. My writing is often nothing but 'stammering.'' (Wittgenstein, op. cit., p. 16e). Stammering, the speaker touches on what can be said about the role of language in a zone between meaningful and material extremes, by doing it with language in a particular way, in a particular form.

[45] Happé, op. cit., p. 239.

[46] A complicating factor here is the dual role that language plays in this chapter: language is at the same time the vehicle and the object of study. It is precisely at the level of meta-description language that the transparent connotation of the window metaphor becomes closely intertwined with our manner of speaking and is thus largely concealed from sight as a structuring principle.

[47] Murray, op. cit., pp. 32-33. Following on from this, Murray comes to a predominantly positive judgment of Biklen's work, which does everything possible to allow an autistic voice to be heard and points to the possibility of subjective expression in the face of the dominant expectations in medical and other institutional contexts.

[48] Murray, op. cit., p. 34. Cf. A. M. Baggs, 'In My Language,' <http://www.youtube.com/watch?v=JnylM1hI2jc>, Last accessed, June 16 2010.

[49] Murray, op. cit., p. 34. The author points out that, according to many other bloggers on autism sites, Baggs's provocative presence detracts attention from the damage autism causes in many lives.

[50] Ibid., p. 49.

[51] When discussing the publicity surrounding the work of the autistic celebrity Tito Rajarshi Mukhopadhyay, Murray points out that the *substance* of what this author has to say has largely been lost sight of: 'his writing is read not as an account of living with autism, but rather as a *product*, an uninterrogated (and in fact *unread*) achievement of someone who should not be able to write in the first place' (Ibid., p. 148).

[52] Cf. the 'stammering' in Wittgenstein, op. cit., p. 16e.

[53] See chapter 4. After trying for years to make a 300 km challenge flight, in the spring of 1994 Momma gained his long-distance certificate.

[54] Momma, op. cit., p. 167.

[55] Ibid., p. 160.

[56] Ibid., pp. 167-68.

[57] Gerland, op. cit., p. 35.

[58] Ibid., p. 24.

[59] Ibid., p. 53.

[60] Ibid., p. 24.

[61] Ibid., p. 93.

[62] D. M. Ricks and L. Wing, 'Language, Communication and the Use of Symbols,' in L. Wing (ed), *Early Childhood Autism* (2nd edition), Pergamon, Oxford [etc.], 1976, p. 93.

[63] Gerland, op.cit., p. 105.

[64] Ibid., p. 125.

[65] Ibid., p. 125.

[66] Momma, op. cit., pp. 83-84.

[67] Ibid., p. 84.

[68] Ibid., p. 84.

[69] Ibid., p. 84.

[70] Ibid., p. 85.

[71] The autist thus shows himself to be extremely adept at translation work in the Latourian sense, where the concept gets both a geometric and a linguistic connotation (see chapter 3). Actor network theoreticians use this concept in an attempt to provide scope for diverse forms of representation, ranging from meaningful words to material forms. 'We need to drive a wedge between re-presentation and language. Between making present again, and its linguistic form. Sometimes re-presentation comes in the shape and form of words. But often it does not. . . . Chains of re-presentations *may* lead to words. May come to take the form of words. But they may equally well lead to, or take the form of, technical objects - for instance, instruments, or diagrams, or skills embodied in human beings' (M. Callon and J. Law, 'Agency and the Hybrid *Collectif,' South Atlantic Quarterly*, Vol. 94, No. 2, 1995, p. 501). My reading of the autistic autobiography, however, departs from this view in a crucial respect: for the autist, language embraces a spectrum of both linguistic and physical ordering; as such it covers on its own the whole centre ground that actor network theory endeavours to span.

[72] Wittgenstein, op. cit., p. 25e.

[73] The dictionary defines numerous meanings for 'passage,' some of them particularly appropriate, including 'part of a discourse or piece of writing' and 'a way affording communication from one place to another.'

[74] Momma, op. cit., p. 140.

[75] Park, op. cit., p. 223.

[76] Ibid., p. 245-246.

[77] Quote from the brochure in which Momma advertises his services as a calligrapher. Collins and Kusch point out that calligraphy as an art form can range from copying the prescribed geometric standard with a steady hand and as accurately as possible (identified by the authors as mimeomorphic actions) making variations on existing letters and designing new ones (a combination of mimeomorphic and polimorphic actions), to work that specifically aims to avoid repetition of existing forms and always tries to find a new way of making a letter unique (because of the social conventions that are the guiding principle here, this would chiefly involve polimorphic actions). See H. M. Collins and M. Kusch, *The Shape of Actions: What Humans and Machines Can Do*, MIT Press, Cambridge, MA and London, 1998. Cf. chapter 5, note 24.

[78] B. Sellin in J. Vogelaar, 'Onrust: een serenadezanger zonder ziel,' *De Groene Amsterdammer*, Vol. 118, 12 January, 1994, p. 2.

[79] Momma, op. cit., p. 9.

[80] My position is thus the reverse of Goode's thesis, which I paraphrased in the first part of this sentence: 'Verbal communication is part of a 'total communicational act.' . . . To treat communication as essentially linguistic is to fall victim to the 'ruse of language' (D. Goode, 'Understanding Without Words: Communication Between an Alingual Deaf-Blind Child and her Mother,' *Journal of Human Studies*, Vol. 13, No. 1, 1990, p 30). Goode takes a radical step towards a better understanding of physical and material harmonization in communicating with deaf-blind children, where language cannot be made productive. However, his plea for an expansion of our concept of communication diverts attention away from needs other than communicational ones that language can address in people with autism.

[81] I. Hacking, 'Autistic Autobiography,' *Philosophical Transactions of the Royal Society Biological Sciences*, nr. 364, 2009, p. 1472.

[82] Ibid.

[83] Cf. the cognitive-psychological explanation for the human tendency to seek central coherence (see chapter 2). See also Wittgenstein's observation and criticism of the fact that for us the mind has become the seat of everything that we regard as important in language: meaning, interpretation, thought processes, etc. (M. Derksen, 'Onwetenschappelijke filosofie,' *KandM*, Vol. XXI, No. 4, 1997, pp. 368-376).

[84] Cf. Kanner, who noted that the lack of other possibilities and the excellent mechanical memories of their children 'often led the parents to stuff them with more and more verses, zoologic and botanic names, titles and composers of victrola record pieces, and the like' (Kanner, 'Autistic Disturbances of Affective Contact,' p. 243). As justified as this criticism was and is, Kanner

neglects to subject to closer scrutiny things that seem worthless from a non-autistic point of view.

[85] The Dutch writer and publicist Wiel Kusters talks about chewing and tasting words, the desire for language that science seldom addresses, 'because the sound of words, their materiality, is only of moderate interest to us. We take words as given and focus our interest on their 'meaning.' But language also has something to say for itself, asserts Kusters, albeit in a different, physical, sensory way. 'It is always the 'meat' of the language that we take into our mouths as we speak. . . . In 'true' language the words have bite and flavour; they don't pass across the table like clammy hamburgers in cardboard cartons.' (W. Kusters, *Honingraten: over de smaak van lezen*, Universitaire Pers Maastricht, Maastricht, 1994, p. 7)

[86] Kees Momma on this habit of Dustin Hoffman's character in Rain Man. (cited in F. Abrahams, 'De mens blijft voor mij onvoorspelbaar: Kees Momma over zijn autistische leven,' *NRC Handelsblad*, 20 January, 1996, p. 3.)

### Autistic Company

[1] O. Sacks, *An Anthropologist on Mars: Seven Paradoxical Tales*, Alfred A. Knopf, New York, 1995, p. 246.

[2] D. J. Cohen and F. R. Volkmar (eds), *Handbook of Autism and Pervasive Developmental Disorders*, 2nd edn, John Wiley and Sons, New York [etc.], 1997, xv.

[3] L. Wing, *In zichzelf gekeerd: voor ouders en opvoeders van het autistische kind,* Lemniscaat, Rotterdam, 1981, p. 48.

[4] Ibid., p. 48.

[5] Cohen and Volkmar, op. cit., p. 509.

[6] S. Baron-Cohen and P. Bolton, *Autism: The Facts*, Oxford University Press Oxford, New York, Tokyo, 1993, p. 81.

[7] T. Peeters, Interview, Opleidingsinstituut Autisme, Antwerp, 23 June 1995.

[8] R. P. Hobson, 'Social Perception in High-Level Autism,' in E. Schopler and G. B. Mesibov (eds), *High Functioning Individuals with Autism*, Plenum Press, New York and London, 1992, p. 157. Cf. chapter 2.

[9] Member of the autism team, taken from my ethnographic fieldwork at W.

[10] T. Peeters, *Autisme: van begrijpen tot begeleiden*, Hadewijch, Antwerp and Baarn, 1994, p. 62.

[11] Team member working at W., taken from my fieldwork.

[12] C. C. Park, *The Siege: The First Eight Years of an Autistic Child. With an Epilogue, Fifteen Years Later*, Little, Brown and Company, Boston and Toronto, 1982, p. 15.

[13] G. B. Mesibov, 'Treatment Issues with High-Functioning Adolescents and Adults with Autism,' in E. Schopler and G. B. Mesibov (eds), *High Functioning Individuals with Autism*, Plenum Press, New York and London, 1992, p. 140.

[14] E. A. Burtt, *The Metaphysical Foundations of Modern Science: The Scientific Thinking of Copernicus, Galileo, Newton and their Contemporaries*, 2nd revised edition, Routledge and Kegan Paul, London and Henley, 1980, p. 15.

[15] L. Wittgenstein, *Culture and Value: a Selection from the Posthumous Remains*, Basil Blackwell, Oxford, 1998, p. 25e. Cf. 'Die Sprache hat für Alle die gleichen Fallen bereit; das ungeheure Netz gut gangbarer Irrwege. Und so sehen wir also Einen nach dem Andern die gleichen Wege gehn, und wissen schon, wo er jetzt abbiegen wird, wo er geradeaus fortgehen wird, ohne die Abzweigung zu bemerken, etc. etc. Ich sollte also an allen Stellen, wo falsche Wege abzweigen, Tafeln aufstellen, die über die gefährlichen Punkte hinweghelfen.'

[16] Peeters, op. cit. 1994, p. 208.

[17] The notion of object-centred forms of sociality is derived in part from Knorr-Cetina, who presents this 'to supplement the purely interpersonal relationships which we generally assume in sociology. You could imagine that we are witnesses of the transition from objects conceived of as things to use (with which we have an external, instrumental relationship), to objects conceived of as 'companions' (Schütz) in current everyday life . . . The notion of object-centred sociality refers . . . to forms of togetherness that manifest themselves in time.' (K. Knorr-Cetina, 'De epistemische samenleving: hoe kennisstructuren zich nestelen in sociale structuren,' *KandM*, Vol. XXI, No. 1, 1997, p. 15).

[18] W. E. Bijker, T. Hughes and T. Pinch (eds), *The Social Construction of Technological Systems: New Directions in the Sociology and History of Technology*, MIT Press, Cambridge, MA and London, 1987.

[19] For related ideas on the construction of subjectivity see E. Gomart and A. Hennion, 'A Sociology of Attachment: Music Amateurs, Drug Users,' in J. Law and J. Hassard (eds), *Actor Network Theory and After*, Blackwell Publishers/The Sociological Review, Oxford, 1999, pp. 220-247. By means of a comparison between two forms of dependence (being mad about music and methadone treatment) they make it clear that a subject is constituted in relation to the context.

[20] Peeters, op. cit., 23 June 1995.

[21] See: I. Hacking, 'Humans, Aliens and Autism,' *Dædelus*, Summer 2009, p. 53.

[22] Ibid., p. 55.

[23] Ibid.
[24] Ibid., p. 56.
[25] Ibid.
[26] J. Bernlef, 'Walker Evans: archeoloog van de oppervlakte,' *Op het Noorden: Essays*, Querido, Amsterdam, 1987, pp. 84-85.
[27] Ibid., p. 84.
[28] Ibid., p. 85.

# Bibliography

Abrahams, F., 'De mens blijft voor mij onvoorspelbaar: Kees Momma over zijn autistische leven.' *NRC Handelsblad*. 20 January 1996, p. 3.

Akrich, M. and B. Latour, 'A Summary of a Convenient Vocabulary for the Semiotics of Human and Nonhuman Assemblies.' In W. E. Bijker and J. Law (eds), *Shaping Technology/Building Society: Studies in Socio-Technical Change*. MIT Press, Cambridge, MA and London, 1992, pp. 259-264.

Albury, W. R., 'Autism: The Experts Still Differ.' *Australian Doctor*. 2 April 1993, pp. 65-66.

————, 'Metaphorical Dimensions of Childhood Autism.' In S. Atkins, K. Kirkby, Ph. Thomson and J. Pearn (eds), *'Outpost Medicine' Australasian Studies on the History of Medicine: Third National Conference of the Australian Society of the History of Medicine*. ASHM/University of Tasmania, Hobart, 1994, pp. 311-319.

————, 'From Changeling to Space Alien: Popular Culture and the 'Otherness' of the Autistic Person.' *Building Bridges: Proceedings of the 1995 National Autism Conference*. Autistic Children's Association of Queensland, Brisbane, 1995, pp. 1-6.

American Psychiatric Association, *Diagnostic and Statistical Manual of Mental Disorders*. Author, Washington DC, 2000.

Asperger, H., 'Die Autistischen Psychopathen im Kindesalter.' *Archiv für Psychiatrie und Nervenkrankheiten*. Vol. 117, 1944, pp. 76-136.

Baggs, A. M., *In My Language*. Retrieved 16 June 2010. <http://www.youtube.com/watch?v=JnylM1hI2jc>.

Bakhtin, M. M., 'Forms of Time and Chronotope in the Novel: Notes Toward a Historical Poetics.' In M. Holquist (ed), *The Dialogic Imagination: Four Essays*. Trans. C. Emerson and M. Holquist, University of Texas Press, Austin, 1981, pp. 84-258.

Bance, A. F., 'The Kaspar Hauser Legend and its Literary Survival.' *German Life and Letters*. Vol. 28, No. 3, 1975, pp. 199-210.

Barnes, H. E., 'Sartre's Ontology: the Revealing and Making of Being.' In C. Howells (ed), *The Cambridge Companion to Sartre*, Cambridge University Press, Cambridge, 1992, pp. 13-38.

Baron-Cohen, S., 'Are Autistic Children 'Behaviourists'? An Examination of Their Mental-Physical and Appearance-Reality Distinctions.' *Journal of Autism and Developmental Disorders*. Vol. 19, No. 4, 1989, pp. 579-600.

———, 'Instructed and Elicited Play in Autism: A Reply to Lewis and Boucher.' *British Journal of Developmental Psychology*. Vol. 8, 1990, p. 207.

———, *Mindblindness: An Essay on Autism and Theory of Mind*. MIT Press, Cambridge, MA and London, 1995.

Baron-Cohen, S. and P. Bolton, *Autism: The Facts*. Oxford University Press, Oxford, New York and Tokyo, 1993.

Baron-Cohen, S., A. M. Leslie and U. Frith, 'Does the Autistic Child Have a Theory of Mind?' *Cognition*. Vol. 21, No. 1, 1985, pp. 37-46.

Baron-Cohen, S. and J. Swettenham, 'Theory of Mind in Autism: Its Relationship to Executive Function and Central Coherence.' In D. J. Cohen and F. R. Volkmar (eds), *Handbook of Autism and Pervasive Developmental Disorders*. John Wiley and Sons, New York, 1997, pp. 880-893.

Baron-Cohen, S., H. Tager-Flusberg and D. J. Cohen, *Understanding Other Minds: Perspectives From Developmental Cognitive Neurosciences*. Oxford University Press, Oxford [etc.], 2000.

Bemporad, J. R., 'Adult Recollections of a Formerly Autistic Child.' *Journal of Autism and Developmental Disorders*. Vol. 9, No. 2, 1979, pp. 179-197.

Benschop, R. J., *Unassuming Instruments: Tracing the Tachistoscope in Experimental Psychology*. ADNP, Groningen, 2001.

Benschop, R. and D. Draaisma, 'In Pursuit of Precision: The Calibration of Minds and Machines in Late Nineteenth-Century Psychology.' *Annals of Science*. Vol. 57, No. 1, 2000, pp. 1-25.

Berckelaer-Onnes, I. A. van, 'Leven naar de letter.' *Tijdschrift voor Orthopedagogiek*. Vol. 31, No. 9, 1991, pp. 413-424.

Berckelaer-Onnes, I. A. van and H. Engeland, *Kinderen en autisme: onderkenning, behandeling en begeleiding*. Boom, Meppel and Amsterdam, 1992.

Bernlef, J., 'Twee heren zonder verleden: over Stan Laurel en Oliver Hardy.' *Op het Noorden: essays*. Querido, Amsterdam, 1987, pp. 118-123.

————, 'Walker Evans: archeoloog van de oppervlakte.' *Op het Noorden: essays*. Querido, Amsterdam, 1987, pp. 79-88.

————, *Out of Mind*. trans. A. Dixon, Faber and Faber, London, 1988.

————, *Vallende ster*. Querido, Amsterdam, 1989.

————, 'Er valt niets te lachen. Over Buster Keaton.' *Ontroeringen: essays*. Querido, Amsterdam, 1990, pp. 128-137.

————, Studium Generale, Rijksuniversiteit Limburg, Maastricht, 2 March 1994.

Bettelheim, B., *The Empty Fortress: Infantile Autism and the Birth of the Self*. Free Press, New York, 1967.

Bijker, W., T. Hughes and T. Pinch (eds), *The Social Construction of Technological Systems: New Directions in the Sociology and History of Technology*. MIT Press, Cambridge, MA and London, 1987.

Biklen, D., *Communication Unbound: How Facilitated Communication is Challenging Traditional Views of Autism and Ability/Disability*. Teachers College Press, New York, 1993.

Boucher, J. and V. Lewis, 'Guessing or Creating? A Reply to Baron-Cohen.' *British Journal of Developmental Psychology*. Vol. 8, 1990, pp. 205-206.

Bromet, J., 'Kinderen die van onze wereld niets begrijpen.' *Margriet*. Vol. 39, 12 June 1976, pp. 70-73, 76.

Bryson, S. E., 'Epidemiology of Autism: Overview and Issues Outstanding.' In D. J. Cohen and F. R. Volkmar (eds), *Handbook of Autism and Pervasive Developmental Disorders*. John Wiley and Sons, New York, 1997, pp. 41-46.

Burtt, E. A., *The Metaphysical Foundations of Modern Science: The Scientific Tthinking of Copernicus, Galileo, Newton and Their Contemporaries* [1932]. Rev. 2nd Edn. Routledge and Kegan Paul, London and Henley, 1980.

Buten, H., *Through the Glass Wall: Journeys Into the Closed-Off Worlds of the Autistic*. Bantam Books, New York, 2004.

Callon, M. and B. Latour, 'Don't Throw the Baby out With the Bath School! A Reply to Collins and Yearley.' In A. Pickering (ed), *Science as Practice and Culture*. University of Chicago Press, Chicago, 1992, pp. 343-368.

Callon, M. and J. Law, 'Agency and the Hybrid *Collectif.*' *South Atlantic Quarterly*. Vol. 94, No. 2, 1995, pp. 481-507.

Cantwell, D., L. Baker and M. Rutter, 'Family Factors.' In M. Rutter and E. Schopler (eds), *Autism: A Reappraisal of Concepts and Treatment*. Plenum Press, New York and London, 1978, pp. 269-296.

Cesaroni, L. and M. Garber, 'Exploring the Experience of Autism through Firsthand Accounts.' *Journal of Autism and Developmental Disorders*. Vol. 21, No. 3, 1991, pp. 303-313.

Chakrabarti, S. and E. Fombonne, 'Pervasive Developmental Disorders in Preschool Children.' *JAMA: The Journal of the American Medical Association*. Vol. 285, No. 24, 2001, pp. 3093-3099.

Cohen, D. J. and F. R. Volkmar (eds), *Handbook of Autism and Pervasive Developmental Disorders*. 2nd Edn. John Wiley and Sons, New York, 1997.

Collins, H. M., *Artificial Experts: Social Knowledge and Intelligent Machines*. MIT Press, Cambridge, MA and London, 1990.

————, 'Dissecting Surgery: Forms of Life Depersonalized.' *Social Studies of Science.* Vol. 24, No. 2, 1994, pp. 311-333.

————, 'Scene from Afar (Reply).' *Social Studies of Science.* Vol. 24, No. 1, 1994, pp. 369-389.

————, 'Socialness and the Undersocialized Conception of Society.' *Science, Technology, and Human Values.* Vol. 23, No. 4, 1998, pp. 494-516.

Collins, H. M. and M. Kusch, *The Shape of Actions: What Humans and Machines Can Do.* MIT Press, Cambridge, MA and London, 1998.

Collins, H. M., G. H. de Vries and W. E. Bijker, 'Ways of Going On: An Analysis of Skill Applied to Medical Practice.' *Science, Technology, and Human Values.* Vol. 22, No. 3, 1997, pp. 267-285.

Collins, H. M. and S. Yearley, 'Epistemological Chicken.' In A. Pickering (ed), *Science as Practice and Culture.* University of Chicago Press, Chicago, 1992, pp. 301-326.

Daru, M., 'Technologie aan tafel: de opkomst van de gezelligheidstechnologie.' In R. Oldenziel and C. Bouw (eds), *Schoon genoeg: huisvrouwen en huishoudtechnologie in Nederland 1898-1998.* SUN, Nijmegen, 1998, pp. 175-196.

Davies, M. and L. Kommandeur, *Anders dan anderen: vragen en antwoorden over de opvoeding van autistische kinderen.* Donker, Rotterdam, 1982.

Davis, L. J. (ed), *The Disability Studies Reader.* Routledge, London and New York, 1997.

Derksen, M., 'Onwetenschappelijke filosofie' [Review of L .Wittgenstein, Het blauwe en het bruine boek]. Trans. W. van Oranje, *KandM: Tijdschrift voor Empirische Filosofie.* Vol. XXI, No. 4, 1997, pp. 368-376.

Draaisma, D., *Why Life Speeds Up as You Get Older: How Memory Shapes Our Past.* Trans. A. and E. Pomerans, Cambridge University Press, Cambridge, 2004.

Editorial Commentary, *Journal of Autism and Developmental Disorders.* Vol. 22, No. 3, 1992, pp. 337-338.

Ehlers, S. and C. Gillberg, 'The Epidemiology of Asperger Syndrome: A Total Population Study.' *Journal of Child Psychology and Psychiatry.* Vol. 34, 1993, pp. 1327-1350.

Eisenberg, L. and L. Kanner, 'Early Infantile Autism, 1943-1955.' *American Journal of Orthopsychiatry.* Vol. 26, 1956, pp. 556-566.

Frith, U. (ed), *Autism and Asperger Syndrome.* Cambridge University Press, Cambridge, 1991.

————, 'Autism.' *Scientific American.* Vol. 268, June 1993, pp. 78-84.

————, *Autism: Explaining the Enigma.* 2nd Edn. Blackwell Publishers, Malden MA/Oxford UK, 2003.

Gaylord-Ross, R. J., T. G. Haring, C. Breen and V. Pitts-Conway, 'The Training and Generalization of Social Interaction Skills with Autistic Youth.' *Journal of Applied Behaviour Analysis.* Vol. 17, 1984, pp. 229-247.

Geest, S. van der, 'Zin en zintuig in gezondheid en ziekte: voorbeschouwing op een symposium.' *Medische Antropologie.* Vol. 5, No. 1, 1993, pp. 63-69.

Gerland, G., *A Real Person-Life on the Outside.* Trans. J. Tate. Souvenir Press, London, 1997.

————, *Een echt mens.* Trans. L. Keustermans. Houtekiet, Antwerpen/Baarn, 1998.

Gillberg, C., 'Autism and Autistic-Like Conditions: Subclasses Among Disorders of Empathy.' [The Emanuel Miller Memorial Lecture 1991]. *Journal of Child Psychology and Psychiatry.* Vol. 33, No. 5, 1992, pp. 813-842.

Gillberg, I. and C. Gillberg, 'Asperger Syndrome, Some Epidemiological Considerations: A Research Note.' *Journal of Child Psychology and Psychiatry.* Vol. 30, 1989, pp. 631-638.

Ginzburg, C., 'Clues: Roots of an Evidential Paradigm.' In *Clues, Myths, and the Historical Method.* Trans. J. and A. C. Tedeschi. Johns Hopkins University Press. Baltimore, MD, 1989, pp. 96-125.

Gomart, E. and A. Hennion, 'A Sociology of Attachment: Music Amateurs, Drug Users.' In J. Law and J. Hassard (eds), *Actor Network Theory and After*. Blackwell Publishers/The Sociological Review, Oxford, 1999, pp. 220-247.

Goode, D., 'Understanding without Words: Communication Between an Alingual Deaf-Blind Child and Her Mother.' *Journal of Human Studies*. Vol. 13, No. 1, 1990, pp. 1-38.

Grandin, T., 'My Experiences as an Autistic Child and Review of Selected Literature.' *Journal of Orthomolecular Psychiatry*. Vol. 13, 1984, pp. 144-174.

————, 'An Inside View of Autism.' In E. Schopler and G. B. Mesibov (eds), *High-Functioning Individuals with Autism*. Plenum Press, New York and London, 1992, pp. 105-126.

Grandin, T. and M. M. Scariano, *Emergence: Labelled Autistic*. Arena Press, Novato, 1993.

Grinker, R. R., *Unstrange Minds: Remapping the World of Autism*. Basic Books Inc., New York, 2007.

Hacking, I., *The Social Construction of What?* Harvard University Press, Cambridge, MA/London, England, 1999.

————, 'Autistic Autobiography.' *Philosophical Transactions of the Royal Society Biological Sciences*. No. 364, 2009, pp. 1467-1473.

————, 'Humans, Aliens and Autism.' *Dædelus*. Summer 2009, pp. 44-59.

Haddon, M., *The Curious Incident of the Dog in the Night-Time*. Jonathan Cape, London, 2003.

Hammersley, M. and P. Atkinson, *Ethnography, Principles in Practice*.2nd Ext. Edn. Routledge, London and New York, 1995.

Happé, F. G., 'The Autobiographical Writings of Three Asperger Syndrome Adults: Problems of Interpretation and Implications for Theory.' In U. Frith (ed), *Autism and Asperger Syndrome*. Cambridge University Press, Cambridge, 1991, pp. 207-242.

————, *Autism: An Introduction to Psychological Theory*. Harvard University Press, Cambridge, MA, 1995.

Harbers, H. and S. Koenis (eds), 'De bindkracht der dingen' [Themanummer]. *KandM: Tijdschrift voor Empirische Filosofie*. Vol. XXIII, No. 1, 1989.

Harbers, H. and A. Mol (eds), 'De aard der dingen' [Themanummer]. *Kennis en Methode: Tijdschrift voor Wetenschapsfilosofie en Wetenschapsonderzoek*. Vol. XVIII, No. 1, 1994.

Hendriks, R., 'Egg Timers, Human Values and the Care of Autistic Youths.' *Science, Technology, and Human Values*. Vol. 23, No. 4, 1998, pp. 399-424.

————, *Autistisch gezelschap: een empirisch-filosofisch onderzoek naar het gezamenlijk bestaan van autistische en niet-autistische personen*. Swets and Zeitlinger, Lisse, 2000.

————, 'De autist, de komiek en de detective.' *Wetenschappelijk Tijdschrift Autisme*. Vol. 5, No. 2, 2006, pp. 60-70.

————, 'Tackling Indifference: Clowning, Dementia and the Articulation of a Sensitive Body.' *Medical Anthropology*. Forthcoming, 2012. DOI 10.1080/01459740.2012.674991

Hermelin, B. and N. O'Connor, *Psychological Experiments with Autistic Children*. Pergamom Press, Oxford, 1970.

Hirschauer, S., 'The Manufacture of Bodies in Surgery.' *Social Studies of Science*. Vol. 21, No. 2, 1991, pp. 279-319.

————, 'Towards a Methodology of Investigations into the Strangeness of One's Own Culture: A Response to Collins.' *Social Studies of Science*. Vol. 24, No. 1, 1994, pp. 335-346.

Hirschman, A. O., *Crossing Boundaries: Selected Writings*. Zone Books, New York, 1998.

Hobson, R. P., 'On Psychoanalytic Approaches to Autism.' *American Journal of Orthopsychiatry*. Vol. 60, No. 3, 1990, pp. 324-336.

————, 'Against the Theory of Theory of Mind.' *British Journal of Developmental Psychology*. Vol. 9, No. 1, 1991, pp. 33-51.

————, 'Social Perception in High-Level Autism.' In E. Schopler and G. B. Mesibov (eds), *High Functioning Individuals with Autism*. Plenum Press, New York and London, 1992, pp. 157-184.

Hof, S. van 't, *Anorexia Nervosa, The Historical and Cultural Specificity: Fallacious Theories and Tenacious Facts*. Swets and Zeitlinger, Lisse, 1994.

Holroyd, S. and S. Baron-Cohen, 'Brief Report: How Far Can People with Autism Go in Developing a Theory of Mind?' *Journal of Autism and Developmental Disorders*. Vol. 23, No. 2, 1993, pp. 379-385.

Howlin, P. and M. Rutter, *Treatment of Autistic Children*. John Wiley and Sons, Chichester, 1987.

Hughes, C. and J. Russell, 'Autistic Children's Difficulty with Mental Disengagement from an Object: Its Implications for Theories of Autism.' *Developmental Psychology*. Vol. 29, No. 3, 1993, pp. 498-510.

Hutchins, E., *Cognition in the Wild*. MIT Press, Cambridge, MA and London, 1995.

Itard, J.-M. G., 'The Wild boy of Aveyron.' In L. Malson, *Wolf Children and the Problem of Human Nature*. Monthly Review Press, New York, 1972.

Kanner, L., 'Autistic Disturbances of Affective Contact.' *The Nervous Child: Quarterly Journal of Psychopathology*. Vol. 2, 1943, pp. 217-253.

————, 'Irrelevant and Metaphorical Language in Early Infantile Autism.' *The American Journal of Psychiatry*. Vol. 103, No. 2, 1946, pp. 242-246.

————, 'Problems of Nosology and Psychodynamics in Early Infantile Autism.' *American Journal of Orthopsychiatry*. Vol. 19, 1949, pp. 416-426.

————, 'Problems of Nosology and Psychodynamics in Early Infantile Autism.' *Childhood Psychosis: Initial Studies and New Insights*. Winston and Sons, Washington, 1973, pp. 51-62.

Kayzer, W., *A Glorious Accident: Understanding Our Place in the Cosmic Puzzle: Wim Kayzer: Featuring Oliver Sacks, Stephen Jay Gould, Daniel C. Dennett, Freeman Dyson, Rupert Sheldrake, Stephen Toulmin*. Freeman, New York, 1997.

Klin, A. and F. R. Volkmar, 'Asperger's Syndrome.' In D. J. Cohen and F. R. Volkmar (eds), *Handbook of Autism and Pervasive Developmental Disorders*. 2$^{nd}$ Edn. John Wiley and Sons, New York, 1997, pp. 94-122.

Knorr-Cetina, K., 'De epistemische samenleving: hoe kennisstructuren zich nestelen in sociale structuren,' *KandM: Tijdschrift voor Empirische Filosofie*. Vol. XXI, No. 1, 1997, pp. 5-28.

Kok, I. and P. Koedoot, *Hulpverlening bij autisme in Nederland*. Trimbos-instituut, Utrecht, 1998.

Kolk-Wolthaar, S. van der, 'Taalstoornissen bij kinderen met autism.' *Logopedie en Foniatrie*. Vol. 56, No. 2, 1984, pp. 12-16.

Kusters, W., 'Autisme: over Vallende Ster van J. Bernlef.' *Tijdschrift voor Gezondheidszorg en Ethiek*. Vol. 1, No. 1, 1991, pp. 20-23.

———, *Honingraten: over de smaak van lezen*, Universitaire Pers Maastricht, Maastricht, 1994.

Lamettrie, J. de, *De mens een machine*. Trans. and Introduction H. Bakx, Boom, Meppel, 1978.

Latour, B., *Science in Action: How to Follow Scientists and Engineers Through Society*. Harvard University Press, Cambridge MA, 1987.

———, *The Pasteurization of France: War and Peace of Microbes, Irreductions*. Trans. A. Sheridan and J. Law. Harvard University Press, Cambridge, MA, 1988.

———, 'A Relativistic Account of Einstein's Relativity.' *Social Studies of Science*. Vol. 18, No. 1, 1988, pp. 3-44.

———, 'Pasteur on Lactic Acid Yeast: A Partial Semiotic Analysis.' *Configurations*. Vol. 1, No. 1, 1992, pp. 129-145.

————, 'Where Are the Missing Masses? The Sociology of a Few Mundane Artifacts.' In W. E. Bijker and J. Law (eds), *Shaping Technology/Building Society: Studies in Socio-Technical Change*. MIT Press, Cambridge, MA and London, 1992, pp. 225-258.

————, 'De antropologisering van het wereldbeeld - een persoonlijk verslag.' *Krisis*. Vol. 15, No. 58, 1995, pp. 29-37.

————, 'The 'Pedofil' of Boa Vista: A Photo-Philosophical Montage.' *Common Knowledge*. Vol. 4, No. 1, 1995, pp. 144–187.

————, 'The Berlin Key or How to Do Words With Things.' In P. M. Graves-Brown (ed), *Matter, Materiality and Modern Culture*. Routledge, London, 2000, pp. 10-21.

Latour, B. and F Bastide, 'Writing Science: Fact and Fiction.' In M. Callon, J. Law and A. Rip (eds), *Mapping the Dynamics of Science and Technology: Sociology of Science in the Real World*. Macmillan, Basingstroke, UK and London, 1986, pp. 51-66.

Lebert, A., 'Howard Buten: Ohne Worte die richtige Sprache finden.' *Süddeutsche Zeitung Magazin*. 5 July 1991, pp. 11-14.

Leslie, A. M., 'Pretence and Representation: The Origins of Theory of Mind.' *Psychological Review*. Vol. 94, 1987, pp. 412-426.

Lewis, V. and J. Boucher, 'Spontaneous, Instructed and Elicited Play in Relatively Able Autistic Children.' *British Journal of Developmental Psychology*. Vol. 6, 1988, pp. 325-339.

Lord, C. and R. Paul, 'Language and Communication in Autism.' In D. J. Cohen and F. R. Volkmar (eds), *Handbook of Autism and Pervasive Developmental Disorders*. 2nd Edn. John Wiley and Sons, New York, 1997, pp. 195-225.

Lynch, M. and H. M. Collins (eds), 'Humans, Animals, and Machines [Special Issue].' *Science, Technology and Human Values*. Vol. 23, No. 4, 1988.

Marchant, R., P. Howlin, W. Yule and M. Rutter, 'Graded Change in the Treatment of the Behaviour of Autistic Children.' *Journal of Child Psychology and Psychiatry*. Vol. 15, No. 3, pp. 211-227.

McDonnell, J. T., 'Mothering an Autistic Child: Reclaiming the Voice of the Mother.' In B. A. Daly and M. T. Reddy (eds), *Narrating Mothers: Theorizing Maternal Subjectivities*. The University of Tennessee Press, Knoxville, 1991, pp. 58-75.

Mertens, A., 'Het fonetisch serveersysteem,' *De Groene Amsterdammer*. Vol. 118, No. 19, 11 May 1994, pp. 26-27.

Mesibov, G. B., 'A Cognitive Program for Teaching Social Behaviours to Verbal Autistic Adolescents and Adults.' In E. Schopler and G. B. Mesibov (eds), *Social Behaviour in Autism*. Plenum Press, New York and London, 1986, pp. 265-283.

———, 'Treatment Issues with High-Functioning Adolescents and Adults With Autism.' In E. Schopler and G. B. Mesibov (eds), *High-Functioning Individuals with Autism*. Plenum Press, New York and London, 1992, pp. 143-155.

Mol, A., 'Decisions No One Decides About: Anaemia in Practice.' [Paper presentation at Ethics in the Clinic: An International Conference on Normative and Sociological Aspects of Clinical Decision-Making], Rijksuniversiteit Limburg, Maastricht, 1993.

———, *The Body Multiple: Ontology in Medical Practice*. Duke University Press, Durham, 2000.

Mol, A. and J. Law, 'Regions, Networks and Fluids: Anaemia and Social Topology.' *Social Studies of Science*. Vol. 24, No. 4, 1994, pp. 641-671.

Mol, A. and J. Mesman, 'Neonatal Food and the Politics of Theory: Some Questions of Method.' *Social Studies of Science*. Vol. 26, No. 1, 1996, pp. 419-444.

Momma, K., *En toen verscheen een regenboog: hoe ik mijn autistische leven ervaar*. Prometheus, Amsterdam, 1996.

———, *Achter de onzichtbare muur: een autist op reis door het leven*. Bakker, Amsterdam, 1999.

Murray, S., *Representing Autism: Culture, Narrative, Fascination*. Liverpool University Press, Liverpool, 2008.

Nadesan, M., *Constructing Autism: Unravelling the 'Truth' and Understanding the Social*. Routledge, London and New York, 2005.

National Society for Autistic Children, 'Definition of the Syndrome of Autism.' *Journal of Autism and Childhood Schizophrenia*. Vol. 8, No. 2, 1978, pp. 162-167.

Nauta, L. W., *Jean-Paul Sartre*. Het Wereldvenster, Baarn, 1966.

―――, 'Exemplarische bronnen van het westers autonomie-begrip.' *Kennis en Methode: Tijdschrift voor Wetenschapsfilosofie en Methodologie*. Vol. VIII, No. 3, 1984, pp. 190-208.

―――, 'Notities.' *Kennis en Methode: Tijdschrift voor Wetenschapsfilosofie en Wetenschapsonderzoek*. Vol. XVIII, No. 1, 1994, pp. 64-68.

Nijhof, G. J., *Herhaalgedrag bij mensen met autisme en een verstandelijke beperking*, Pons and Looijen, Wageningen, 1999.

Noske, B., *Humans and other Animals: Beyond the Boundaries of Anthropology*. Pluto Press, London, 1989.

O'Connor, N. and B. Hermelin, 'Low Intelligence and Special Abilities: Annotation.' *Journal of Child Psychology and Psychiatry*. Vol. 29, No. 4, 1988, pp. 391-396.

Ornitz, E. and E. Ritvo, 'Perceptual Inconstancy in Early Infantile Autism.' *Archives of General Psychiatry*. Vol. 18, 1968, pp. 76-98.

Osteen, M., *Autism and Representation*. Routledge, London and New York, 2008.

Paedologisch Instituut Nijmegen, *Verslag over de jaren 1937-1938*. Author, Nijmegen, 1938.

―――, *Verslag over de jaren 1939-1940*. Author, Nijmegen, 1940.

Park, C. C., *The Siege: The First Eight Years of an Autistic Child. With an Epilogue, Fifteen Years Later*. Little, Brown and Company, Boston and Toronto, 1982.

Peters, A., 'Echt gebeurd als amputatie van de verbeelding: J. Bernlef verdedigt de literatuur tegen modieuze beperkingen.' *De Volkskrant*. 17 April 1998, p. 35.

Peeters, T., *Over autisme gesproken: een serie vraaggesprekken met Engelse deskundigen over autism*. Dekker and V.d. Vegt, Nijmegen, 1980.

————, *Uit zichzelf gekeerd: leerprocesen in de hulpverlening aan kinderen met autisme en verwante communicatiestoornissen*. Dekker and Van de Vegt, Nijmegen, 1984.

————, *Autisme: van begrijpen tot begeleiden*. Hadewijch, Antwerpen and Baarn, 1994.

Plessner, H., *Lachen en wenen: een onderzoek naar de grenzen van het menselijk gedrag*. Trans. J. van Helmond, Aula, Utrecht, 1965.

Premack, D. and G. Woodruff, 'Does the Chimpanzee Have a Theory of Mind?' *Behaviour and Brain Sciences*. Vol. 1, No. 4, 1978, pp. 515-526.

Prior, M. and R. Cummins, 'Questions about Facilitated Communication and Autism.' *Journal of Autism and Developmental Disorders*. Vol. 22, No. 3, 1992, pp. 331-338.

Rang, B., 'When the Social Environment of a Child Approaches Zero: Wolfskinderen en de ontwikkeling van de menswetenschappen.' *Comenius*. Vol. 27, No. 3, 1987, pp. 316-343.

Ricks, D. M. and L. Wing, 'Language, Communication and the Use of Symbols.' In L. Wing (ed), *Early Childhood Autism*. 2nd Edn. Pergamom, Oxford, 1976, pp. 93-134.

Rimland, B., *Infantile Autism: The Syndrome and Its Implications for a Neural Theory of Behavior*. Meredith Publishing Company, New York, 1964.

Roeck, A. de, 'Taal als troebel venster op autistisch denken.' *Studium Generale*. Universiteit Maastricht, Maastricht, 21 January 1997.

Rood, L., *Het boek Job*. Prometheus, Amsterdam, 1994.

Rose, I., 'Autistic Autobiography: Introducing the Field.' October, 2005. <http://www.cwru.edu/affil/sce/Texts_2005/Autism%20and%20Representati on%20Rose.doc>.

Runia, E., *De pathologie van de veldslag: geschiedenis en geschiedschrijving in Tolstoj's Oorlog en Vrede*. Meulenhoff, Amsterdam, 1995.

Russell, J., N. Mauthner, S. Sharpe and T. Tidswell, 'The Windows Task as a Measure of Strategic Deception in Preschoolers and Autistic Subjects.' *British Journal of Developmental Psychology*. Vol. 9, 1991, pp. 331-349.

Rutter, M., 'Behavioural and Cognitive Characteristics of a Series of Psychotic Children.' In J. Wing (ed), *Early Childhood Autism*. Pergamom, Oxford, 1966, pp. 51-82.

————, 'Diagnosis and Definition of Childhood Autism.' *Journal of Autism and Childhood Schizophrenia*. Vol. 8, No. 2, 1978, pp. 139-161.

Rutter, M. and L. Lockyer, 'A Five to Fifteen Year Follow-Up Study of Infantile Psychosis: I. Description of Sample.' *British Journal of Psychiatry*. Vol. 113, No. 504, 1967, pp. 1169-1182.

Rutter, M. and E. Schopler (eds), *Autism: A Reappraisal of Concepts and Treatment*. Plenum Press, New York and London, 1978.

Sacks, O., *Seeing Voices: A Journey Into the World of the Deaf.* University of California Press, Berkeley, 1989.

————, *A Leg to Stand On*. Duckworth, London, 1984.

————, *The Man Who Mistook His Wife for a Hat*. Simon and Schuster, New York, 1985.

————, *An Anthropologist on Mars: Seven Paradoxical Tales*. Alfred A Knopf, New York, 1995.

Sartre, J.-P., *L'être et le néant: essai d'ontologie phénoménologique*. Gallimard, Paris, 1943.

Sass, L. A., J. Parnas and J. Whiting, 'Mind, Self and Psychopathology: Reflections on Philosophy, Theory and the Study of Mental Illness.' *Theory and Psychology*. Vol. 10, No. 1, 2000, pp. 87-98.

Schopler, E., C. A. Andrews and K. Strupp, 'Do Autistic Children Come From Upper-Middle-Class Parents?' *Journal of Autism and Developmental Disorders*. Vol. 9, No. 2, 1979, pp. 139-152.

Schopler, E. and G. B. Mesibov (eds), *Communication Problems in Autism*. Plenum Press, New York and London, 1985.

Schopler, E., M. Rutter and S. Chess, 'Change of Journal Scope and Title' [Editorial]. *Journal of Autism and Developmental Disorders*. Vol. 9, No. 1, 1979, pp. 1-10.

Schrameijer, F., *Een wankele wereld. In het Workhome, een woon-werkgemeenschap voor mensen met autism*. Leo Kannerhuis, Doorwerth, 2007.

Schuler, A. and B. Prizant, 'Echolalia.' In E. Schopler and G. B. Mesibov (eds), *Communication Problems in Autism*. Plenum Press, New York and London, 1985, pp. 163-184.

Searle, J., *Mind, Language, and Society: Doing Philosophy in the Real World*. Weidenfeld and Nicolson, London, 1999.

Sellin, B., *I Don't Want to Be Inside Me Anymore: Messages from an Autistic Mind*. Transl. A. Bell. Basic Books, New York, 1995.

Serres, M., 'De doorgang van het Noord-Westen.' *Kennis en Methode: Tijdschrift voor Wetenschapsfilosofie en Wetenschapsonderzoek*. Vol. XVI, No. 3, 1992, pp. 257-265.

Shapin, S., *The Scientific Revolution*. The University of Chicago Press, Chicago and London, 1998.

Siccama, W., 'De filosofische clou van een komedie: Samuel Becketts Film.' In E. Mulder and H. Ester (eds), *De schone waarheid en de steen der dwazen: transartistieke studies*. Ambo, Baarn, 1996, pp. 185-201.

Simmel, G., 'Exkurs über den Fremden.' *Soziologie: Untersuchungen über die Formen der Vergesellschaftung*. Duncker and Humblot, Berlin, 1983, pp. 509-512.

———, 'Die Geselligkeit.' In *Grundfragen der Soziologie (Individuum und Gesellschaft)*. Walter de Gruyter, Berlin and New York, 1984, pp. 48-68.

———, 'Sociologie van de maaltijd.' In JMM de Valk (Choice and introduction), *Brug en deur: een bloemlezing uit de essays*. Trans. C. Govaart. Kok Agora, Kampen, 1990, pp. 69-79.

Sinclair, J., 'Bridging the Gaps: An Inside-Out View of Autism (Or, Do You Know What I Don't Know?).' In E. Schopler and G. B. Mesibov (eds), *High-Functioning Individuals With Autism*. Plenum Press, New York and London, 1992, pp. 294-302.

———, 'Don't Mourn For Us.' *Our Voice: Newsletter of Autism Network International*. Vol. 1, No. 3, 1993.

Somers, M., 'The Narrative Constitution of Identity: A Relational and Network Approach.' *Theory and Society*. Vol. 23, No. 5, 1994, 605-649.

Sontag, S., *Ilness as a Metaphor and AIDS and its Metaphors*. Anchor, Doubleday [etc.], 1990.

Steerneman, P., *Leren denken over denken en leren begrijpen van emoties*. 3rd Rev. Edn. Garant, Leuven and Apeldoorn, 2004.

Tager-Flusberg, H., 'On the Nature of Linguistic Functioning of Early Infantile Autism.' *Journal of Autism and Developmental Disorders*. Vol. 11, No. 1, 1981, pp. 45-56.

Tammet, D., *Born on a Blue Day: A Memoir of Asperger's and an Extraordinary Mind*. Hodder and Stoughton, London, 2006.

Theisz, R. D., 'Kaspar Hauser im zwanstigsten Jahrhundert: der Aussenseiter und die Gesellschaft.' *The German Quarterly*. Vol. 49, No. 2, 1976, pp. 168-180.

Tinbergen, E. A. and N. Tinbergen, *Early Childhood Autism: An Ethological Approach*. Verlag Paul Parey, Berlin and Hamburg, 1972.

————, *Autistic Children: New Hope for Cure*. Allen and Unwin, London, 1983.

Treffert, D. A., *Extraordinary People: Understanding Idiot Savants*. Harper and Row, New York, 1989.

Turkle, S., *The Second Self: Computers and the Human Spirit*. Simon and Schuster, New York, 1984.

Vogelaar, J., 'Onrust: een serenadezanger zonder ziel.' *De Groene Amsterdammer*. Vol. 118, 12 January 1994, pp. 22-23.

Volkmar, F., A. Carter, J. Grossman and A. Klin, 'Social Development in Autism.' In D. J. Cohen and F. R. Volkmar (eds), *Handbook of Autism and Pervasive Developmental Disorders*. 2$^{nd}$ Edn. John Wiley and Sons, New York, 1997, pp. 173-194.

Volkmar, F. R. and D. J. Cohen, 'The Experience of Infantile Autism: A First Person Account by Tony W.,' *Journal of Autism and Developmental Disorders*. Vol. 15, No. 1, 1985, pp. 47-54.

Volkmar, F. R., A. Klin and D. J. Cohen, 'Diagnosis and Classification of Autism and Related Conditions: Consensus and Issues.' In D. J. Cohen and F. R. Volkmar (eds), *Handbook of Autism and Pervasive Developmental Disorders*. 2$^{nd}$ Edn. John Wiley and Sons, New York, 1997, pp. 5-40.

Vries, G. H. de, 'Wittgensteins afscheid van de epistemologie.' In E. L. G. E. Kuypers (ed), *Wittgenstein in meervoud*. Garant, Leuven and Apeldoorn, 1991, pp. 17-28.

————, 'Bewogen bewegers: ironie in het intellectuele bestaan.' In L. Nauta, G. de Vries, H. Harbers, S. Koenis, A. Mol, D. Pels and R. de Wilde (eds), *De rol van de intellectueel: een discussie over distantie en betrokkenheid*. Van Gennep, Amsterdam, 1992, pp. 111-127.

————, 'Should We Send Collins and Latour to Dayton, Ohio?' *EASST Review*. Vol. 14, No. 1, 1995, pp. 3-10.

————, *Zeppelins: over filosofie, technologie en cultuur*. Van Gennep, Amsterdam, 1999.

Weeks, S. J. and R. P. Hobson, 'The Salience of Facial Expression for Autistic Children.' *Journal of Child Psychology and Psychiatry*. Vol. 28, No. 1, 1987, pp. 137-151.

Wellman, H. and D. Estes, 'Early Understanding of Mental Entities: A Reexamination of Childhood Realism.' *Child Development*. Vol. 57, 1986, pp. 910-923.

Williams, D., *Nobody, Nowhere: The Extraordinary Autobiography of an Autistic*. Avon Books, New York, 1992.

Winch, P., *The Idea of a Social Science*. Routledge and Kegan Paul, London, 1958.

Wing, L., *Autistic Children: A Guide for Parents*. Constable, London, 1971.

———— (ed), *Early Childhood Autism*. 2$^{nd}$ Edn. Pergamom, Oxford [etc.], 1976.

————, 'Review of H. Lane, The Wild Boy of Aveyron.' *Journal of Autism and Developmental Disorders*. Vol. 8, No. 1, 1978, pp. 119-123.

————, *In zichzelf gekeerd: voor ouders en opvoeders van het autistische kind*. 2$^{nd}$ Rev. Edn. Trans. S. van Vliet. Lemniscaat, Rotterdam, 1981.

————, 'Language, Social, and Cognitive Impairments in Autism and Severe Mental Retardation.' *Journal of Autism and Developmental Disorders*. Vol. 11, No. 1, 1981, pp. 31-44.

————, 'The Continuum of Autistic Characteristics.' In E. Schopler and G. B. Mesibov (eds), *Diagnosis and Assessment in Autism*. Plenum Press, New York and London,' 1981, pp. 91-110.

————, 'The Relationship Between Asperger's Syndrome and Kanner's Autism.' In U. Frith (ed), *Autism and Asperger Syndrome*. Cambridge University Press, Cambridge, 1991, pp. 93-121.

————, 'Manifestations of Social Problems in High-Functioning Autistic People.' In E. Schopler and G. B. Mesibov (eds), *High-Functioning Individuals With Autism*. Plenum Press, New York and London, 1992, pp. 129-142.

————, *The Autistic Spectrum: A Guide for Parents and Professionals.* Constable, London, 1996.

————, 'Syndromes of Autism and Atypical Development.' In D. J. Cohen and F. R. Volkmar (eds), *Handbook of Autism and Pervasive Developmental Disorders.* 2$^{nd}$ Edn. John Wiley and Sons, New York, pp 148-169.

Wing, L. and J. Gould, 'Systematic Recording of Behaviours and Skills of Retarded and Psychotic Children.' *Journal of Autism and Childhood Schizophrenia.* Vol. 8, No. 1, 1978, pp. 79-97.

————, 'Severe Impairments of Social Interaction and Associated Abnormalities in Children: Epidemiology and Classification.' *Journal of Autism and Developmental Disorders.* Vol. 9, No. 1, 1979, pp. 11-29.

Wing, L., J. Gould, S. R. Yeates and L. M. Brierley, 'Symbolic Play in Severely Mentally Retarded and in Autistic Children.' *Journal of Child Psychology and Psychiatry.* Vol. 18, No. 2, 1977, pp. 167-178.

————, *Philosophical Investigations.* Basil Blackwell, Oxford UK/ Cambridge USA, 1994.

Wulff, S. B., 'The Symbolic and Object Play of Children With Autism: A Review.' *Journal of Autism and Developmental Disorders.* Vol. 15, No. 2, 1985, pp. 139-148.

**Personal Communications**

Buten, H., Correspondence. 22 April 1999.

Buten, H., Interview. Centre Adam Shelton, Saint Denis, 27 May 1999.

Buten, H., Correspondence. 12 January 2000.

Peeters, T., Interview. Opleidingsinstituut Autisme, Antwerp, 23 June 1995.

Roeck, A. de, Interview. Antwerp, 7 August 1997.

## Audiovisual Sources

KRO, 'Als een loden last: een roep uit de wereld van een autist.' *Sporen*. 6 May 1994.

HOS, 'Mijn eigen wereld.' *Yoy*. 22 February 1996.

VARA, 'Kleding voor autisten.' *Spijkers met koppen*. 1 February 1998.

NPS, 'Trainman.' *Tijdcodes*. 10 March 1998.

VPRO/BBC, 'Gedachtenlezers.' *Noorderlicht*. 13 March 1998.

NPS/VARA, 'Autisme: de wereld in fragmenten.' *Zembla*. 7 May 1998.

VPRO/BBC, 'Rage for Order.' *The Mind Traveller*. Part 4, 11 June, 1998.

## List of Illustrations

*Figure 1.* Christian Murphy. NEC Advertisement. WIRED, July 1997.

*Figure 2.* Clock Dial with Moon Phase Disc. Poster Paint on Paper. © Kees Momma. July 1999.

*Figure 3.* 'With Lacelike Precision.' Calligraphy. © Kees Momma. July 1999.